T0261733

Continuing Medical Education

CONTINUING MEDICAL EDUCATION

Looking Back, Planning Ahead

Edited by

Dennis K. Wentz, MD

Dartmouth College Press *Hanover, New Hampshire*
Published by University Press of New England
Hanover and London

Dartmouth College Press
Published by University Press of New England
www.upne.com
© 2011 Trustees of Dartmouth College
Manufactured in the United States of America

For permission to reproduce any of the material in
this book, contact Permissions, University Press
of New England, One Court Street, Suite 250,
Lebanon NH 03766; or visit www.upne.com

Library of Congress Cataloging-in-Publication
Data appear on the last printed page of this book.

5 4 3 2 1

Contents

Foreword

When I graduated from Cornell University Medical College in 1941, I thought I was brimful of knowledge, ready to be a doctor and to bring my skills to patients. Little did I know that my learning had just begun and, even more important, that much that I had been taught would soon become obsolete if in fact it hadn't been wrong in the first place.

I am now ninety-three years old and, after sixty-nine years in medicine, I continue to be astounded about how medicine has changed in my lifetime. I also continue to be blessed by associating with young colleagues who are bringing about changes that I could have never dreamed of in practice and in the understanding of disease, sometimes utilizing fields of inquiry and discovery that didn't even exist when I began to practice.

I have also been blessed to have been a surgeon at a time when I had the privilege to help shape the new and evolving field of pediatric surgery. My colleagues and I learned daily, especially from our patients and their families, as we pushed boundaries and shaped and marveled at the incredible progress being achieved. Those were exciting and meaningful times for medicine and for me personally. Later in my career, I had the wonderful opportunity to move from the field of surgery (caring mostly for individual patients) to a whole new world of public health when I became your surgeon general for two terms. It was then that I saw firsthand the power of prevention and the fruits of teamwork between doctors and other professionals to bring about important transformations in health and health care. I came to appreciate, as never before, the

social and cultural determinants of illness and the fact that indeed it does take a village as the best way to bring about effective and lasting change. Many of these villages of change were inhabited by courageous and forward-thinking heroes—pioneers who would not accept the status quo and bravely led us to better futures.

Now in my retirement at Dartmouth, where I founded the Koop Institute to help inspire young people entering medicine as I had been inspired, I continue to be astounded by the bright young people I encounter and the progress they are making. I learn something new every day, and I think that fact in itself is one of the most appealing aspects of my journey in this profession. We have come so far and are poised on the cusp of so much more progress. It has been an incredible journey since my medical school days, and I treasure the memories of all my teachers who inspired me along the way.

When I started out, the formal discipline of continuing medical education (CME) did not even exist. Yet, as I think of a physician's life, I realize that medical school and residency/fellowship training, which do have a very important role in the formation of physicians and receive a lot of attention by educators and leaders in medicine, do not represent the conclusion to one's medical education. So much of how medicine is practiced is learned in the years beyond residency. My most important educational experiences occurred in practice, and they happened every single day. They shaped me, my practice, and medicine in general more than I would have ever imagined from the vantage point of medical school or residency. Most of my real education came in those years that CME should have been the most important resource.

But, even with this realization and all of the important developments that have formed the field of continuing medical education, it is not enough—yet. This is why I think *Continuing Medical Education: Looking Back, Planning Ahead,* by Dennis Wentz and colleagues, will be an important milestone document in the field. The work in this book reminds me of a painting, Gauguin's famous triptych *Where Do We Come From? What Are We? Where Are We Going?* This book describes those three spaces or phases of CME, with the most important and exciting being where we will go. In these times of rapid change, we need effective continuing education to bring discoveries to the bedside, to the community, and to the fostering of health in general. In this era of health-care reform, CME will help us to learn to do it wisely, well, safely, and right. Discovery is happening at a rapid and ever accelerating pace; no one person can keep up and stay current without an effective system of what Dave Davis calls "knowledge management" and the ability to put such into effective action through "knowledge transfer."

The history of where we have come from has important lessons. CME, despite its importance in changing practice and doing things right, has been the poor stepchild of undergraduate medical education and graduate medical education. It has been dominated by the talking-at-you, lecture-based mode as the predominant vehicle for the transfer of information; but in reality, this strategy has not been effective in changing the behaviors of physician participants. Now armed with more information of how people learn and how behavior may be changed and new pedagogies to better engage the learner and foster real change, we enter a new and exciting era for CME that is documented in this book.

I almost can't believe the things that are done now or talked about—like the field of robotics and how it is revolutionizing surgical proce-

dures or the developments in nanotechnology that seemed more like science fiction than reality a few years ago—but these types of things are having profound impact. The other revolutions that intrigue me are in the fields of informatics and genetics. We are entering an era of individualized, personalized medicine that I never could have dreamed of in my days of practice, and the new informatics tools for accessing, evaluating, managing, and even creating information are mind boggling. How can one keep up? How does one acquire new skills? How do we learn to use the new tools effectively?

Another trend I see is what is being called *disruptive technologies.* Who could have imagined that angioplasty could almost replace coronary artery surgery? Or that kidney stones could be pulverized by sound waves? Or that surgery could be done through such small openings using laparoscopes? And that is the present. What will lasers be able to do? What will molecular techniques tell us about such things as disease susceptibility and therapeutic vulnerabilities of wayward cells?

I am delighted that this book addresses that the future of health care will be multidisciplinary and that we must escape from the silos we educate practitioners in now to truly embrace those multidisciplinary programs. This is how medicine is, should be, and will be practiced. For the reader, my strong advice is to develop or expect such programs.

I have been thrilled to see the evolution of the competency movement and the trend to teach for, measure, and expect more than just knowledge. As a matter of fact, I see this movement as one of the most helpful things that will change the world of CME. The Accreditation Council for Graduate Medical Education has defined six competencies that include medical knowledge, skills for patient care, communication, professionalism, practice-based learning, and system-based practice. I think this is a great improvement in conceptualizing growth in medicine and providing realistic assessments that will change outcome for both learners and patients. All have great potential in the CME world, but the one that most excites me is practice-based learning, which brings a systematic and intentional approach to what doctors have done for years as they learn in their practice. Bringing rigor, methods, and tools to this can revolutionize CME.

I foresee that we will be able to define and expect competencies for individual practitioners and assess if these competencies are being met. This approach will help lead a true revolution in which individuals can measure what they need to be doing for their patients and learn how to do it better. For example, a physician managing a panel of diabetics will be assessed by the values of the panel's hemoglobin A1C levels, and, if levels are not optimal, a focused continuing education program can be provided after which the diabetic control measures will be reassessed. This type of process will lead to true quality and safely, more evidence-based practice, and better medical care for everyone. The trick will be to frame this type of evaluation and learning as a learning process—not a punitive process—that everyone in medicine will use to improve themselves.

This book is a gem and a starting place for a world of change as we continuously learn how to implement better CME methods for the benefits of our patients and our profession. Thank you, Dr. Wentz. I wish I had another 93 years to see the changes this book will promote. I thank all of the contributors for their wisdom and urge them all to stay the course. What they say here and do is important to the future of medicine.

Acknowledgments

On behalf of the contributors, I wish to extend an important and warm thank you to those numerous individuals who aided us in writing this comprehensive history of continuing medical education and continuing professional development. Your valuable knowledge, time, and help made this book possible.

Continuing Medical Education

.

David Price, Carol Havens, and
Mary Jane Bell

INTRODUCTION

*Continuing Professional Development and Improvement to
Meet Current and Future Continuing Medical Education
Needs of Physicians*

Friday evening, after a long day of patient care, a physician sits down to complete some paperwork before heading home for a quick dinner and going to see her children in a school play. She has seen several patients with complex medical problems, prompting several questions she is unable to answer. Rifling through her mail, she sees a letter from her hospital asking for verification of continuing medical education (CME) activities as part of her re-credentialing, an application from her state medical board requesting documentation of CME in several state-mandated content areas, and a reminder from her specialty board to complete her next set of maintenance of certification activities. She also sees her quality report card from a major insurance carrier, highlighting several areas for improvement. Scattered throughout the pile of mail are several journals and four different post cards advertising CME meetings at various locations throughout the country. Feeling totally overwhelmed about addressing her patients' unanswered needs, improving her quality report card, and meeting all of her CME requirements, she leaves for the evening, knowing that she will spend a good portion of her scheduled day off trying to catch up.

What will CME look like in the future? We believe that the CME enterprise will evolve, guided by changing social and economic forces, to having greater value to physicians, other health-care providers, patients, and society. Emerging evidence demonstrates that CME is a vehicle for change. Done correctly, it can alter clinical practice behaviors and improve health-care delivery and patient outcomes. By advancing clinical practice among all health-care providers, CME can transform the health-care system to better meet the expectations of patients and society at large.

CME professionals must continue to attend to the wants and needs of our main consumers, while engaging our physician colleagues in designing future CME. However, just as performance improvement CME (PICME) programs assess gaps in care and patient outcomes and not just physician self-expressed needs, we believe the CME enterprise must look beyond physician wants. It should be guided by the population health needs of communities, regions, states, and the nation. Thus, the future of CME will be determined not only by physician wants but by other forces and expectations. In addition to providers, stakeholders committed to creating healthy communities (i.e., citizens, payers, governments, and regulatory agencies) will shape the future directions of CME.

The term *continuing medical education* is

somewhat limiting. *Continuing* remains appropriate because it suggests a lifelong commitment to learning and performance improvement. *Medical* potentially constrains the content of CME to doctor-targeted, disease-specific updates at the expense of organizational as well as interprofessional education and practice learning opportunities. *Medical* also neglects the psychosocial and humanitarian aspects of the physician role and ignores the necessity for us to gain competencies in communication skills and cultural awareness. *Education* implies a learning process with an endpoint, just as one graduates from high school or college. *Lifelong learning,* another commonly proposed term for CME, may constrain the implied intent of our efforts by suggesting that learning (knowledge), rather than doing, changing, or discovering, is the endpoint. *Continuing professional development* (CPD), a more inclusive term, better reflects where CME is going and will replace our outdated terminology. Even this term does not adequately reflect the scope of our future efforts. No doubt, the terminology of what we call that which we do will evolve. We have chosen to use the term *continuing professional development and improvement* (CPDI) to describe the CME of the future.

In this chapter, we will identify external trends in society, general education, and health care that define the future of CPDI. We will then hypothesize about what physicians will want and need from their CPDI activities, and we will discuss briefly the expectations of our colleagues of us, their future CPDI leaders. We will conclude with some predictions (or hopes) of what CPDI will look like 20 years from now. When the next CPDI retrospective occurs, we trust that the CPDI field will have progressed significantly and become an enterprise that aids physicians in personal and professional development and improvement, resulting in the transformation of the health-care system toward the delivery of patient-centered, humanistic, cost-effective health care.

Factors Impacting Future CPDI

Many forces—including population demographics, physician supply, the continued and rapid growth of medical knowledge and new technology, a growing emphasis on gap analysis and quality improvement in medicine, trends in adult and medical education design and delivery, and physician educational desires and needs (which are not necessarily synonymous)—are shaping the future of CPDI. Discussion of each of these factors follows.

Societal Demographic Issues

As the population ages, progressively more patients will be living with one or more chronic diseases. While chronic disease management is often reflected in CPDI programs, additional shifts will need to occur to address the care for patients with multiple, simultaneous comorbidities. Factors such as global economies and culturally heterogeneous societies will demand that communication and treatment be tailored to meet the needs of the individual patient. Patients have increasing access to open source medical information via communications technology, and CPDI needs to help physicians guide patients to reliable, evidence-based resources. We, as physicians, also need to be prepared to engage in discussion with patients who might know (or believe they might know) more about a condition than we do.

Advances in knowledge production and technology have important implications for the way we interact with patients. As social and economic trends shift, we may see changes in the number of single-parent households, dual-income households, individuals who hold multiple jobs and, unfortunately, more patients with limited access to the health-care system. These changes may result in patients having less access to care through a traditional doctor's office visit, and health-care providers may need to communicate with their patients through alternate means (telephone, e-mail, text messaging, videoconference, Skype, etc.). In addition, patients may demand alternatives to doctor office visits. Younger patients, in particular, may prefer to obtain information or contact their health-care provider through technology instead of in person.

Physician Workforce Issues

Shortages of primary care physicians in North America have resulted from a reduction of medical school positions, decreasing numbers of trainees entering primary care postgraduate training, and increasing proportions of internal medicine residents who enter subspecialty or hospitalist positions.[1] The geographic misdistribution of physicians continues to be a concern, as many rural areas remain health-care shortage areas.[2] In addition, rural physicians have less access to traditional CPDI, highlighting the need for further expansion of distance training opportunities (videoconference, webinar, asynchronous learning, etc.).

Demographic trends among physicians are also likely to influence future CPDI. Younger adults tend to be more familiar with instructional technology; younger physicians, therefore, may increasingly prefer asynchronous, technology-driven methods of professional development delivered through computers, handheld devices, blogs, blackboards, and podcasts.[3] Progressively more women are entering the medical profession, many of whom must balance work and family responsibilities. Younger male medical graduates may prefer part-time work arrangements as well.[4] Current and future physicians are increasingly interested in activities outside of medicine, which may include family responsibilities (both children and parents) as well as other interests such as music, sports, or travel. These physicians may look to self-directed and/or local CPDI opportunities to allow time for these other pursuits.

Recent studies highlight the potential risk of substandard health-care delivery by older physicians, due to an over reliance on practice experience, lack of engagement in formal CPDI activities, and cognitive decline.[5] As recent economic downturns may delay planned retirement of older physicians, CPDI professionals may have to take steps to re-engage these physicians in educational and performance improvement (PI) activities.

Expanded Medical Content Issues

The continued rapid rate of growth of medical knowledge makes it difficult for most physicians to remain current in their field through reading and traditional CPDI activities alone. There is often a significant time lag before new, evidence-based, cost-effective medical knowledge is applied consistently in practice.[6] Identifying, adapting, and applying new knowledge requires the ability to access high quality (evidence-based, unbiased) sources of information, appraise the information, adapt the information to one's own patient population, and introduce new practice workflows. Physicians need continuous support from CPDI providers in all of these areas, especially to access and use effectively evidence-based medical information, just in time, at the point of care.

The changing landscape of health care, societal expectations, and extended roles for health-care providers will necessitate advanced training for physicians. As more care is delivered in teams, physicians will need to be able to work in teams and lead them, leveraging team members' skills and capabilities within the limits of their licensure. Other roles physicians will need to fill include manager, patient advocate, health-care policy leader, teacher, and mentor for newer colleagues and other health-care providers.

Other General Health-Care Trends

As the gross national product for health-care delivery increases, CPDI programs will have to address more rigorously the issue of cost effectiveness and help physicians ask hard questions about value: Is the added cost of something new worth the improvement in quality? As employers shift the responsibility for health-care costs to their employees through policy changes and high-deductible plans with medical savings accounts, the ranks of the un- and underinsured continue to increase. Patients may be asking questions about the value of health-care interventions and some patients may elect to gamble with and/or defer important aspects of their health care. With health-care spending representing increasing percentages of governmental budgets, changes or limitations in currently covered interventions may drive patients covered by private insurance, Medicare, and Medicaid to engage physicians in discussions of value. At the same time, advances in genomics has increased the need to address societal expectations of personalized medicine by increasing our attention to risk/benefit assessments (including the potential for genetic tailoring of diagnostic and treatment strategies).

Quality-improvement (QI) and benchmarking initiatives in health care have uncovered marked variation in the outcomes of care. Work by Fisher and others[7] has revealed wide regional variation in the utilization and cost of health-care services, often without appreciable differences in overall quality of care. These data will be increasingly available as electronic medical records (EMRs), quality report cards, and patient registries become more widespread. In addition to providing objective needs assessment data for targeting CPDI and quality initiatives, CPDI professionals have an opportunity to help physicians utilize EMRs as both a PI and quality assurance tool for their practices. CPDI professionals can also assist physicians in setting personal learning priorities and improvement opportunities from the increasing amount of available practice data. With the increasing recognition that quality care is dependent on effective interdisciplinary working relationships (even in small office settings), CPDI can help prepare physicians to function better as members of a health-care delivery team.

Trends in Adult Education Design and Delivery

Trends in adult education continue to affect the delivery of CPDI programs. Younger physicians are increasingly accustomed to and familiar with computer-based education delivered synchronously and asynchronously over the Internet in both individual and group formats, and they are frequent users of other technology such as hand held computers, MP3 players, videoconferencing, and social networking sites. Thus, while social and constructivist learning theories continue to inform CPDI activities (physicians, building on previous knowledge and experience, can vet new knowledge with their peers, try out applying it, seek peer feedback, and learn practical tips on how their peers apply the knowledge), interaction and learning are likely to increasingly occur in virtual settings, relying less on face-to-face peer interaction. Additionally, younger generations of adult learners familiar with quickly looking up facts may be more interested in problem solving and learning how to learn in order to develop heuristics for future use; whereas older, more established and busy learners may be interested in key points, facts, and knowing what to do.[8]

Explicit knowledge—formal, conscious, codified information—is used to address simple tasks. It is relatively easy to explain or look up, is formally taught, and is amenable to change or modification in the short term. Without reinforcement or rehearsal, it is short lived. For example, the correct dose of antibiotic to use in an elderly patient with pneumonia and renal insufficiency is a form of explicit knowledge. It is often used to answer questions of what to do (i.e., the dose of antibiotic) or how to do something (i.e., the way to perform a new office or surgical procedure). Implicit knowledge—tacit, uncodified, experiential, unconscious information—is accu-

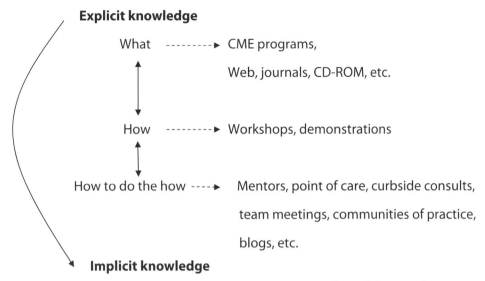

Figure A-1 Examples of CME Formats Based on the Desired Type of Knowledge Transfer

mulated over years of experience. It is used to address complex tasks, is built on prior experience and pattern recognition, is heuristically based, and is often difficult to articulate. Implicit memory is harder to change and more durable than explicit memory.[9] Implicit knowledge is often learned informally and socially from peers. It is the knowledge of how to do the how, that is, what physicians do in daily practice to get through their day or how they incorporate new knowledge or new workflows into their practices. New knowledge is created when explicit knowledge becomes unconscious (implicit) and when implicit knowledge leads to new challenges that physicians need to solve, generating new explicit-knowledge questions. CPDI providers can use this framework to choose formats for CME interventions based on the desired type of knowledge transfer (see Figure A-1).

The collapsing hierarchy between the teacher as oracle of knowledge and the student as passive recipient of wisdom will increasingly lead to medical educators serving as coaches, facilitators, and mentors rather than imparters of knowledge; indeed, medical educators will often learn with CPDI participants.

Trends in Medical Education in Particular

Recent efforts by the American Medical Association (AMA), Canadian College of Family Physicians (CCFP), Royal College of Physicians and Surgeons of Canada (RCPSC), and the Accreditation Council for Continuing Medical Education (ACCME) to encourage and accredit point-of-care learning is an acknowledgment of the fact that most adults learn in the work setting based on real and current patient problems. This is particularly important to meet immediate learning needs in times of crises (i.e., public health dilemmas like the SARS outbreak of 2003, anthrax infections in 2001–2002, and the H1N1 influenza pandemic of 2009).

There is increasing recognition of the need for the facilitation of seamless, lifelong learning across the continuum from undergraduate and postgraduate medicine to CPDI. Additionally, at both the undergraduate and postgraduate medical education level, several organizations have called for educational interventions to help physicians develop and maintain sets of desirable attributes or competencies (see Table A-1). CPDI providers can align their programming with

TABLE A-1 *Selected Competency Frameworks of Different Medical Organizations in North America*

Accreditation Council for Graduate Medical Education	Institute of Medicine	American Board of Medical Specialties	Royal College of Physicians and Surgeons of Canada*
Medical knowledge	Patient-centered care	Professionalism	Medical expert
Patient care	Interdisciplinary teamwork	Self-assessment and lifelong learning	Communicator
Communication and interpersonal skills	Evidence-based practice	Cognitive expertise	Collaborator
Professionalism	Evaluation of performance in practice	Evaluation of performance in practice	Health advocate
Systems-based practice	Medical informatics		Manager
Practice-based learning and improvement			Scholar
			Professional

*J. R. Frank and others, *Report of the CanMEDS Phase IV Working Groups* (Ottawa: The Royal College of Physicians and Surgeons of Canada, 2005).

these efforts by developing educational activities with needs assessments relating directly to these competency areas; selecting formats for educational activities that are likely to increase competence and performance rather than just knowledge; and assessing outcomes (changes) in competence after their programs.

The Institute of Medicine recommends that "all health professionals should be educated to deliver patient-centered care as members of an interdisciplinary team."[10] Interdisciplinary training is already part of hospice and palliative care fellowship training. Early pilots of interdisciplinary training in QI have been conducted at the graduate medical education level; other residency level pilot programs, such as the Preparing the Personal Physician for Practice (P[4]) program of the American Board of Family Medicine and Association of Family Medicine Residency Directors, are in process.[11] Learnings from these programs could inform interdisciplinary educational efforts at both the postgraduate (CPDI) and undergraduate health professional educational level.

Physicians' Wants

Outside forces and expectations of physicians are changing and increasing. Busy physicians will expect CPDI interventions to provide both maintenance of certification (competence) credits and align with maintenance of licensure requirements. There are natural alignments of CPDI activities with the American Board of Medical Specialties maintenance of certification (MOC) requirement for lifelong learning. The needs assessment-objectives-intervention-evaluation development cycle of CPDI aligns well with many constructs of QI, including Plan-Do-Study-Act;[12] CPDI-QI activities could potentially help satisfy requirements for MOC. Furthermore, CPDI activities could provide assistance to physicians who are engaged in practice re-entry or retraining requirements that may be required by specialty or state medical boards.

Physicians will increasingly want educational credit for the learning they get every day, rather than having to rely on separate activities and checking boxes on a form just to meet educational requirements. While accreditation agencies will (and should) continue to require documentation of improvements in competence, processes, or outcomes resulting from learning activities, physicians will not likely want to engage in detailed documentation; they will want quick, easy ways to document their learnings, either from traditional CPDI activities, from point-of-care education, or from QI activities. Ideally, this documentation will not only serve credit accumulation purposes but also serve as a resource to help physicians in CPDI efforts.

Increasingly busy physicians will want their CPDI activities to be relevant to their real questions, real problems, and real work and less geared toward academic interest. They will also want their education to help them prioritize interventions for individual patients and groups of patients, based upon multiple patient needs, individual patient preferences, and competing demands faced by both physicians and patients. With progressive increases in the cost of care and pressure on physicians to attend to costs, physicians will not only need education about new technologies and interventions but will also require guidance on how to judge the value (quality compared with cost) of new technologies compared with existing treatments. Physicians will want tools to help adapt and implement guidelines (developed on general, broadly based population evidence) to their personal practices and to individual patient circumstances. In other words, physicians will want to know more than just what to do; they will want to know how to do it and where to find it efficiently and practically in a busy, real-world practice environment.

Physicians will also want their CPDI delivered efficiently (i.e., brief and to the point) with time for them to ask clarifying questions. They will expect their education to be based on credible, current, high quality evidence not influenced by commercial interests, with available tools to help them remember and apply their learning in their practice in the immediate future. They will expect

balanced discussions on the strengths and weaknesses of existing evidence underlying practice recommendations. This implies, as noted earlier, the continued need for an informatics curricula on information retrieval—especially at the point of care—and evidence-based medicine curricula for critical appraisal, synthesis, and the application of evidence. It also implies a role for CPDI providers in identifying inconsistencies in the evidence and helping physicians decide if inconsistent, weak, or competing evidence should be applied in practice and how this should be done. Similarly, while physicians will expect faculty or facilitators to be engaging, they will also expect faculty to be credible, free of conflict of interest, and cognizant of the realities of daily practice in the attendee specialty and setting. Physicians will continue to expect high value for their education dollar and time, especially given current controversies around the role of commercial support of CME activities, if they will be paying more for their education than is current practice.

As discussed earlier, demographic changes among physicians will affect the way CPDI programs are delivered. Younger physicians starting families, and perhaps older physicians who may be caring for their parents, will want easy access to CPDI activities to minimize travel time. They will increasingly use instructional technology to access synchronous and asynchronous distance learning but will still desire the opportunity to interact with colleagues, to ask questions for clarification, and to seek practical tips from trusted peers on how to apply new knowledge and skills. For these physicians, convenience is key; although, how they define *convenience* may vary. Interaction will increasingly be virtual (asynchronous and synchronous) as well as face to face, as physicians continue to adopt delivery systems such as blogs, social networking Internet sites, or instant messaging to communicate with colleagues. Purely knowledge-based improvements can occur in a variety of settings; live activities must offer training and information not easily accessible or effective through technology.

Information will need to be delivered (whether in a live format or technology based) in brief sections that provide practical, immediately applicable recommendations with resources available for those who want more detail.

Different generations of physicians learn in different ways; medical educators will need to meet these diverse learning needs. Some evidence suggests that future physicians will learn best in groups by working together in a stimulating environment, while baby-boomer physicians will still prefer auditory learning in a lecture format.[13] Meeting the various needs of these learners will require more opportunities for active learning in various formats.

Finally, physicians will want quick and easy ways to document their learnings and record their earned educational credits, either from traditional CME or from learning from QI activities at the point of care.

Physicians' Needs

We physicians, like most humans, often don't know what we don't know and may not accurately self-assess all of our needs.[14] Thus, CPDI providers must address not only physician wants but also those needs that physicians have but may not realize, acknowledge, or accept. Addressing these needs will involve changes to the way CPDI is conceived, planned, and delivered. Change is unsettling, but as we and others in this book have discussed, change is occurring and must occur in the CPDI enterprise. One role for CPDI professionals is to help bring physicians along and guide them through this change.

For example, to many physicians, the purpose of CPDI is to impart new knowledge through a series of one-and-done updates. Many physicians believe that this traditional model of CPDI is effective because it is part of the historically accepted system; physicians may be unaware or even discount the ample evidence that this type of traditional CPDI is generally ineffective in changing practice behavior or long-term practice outcomes.[15] CPDI providers must help move physicians from the "CME as knowledge in isolated programs" framework toward a continuous process of ongoing, reinforcing learning interventions (i.e., educational campaigns[16]) with the goal of significant, measurable, sustainable improvements in care delivery. Even lectures, which are appropriate for knowledge transfer, can be more effective by the use of interaction, reflection, and repetition.[17]

Physicians tend to be drawn to CPDI activities that are topic specific and disease focused. As expectations of physicians continue to evolve, new competencies in areas such as clinician-patient communication (i.e., brief negotiation skills, coaching rather than directing care, etc.) and cultural awareness and flexibility are needed. While many physicians increasingly acknowledge the importance of these areas, they still tend not to make these areas a priority in seeking educational opportunities.[18] Programs focusing explicitly on these topics may not draw interest from a large number of physicians; alternately, those who attend may be the choir who not only understand the importance of these competencies but are performing reasonably well in them (consistent with Eva and Regher's observations that high performers underestimate their performance and lower performers overestimate their performance). Therefore, we believe that these and other less traditional topics should be embedded within disease-based CPDI opportunities in order to reach a larger audience of physicians. For example, an educational program on diabetes mellitus could include objectives on negotiating behavior change and self care with poorly controlled diabetic patients and tailoring dietary recommendations to Latino patients. Additionally, partly due to expectations of the role of the physician and partly due to the way CPDI is currently financed, CPDI topics tend to focus on disease diagnosis and pharmacologic or procedural treatment;[19] nonpharmacologic interventions (i.e., lifestyle modification) are often not addressed or only mentioned superficially. While prevention topics are common in current CPDI (e.g., cancer screening), other public health prevention topics are not as common; similarly, when these programs do occur, they often focus on procedural treatment (i.e., bariatric surgery for obesity) rather than primary and secondary prevention or lifestyle management. We believe that CPDI professionals should create tighter linkages with both public health and patient education professionals to help better address prevention and lifestyle issues as well as patient self-help skill-building.

Many physicians select educational programs in areas where they are already reasonably comfortable to validate that their current practice is up to date. We may not recognize or may choose to discount topic areas where we have larger personal gaps in care. Even if we are willing to try to pick topic areas where we are underperforming, our own global self-assessments of those areas are inaccurate.[20] EMRs, disease registries, and organizational quality metrics can provide valuable data to help physicians objectively identify and target areas for improvement. CPDI professionals play two important roles: that of helping physicians access and use this data to select effective, meaningful CPDI programs and that of improving access to this data to develop accredited educational activities.

Truly interdisciplinary health-care teams are a different model for many physicians who were trained to be the captain of the ship. While physician leadership is important, the hierarchical metaphor can be counterproductive to the development of highly effective teams. CPDI professionals can help health-care teams to learn about and respect each other's roles and contributions and to communicate clearly, effectively, and respectfully with common, shared language.[21] Group visits—long used in behavioral health care—have shown promise in the both urban and rural medical settings for care of older patients

and patients with chronic disease.[22] Education on group visits may be a critical tool to help busy physicians, who individually or in aggregate are short on appointments, meet the needs of their patients.

Demonstrating the Impact of CPDI

Physicians most often evaluate the personal impact of CME programs using the traditional, immediate postprogram happiness index, such as speaker holding an attendee's interest and presenting content deemed interesting and at an appropriate level. More physicians are completing intent-to-change statements as part of postprogram evaluations, which do serve as a proxy for longer term outcomes,[23] even if physician attendees themselves may not necessarily perceive these statements as a method of assessing impact of education. Because they are reasonable predictors of future changes in practice and are easy to gather, intent-to-change statements will likely remain a staple of CPDI assessment; however, we believe that important work needs to be done to help categorize intent-to-change statements in order to facilitate concise reporting of CPDI program outcomes to faculty, planners, and other key stakeholders. Increasing emphasis will be placed on more objective assessments of changes in competence, practice performance, or patient care outcomes after educational programs,[24] recognizing that—short of a well controlled, randomized trial—causal attributions to the CPDI intervention will be difficult to quantify. Nonetheless, if educational programming can help organizations (as one of many tools) improve the process of care, we believe that exact quantification of the educational program's percent effort or effect size is unnecessary. Furthermore, as educational programming is undertaken in a systems context with the goal of achieving sustainable improvements in health-care team function, organizational quality, population outcomes, and affordability of health care, identification of barriers to

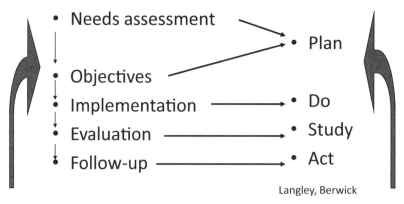

Langley, Berwick

Price D, Medical Teacher 2005

Figure A-2 CME Process vs QI Cycle

intended change in practice can serve as important CPDI outcomes,[25] helping those leading organizational- or population-improvement efforts determine next steps to achieving their goals. Just as physicians must learn to work in teams, so must CME professionals learn to work with other internal partners (QI, pharmacy and therapeutics, etc.) as well as external stakeholders (CME, public health, other providers).

Predictions for the Next 20 Years of CPDI

A multitude of forces are converging on the CPDI, leading to an examination of the role, structure, and function of the whole enterprise. It is clear that more is now expected and needed from us than just knowledge dissemination. Despite the many pressures, inherent uncertainties, and stresses of change, we believe that this is an exciting time to be involved in CPDI. Infrastructure (i.e., multiple collaborations, research funding) and leadership support (i.e., administrative leadership as well as leadership from respected opinion leaders) will be needed to help faculty and learners buy in to a successful paradigm switch in the aims and delivery of future educational interventions. So how will CPDI look 20 years from now? We offer the following predictions and hopes:

- Adult educational and social learning theories will increasingly be applied to the design, implementation, and evaluation of CPDI programs.
- Innovation in CPDI will occur in part due to collaborations and partnerships with other clinicians, quality experts, public health experts, adult educators, sociologists, medical anthropologists, foundations, and governmental and quasi-governmental agencies.
- The linkages and cooperation between undergraduate, graduate, and postgraduate physician education will continue to increase; greater collaboration will occur between medical education and the education of other health-care professionals at each of these levels.
- Educational interventions will increasingly be delivered at the level of the multi-professional team and will include role recognition, respect, and team communication (particularly as it relates to developing a commonly understood and shared lexicon with the aim of improving team cohesiveness in delivering care efficiently.
- Interdisciplinary education will begin earlier in the training of health-care professionals.

- Quality educational interventions will address individual and team learning needs and have elements of self-pacing, self-direction, an opportunity for reflection and practicing of new skills, and quality and quantity of interpersonal interaction (social comfort, educational value, and expert facilitation).
- Educational interventions will focus on quality, affordability, and outcomes of care for populations of patients while incorporating methods of respecting individual patient preferences.
- Clinician-patient communication skills (including patient medical literacy) and cultural competence will increasingly become part of CPDI initiatives.
- While continuing to include evidence-based content, educational programs will increasingly assess the added value (quality divided by cost) of newer interventions over existing interventions.
- The lines between CPDI and QI will become increasingly blurred (see Figure A-2) as health-care systems and physicians continue to search for ways to leverage time, effort, and money.
- Educational programming will move away from a one-and-done conference format toward a continuous, iterative, innovative process using multifaceted educational interventions (some in person, some virtual, some group, some individual). Each intervention will build on and reinforce the learnings of the previous effort.
- EMRs and other medical databases (including disease registries, quality of care dashboards, medical legal claims, patient satisfaction, etc.) will become a valuable source of objective needs assessment data and educational outcomes analysis.

    Limitless virtual libraries (knowledge databases), medical records, and narratives of office visits will help provide structure and content for educational interventions.

- Educational interventions will increasingly be delivered in real time or asynchronously using interactive, easily accessible, distributed delivery systems such as large scale, high bandwidth, multipoint videoconferencing; integrated Web-based imaging tools; computers; and handheld devices that will improve the convenience of educational programming while maintaining important aspects of social learning.
- Collaborative online learning will be international in scope, culturally sensitive, flexible, and responsive to learner needs in real time and will facilitate change in clinical practice behaviors.
- Educational programs will help identify and clarify barriers to improved care and will also help create and disseminate new tacit knowledge (i.e., ways of doing things).

Friday evening, after a long day of patient care, a physician sits down to complete some paperwork. Although she has seen several patients with complex medical problems, she takes pride that her office staff helped her address many patient concerns and she was able to answer quickly several questions by accessing evidence-based information at the point of care. Rifling through her mail, she sees a letter from her hospital asking for verification of CME activities as part of her re-credentialing, an application from her state medical board requesting documentation of CME in several state-mandated content areas, and a reminder from her specialty board to complete her next set of MOC activities. She also sees her quality report card from a major insurance carrier, highlighting several areas for improvement. With a few clicks on her EMR, she produces documentation of her learning at the point of care and the results of an office-based quality improvement project. With another few clicks, she adds this information to her online CME transcript, forwards the transcript to her hospital, state licensing board, and medical specialty board, and sends the CME-accredited QI activity report to the insurance company. Her mind free and clear, she heads home for a quick dinner before going to see her children in a school play, knowing her scheduled day off is free for other pursuits.

Notes

1. T. Bodenheimer, "The Future of Primary Care: Transforming Practice," *New England Journal of Medicine* 359, no. 20 (2008): 2086, 2089; K. E. Hauer, and others, "Factors Associated with Medical Students' Career Choices Regarding Internal Medicine," *Journal of the American Medical Association* 300, no. 10 (2008): 1154–1164; M. H. Ebell, "Future Salary and US Residency Fill Rate Revisited," *Journal of the American Medical Association* 300, no. 10(2008): 1131–1132; A. Steinwald, *Primary Care Professionals: Recent Supply Trends, Projections, and Valuation of Services: Statement to the Committee on Health, Education, Labor, and Pensions, US Senate* (Government Accountability Office, 2008); Council on Graduate Medical Education, "Physician Workforce Policy Guidelines for the United States, 2000–2020," In *US Department of Health and Human Services*, vol. 16 (Health Resources and Services Administration, 2005); R. S. Lipner, and others, "Who Is Maintaining Certification in Internal Medicine—And Why? A National Survey 10 Years after Initial Certification," *Annals of Internal Medicine* 144, no. 1 (2006): 29–36.

2. Primary Care HPSA Maps, Robert Graham Center Web site, http://www.graham-center.org/online/graham/home/tools-resources/maps/maps/hpsamaps.html (accessed May 25, 2009).

3. N. Howe and W. Strauss, "The Next 20 Years: How Customer and Workforce Attitudes Will Evolve," *Harvard Business Review* 85, no. 7 (2007): 41–52; K. Pardue and P. Morgan, "Millennials Considered: A New Generation, New Approaches, and Implications for Nursing Education," *Nursing Education Perspectives* 29, no. 2 (2008): 74–79; S. A. Johnson and M. L. Romanello, "Generational Diversity. Teaching and Learning Approaches," *Nurse Educator* 30, no. 5 (2005): 212–216; D. Billings and K. Kowalski, "Teaching Learners from Varied Generations, *Journal of Continuing Education in Nursing* 35, no. 3 (2004): 104–105.

4. T. Flatt, "Part-time Practice Trends Intensify Physician Shortage according to AMGA and Cejka Search 2007 Physician Retention Survey," *AMGA News*, March 12, 2008, http://www.amga.org/AboutAMGA/News/article _news.asp?k=267 (accessed May 26, 2009); C. Westfall, "Physician Demographics and Turnover Rates," *Physicians News Digest,* May 2007, http://www.physiciansnews .com/business/507westfall.html (accessed May 26, 2009).

5. N. K. Choudhry and others, "Systematic Review: The Relationship between Clinical Experience and Quality of Health Care," *Annals of Internal Medicine* 142 (2005): 260–273; K. W. Eva, "Stemming the Tide: Cognitive Aging Theories and Their Implications for Continuing Education in the Health Professions," *Journal of Continuing Education in the Health Professions* 23 (2003): 133–140; K. W. Eva, "The Aging Physician: Changes in Cognitive Processing and Their Impact on Medical Practice, *Academic Medicine* 77 (2002): S1–S6.

6. E. M. Antman and others, "A Comparison of Results of Meta-Analyses of Randomized Control Trials and Recommendations of Clinical Experts. Treatments for Myocardial Infarction," *Journal of the American Medical Association* 268, no. 2 (1992): 240–248; Institute of Medicine Committee on Quality of Health Care in America, *Crossing the Quality Chasm: A New Health System for the 21st Century* (Washington, DC: National Academies Press, 2001).

7. B. Sirovich and others, "Discretionary Decision Making by Primary Care Physicians and the Cost of US Health Care," *Health Affairs* 27, no. 3 (2008): 813–823; E. S. Fisher and others, "The Implications of Regional Variations in Medicare Spending. Part 1: The Content, Quality, and Accessibility of Care," *Annals of Internal Medicine* 138, no. 4 (2003): 273–287.

8. J. E. Ormrod, *Human Learning,* 3rd ed. (Upper Saddle River, NJ: Prentice-Hall, 1999); L. Vygotsky, *Mind in Society: The Development of Higher Psychological Processes* (Boston: Harvard University Press, 1978); K. Pardue and K. Morgan, "Millennials Considered: A New Generation, New Approaches, and Implications for Nursing Education," *Nursing Education Perspectives* 29, no. 2 (2008): 74–79.

9. U. Lee and D. A. Vahoch, "Transfer and Retention of Implicit and Explicit Learning," *British Journal of Psychiatry* 87 (1996): 637–651; D. Rundus, "Analysis of Rehearsal Process in Free Recall," *Journal of Experimental Psychology* 89 (1971): 63–77.

10. A. Greiner and E. Knebel, eds., *Health Professions Education: A Bridge to Quality* (Washington, DC: National Academies Press, 2003).

11. "ACGME Program Requirements for Graduate Medical Education in Hospice and Palliative Medicine," Accreditation Council for Graduate Medical Education Web site, http://www.acgme.org/acWebsite/down loads/RRC_progReq/540_hospice_and_palliative

_medicine_02122008.pdf (accessed May 25, 2009); P. Varkey and others, "An Experiential Interdisciplinary Quality Improvement Education Initiative," *American Journal of Medical Quality* 21, no. 5 (2006): 317–322, http://www.transformed.com/p4-pdfs/P4ProjectInnovations.pdf (accessed May 1, 2009).

12. D. Price, "Continuing Medical Education, Quality Improvement, and Transfer of Practice," *Medical Teacher* 27, no. 3 (2005): 259–268.

13. S. A. Johnson and M. L. Romanello, "Generational Diversity. Teaching and Learning Approaches," *Nurse Educator* 30, no. 5 (2005): 212–216; D. Billings and K. Kowalski, "Teaching Learners from Varied Generations," *Journal of Continuing Education in Nursing* 35, no. 3 (2004): 104–105.

14. D. A. Davis and others, "Accuracy of Physician Self-assessment Compared with Observed Measures of Competence: A Systematic Review, *Journal of the American Medical Association* 296 (2006): 1094–1102; G. Regehr and M. Mylopoulos, "Maintaining Competence in the Field: Learning about Practice, through Practice in Practice," *Journal of Continuing Education in Health Professions* 28, no. S1 (2008): S19–S23.

15. D. Davis and others, "Impact of Formal Continuing Medical Education. Do Conferences, Workshops Rounds, and Other Traditional Continuing Education Activities Change Physician Behavior or Health Care Outcomes?" *Journal of the American Medical Association* 282 (1999): 867–874; "Getting Evidence into Practice," *Effective Health Care* 5, no. 1 (1999): 1–16, http://www.york.ac.uk/ inst/crd/ehc51.pdf (accessed May 1, 2009); O. Thomsom and others, "Continuing Education Meetings and Workshops: Effects on Professional Practice and Health Care Outcomes," *Cochrane Database of Systematic Reviews* 1 (2004); P. E. Mazmanian and D. A. Davis, "Continuing Medical Education and the Physician as Learner. Guide to the Evidence," *Journal of the American Medical Association* 288 (2002): 1057–1060; S. S. Marinopoulos and others, *Effectiveness of Continuing Medical Education. Evidence Report/Technology Assessment Number 149*, AHRQ Publication No. 07-E006 (Rockville, MD: Agency for Healthcare Research and Quality, 2007).

16. Term coined by Kevin Bunnell, EdD.

17. D. Davis and others, "Impact of Formal Continuing Medical Education. Do Conferences, Workshops Rounds, and Other Traditional Continuing Education Activities Change Physician Behavior or Health Care Outcomes?" *Journal of the American Medical Association* 282 (1999): 867–874; P. E. Mazmanian and D. A. Davis, "Continuing Medical Education and the Physician as Learner. Guide to the Evidence," *Journal of the American Medical Association* 288 (2002): 1057–1060.

18. D. W. Price and others, "Results of the First National Kaiser Permanente Continuing Medical Education Needs Assessment Survey," *The Permanente Journal* 5, no. 4 (2001): 54–62; note that similar results were obtained on a subsequent needs assessment survey.

19. A. S. Relman, "Separating Continuing Medical Education from Pharmaceutical Marketing," *Journal of the American Medical Association* 285 (2001): 2009–2012; R. Steinbrook, "Financial Support of Continuing Medical Education," *Journal of the American Medical Association* 299 (2008): 1060–1062; S. Hensley, "When Doctors Go to Class, Industry often Foots the Bill: Lectures Tend to Feature Pills Made by Course Sponsors; Companies Deny Influence; A Purple Heartburn Brochure," *Wall Street Journal*, East ed., December 4, 2002: A1, A12; R. Van Harrison, "The Uncertain Future of Continuing Medical Education: Commercialism and Shifts in Funding," *Journal of Continuing Education in the Health Professions* 23, no. 4 (2003): 198–209; H. P. Katz and others, "Academia-Industry Collaboration in Continuing Medical Education: Description of Two Approaches," *Journal of Continuing Education in the Health Professions* 22 (2002): 43–54; M. Hager and others, eds., *Continuing Education in the Health Professions: Improving Healthcare through Lifelong Learning* (New York: Josiah Macy, Jr. Foundation, 2008), http://www.josiahmacyfoundation.org.

20. G. Regehr and M. Mylopoulos, "Maintaining Competence in the Field: Learning about Practice, through Practice in Practice," *Journal of Continuing Education in the Health Professions* 28, no. S1 (2008): S19–S23.

21. J. Sargeant and others, "Effective Interprofessional Teams: 'Contact Is Not Enough' to Build a Team," *Journal of Continuing Education in the Health Professions* 28, no. 4 (2008): 228–234.

22. E. A. Coleman and others, "Reducing Emergency Visits in Older Adults with Chronic Illness. A Randomized, Controlled Trial of Group Visits," *Effective Clinical Practice* 4, no. 2 (2001): 49–57; A. Beck and others, "A Randomized Trial of Group Outpatient Visits for Chronically Ill Older HMO Members: The Cooperative Health Care Clinic," *Journal of the American Geriatrics Society* 45, no. 5 (1997): 543–549.

23. J. Wakefield, "Commitment to Change: Exploring Its Role in Changing Physician Behavior through Continuing Education," *Journal of Continuing Education in the Health Professions* 24 (2004): 197–204; J. Wakefield and others, "Commitment to Change Statements Can Predict Actual Change in Practice," *Journal of Continuing Education in the Health Professions* 23 (2003): 81–93; J. L. Dolcourt, "Commitment to Change: A Strategy for Promoting Educational Effectiveness," *Journal of Continuing Education in the Health Professions* 20 (2000): 156–163.

24. Updated Accreditation Criteria, Accreditation Council for Continuing Medical Education Web site, http://www.accme.org (accessed May 25, 2009).

25. L. J. Cochrane and others, "Gaps between Knowing and Doing: Understanding and Assessing the Bar-.riers to Optimal Health Care," *Journal of Continuing Education in Health Professions* 27 (2007): 94–102; D. Price, "Continuing Medical Education, Quality Improvement, and Transfer of Practice," *Medical Teacher* 27, no. 3 (2005): 259–268.

PART I

Reflections at the Beginning

CHAPTER I

Lifelong Medical Education: Past, Present, Future

To ensure quality medical care, the medical profession and society both rely heavily on lifelong learning by physicians. Although many other factors are necessary for optimal patient care, highly informed physicians are essential. Advances in medical research leading to improved diagnosis and treatment require that physicians not only keep abreast of developments but also continually review fundamental concepts. The need for continuing medical education (CME) is, therefore, indispensable.

Organized medicine has always fostered postgraduate education for physicians, which we now associate with formal classroom teaching. In 1906, the American Medical Association (AMA) endorsed a national plan to encourage county medical societies to offer weekly programs on basic medical science and therapy. Most medical specialty societies were founded to enhance continuing education of their members. In 1927, the University of Michigan established the first formal department of postgraduate medicine within a medical school.[1] Eight years later, John Youmans, supported by a grant from the Commonwealth Fund to study CME, visited small-town physicians to determine the effects of courses conducted at Vanderbilt University School of Medicine.[2] Youmans concluded that practical programs focusing on patients were more effective than didactic lectures.

In 1932, the Association of American Medical Colleges (AAMC) declared CME synonymous with *good practice*.[3] In 1940, the Commission on Graduate Medical Education, chaired by Willard C. Rappleye, stated that medical schools did not adequately motivate physicians to continue their medical education.[4]

In a 1955 study sponsored by the American Medical Association, Douglas Vollan recommended the establishment of a national advisory council on postgraduate education to establish CME standards.[5] The study suggested accreditation of CME providers and foresaw mandatory CME and recertification. Multiple attempts to centralize CME or develop a national plan have faltered.

In 1961, Darley and Cain recommended the founding of a National Academy of Continuing Education.[6] The AMA, the AAMC, and the major specialty societies tried to develop a national CME program. Dryer proposed a "university without walls," emphasizing film and television presentations and self-assessment examinations.[7] The AMA appointed Patrick Storey to implement the Dryer Report, but the program was ultimately unsuccessful. Storey later speculated that the project might have succeeded if computers had been available.

The government-initiated Regional Medical Program was designed to bring laboratory advances to the bedside for patients suffering from heart disease, cancer, and stroke.[8] The program, which existed from 1967 through 1973, became diffuse and unwieldy and prompted complaints that tax dollars should not be used for physicians' CME. The Regional Medical Program was the last formal attempt to centralize CME. A central influence did come about when most specialty boards designed recertification tests. In preparing for the recertification examinations, physicians often use sources developed by the individual specialty societies.

Following World War II, formal CME expanded dramatically, with courses sponsored by hospitals, specialty groups, medical schools, and commercial firms. Today, it has become a $2 billion industry, with almost half of the funding derived from industry.[9] Although didactic courses dominate formal CME, other modalities are available such as educational audio-video tapes, CDs, DVDs, short courses via the Internet, and booklets to help physicians prepare for specialty recertification. Most of these rely on the physician's memory in applying accumulated information to patient care.

Mandatory CME

Traditionally a voluntary responsibility of physicians, CME has become a requirement. In 1947, the American Academy of General Practice became the first organization to require attendance in CME activities for membership. In 1965, the Oregon Medical Association established CME requirements for licensure. Gradually, most states and specialty societies required participation in CME.[10]

Accreditation of Providers

As early as 1954, the Vollan Report suggested accreditation of sponsored CME.[5] In 1961 and 1967, the AMA, which has often led the way in the organization of CME, tested a voluntary program to accredit providers of CME. In 1977, the Liaison Committee on CME became the group to accredit CME formally.[11] It consisted of representatives from the AMA, the AAMC, the American Board of Medical Specialties, the Council of Medical Specialty Societies, the American Hospital Association, the Association for Hospital Medical Educators, and the Federation of State Medical Boards. The Accreditation Council for Continuing Medical Education (ACCME) is now the national accreditation agency.

The process of granting institutions the right to offer accredited CME has become increasingly complicated and vigorous. Initially, a CME peer would audit a provider's institution, inspect files, have discussions with the administration and faculty, and attend a course. Most of this was done without a standard protocol to follow and was based on a general impression of the program.

Currently, the accreditation process entails massive preparation documenting compliance with prescribed essentials as defined by the ACCME. Government regulations have led, in some cases, to an emphasis on minutiae that does not enhance the course value. Nevertheless, the ACCME has guided accredited CME institutions to adopt sound educational principles in planning, executing, and evaluating programs. It has properly insisted on disclosure of conflict of interest of institutions and instructors that have received financial or other benefits from industry.

State of the Art in 2009

Today, information sources for physicians are vast and readily available. Medical journals are better than ever. Most newspapers, magazines, and television news programs report recent medical developments. Electronic information sources have increased exponentially, some accessible at the point of care. Fortunately, the National Library of Medicine is a treasure trove of information for clinicians at no cost to the user. Its databases allow instant information at the click of the mouse, refined as the physician narrows and circumscribes his question more precisely.[12] If a physician has time, there is no reason to be uninformed. Despite all these ready resources, physicians seem to be overextended or have distracting obligations that leave little time to seek answers to questions that arise in practice.

Despite the easy accessibility of information, the prevailing theme continues to equate formal CME with attending courses in person or via the Internet, listening to CDs, and studying for recertification.

To be sure, courses and recertification aids are better than ever, with most programs emphasizing needs-assessment and careful course design. Teaching aids, such as PowerPoint and electronic response systems, have greatly enriched programs and have fostered more active participation from the audience. Speakers are also more skilled than they were decades ago. The courses are probably as good as they can be, and further tinkering will result in minor improvements.

Lecture courses have an essential role in keeping physicians aware of the latest medical developments, reviewing basic concepts, and providing contact with experts in the field.

The intrinsic limitation of courses and studying for recertification is that their impact on patient care is dependent on the physician's memory. No amount of changes in course planning, course design, accreditation of providers, or mandatory physician attendance can significantly alter this limitation.

Research

Much of the research in CME has been directed toward testing the efficacy of CME. Most studies agree with the conclusion reached by Haynes and associates: "If the ultimate question in CME is whether patient outcomes can be improved, then the results of these studies are disappointing."[13] This is understandable, since courses are based on group educational needs whereas individual physicians may have specific learning needs that vary from statistical group needs. Since physicians attending courses have different backgrounds and experiences, the measurable "take

home" learned points are variable among the group. Weeks may pass before some physicians use information learned while attending a program. Thus measurement of the effect of most lecture courses on patient outcomes is currently not possible. Physicians do, however, learn, and lectures contribute to this learning. No one limited the treatment of duodenal ulcer to a milk diet and antacids after the availability of proton pump inhibitors and the discovery of helicobacter as a major cause of duodenal ulcer that is treatable with antibiotics.

To complicate matters, patient outcome depends on much more than physician knowledge. At every step, errors and omissions may affect patient outcomes despite the physician's knowledge. A fine example is the classic study by Starfield and Scheff, who found that in only 14 of 53 children with low hemoglobin was the problem recognized, diagnosed, and treated.[14] The low hemoglobin was unrecognized in 24 patients, recognized but undiagnosed in 6, diagnosed but untreated in 1, and treated but not re-examined in 4. Four other patients were diagnosed correctly but did not keep follow-up appointments. This and countless other studies clearly indicate that much more than physician knowledge is responsible for patient outcomes.

So patient care depends not only on a physician's knowledge but perhaps even more on how problems in ambulatory and hospital care settings are handled.

Can current technology address a physician's learning and medical omissions, errors, and patient compliance? Future developments will tell.

Future

Information technology is beginning to broaden physicians' education, permitting the linking of education more directly to practice. This has been a goal for decades. Osler said, "In what may be called the natural method of teaching, the student begins with the patient, continues with the patient, and ends his studies with the patient, using books and lectures as tools . . . as means to an end."[15]

Lawrence Weed pointed out that using information learned depends on memory and the determination to apply the information.[16] He showed that much information at the point of care can be built into electronic medical records. McDonald and coworkers developed an electronic medical record system that includes reminders to physicians, reducing errors of omission and oversight.[17] Various products have been developed that supply information at the point of care, and many physicians carry hand-held devices that supply information when needed.

Further improvements will undoubtedly continue in ease of access and integration of information at the point of care, with electronic tools to preclude oversights. These developments should improve patient outcomes, but more resources will be needed. As demonstrated by the Starfield study, errors and omissions occur at every step in health care.[18] Developing tools to minimize errors and omissions unrelated to physician knowledge and performance offers rich opportunities for research.

Thus, the current methods of CME based on memory are slowly being supplemented by ever-improving information technology that will link education more directly to patient care. With these advances and the possibility of developing more electronic practice tools to identify errors and omissions unrelated to physician knowledge and to improve patient compliance, we will be better able to measure improved patient outcome.

Notes

1. J. D. Bruce, "Postgraduate-Education in Medicine," *Journal of the Michigan State Medical Society* 36 (1937): 369–377.

2. J. B. Youmans, "Experience with a Postgraduate Course for Practitioners: Evaluation of Results," *Journal of the Association of American Medical Colleges* 10 (1935): 154–173.

3. Commission on Medical Education, "Postgraduate Medical Education," *Final Report of the Commission on Medical Education* (New York: Office of the Director of Study, 1932), 136.

4. Commission on Graduate Medical Education, *Graduate Medical Education* (Chicago: University of Chicago Press, 1940), 168.

5. D. D. Vollan, *Postgraduate Medical Education in the United States: A Report of the Survey of Postgraduate Medical Education Carried Out by the Council on Medical Education and Hospitals of the American Medical Association, 1952 to 1955* (Chicago: American Medical Association, 1955).

6. W. Darley and A. S. Cain, "A Proposal for a National Academy of Continuing Medical Education," *Journal of Medical Education* 36 (1961): 33–37.

7. B. V. Dryer, "Lifetime Learning for Physicians: Principles, Practices, Proposals," *Journal of Medical Education* 37 (1962): 89–91.

8. The President's Commission on Heart Disease, Cancer, and Stroke, *A National Program to Conquer Heart Disease, Cancer, and Stroke: Report to the President* (Washington, DC: Government Printing Office, 1964).

9. R. Steinbrook, "Financial Support of Continuing Education in the Health Professions," *Continuing Education in the Health Professions: Improving Health Care through Lifelong Learning* (New York: Josiah Macey, Jr. Foundation, 2007), 104–126.

10. M. W. Breese, *Proceedings of the First National Conference of State Medical Association Representatives on Continuing Medical Education* (Chicago: American Medical Association, 1968).

11. "History of Accreditation of Medical Education Programs," *Journal of the American Medical Association* 250 (1983): 1502–1508.

12. P. R. Manning and L. DeBakey, "The Medical Library," in *Medicine: Preserving the Passion in the 21st Century* (New York: Springer-Verlag New York, Inc., 2004), 191–199.

13. R. B. Haynes and others, "A Critical Appraisal of the Efficacy of Continuing Medical Education," *Journal of the American Medical Association* 251(1984): 61–64.

14. B. Starfield and D. Scheff, "Effectiveness of Pediatric Care: The Relationship between Processes and Outcome," *Pediatrics* 49 (1974): 547–552.

15. W. Osler, *Aequenemitas with Other Addresses to Medical Student, Nurses and Practitioners of Medicine* (Philadelphia: Blackstone Co., 1906), 315.

16. L. L. Weed, *Your Health and How to Manage It* (Essex Junction, VT: Essex Publishing, 1975), 91.

17. C. S. McDonald, "Protocol-based Computer Reminders, the Quality of Care and the Non-perfectibility of Man," *New England Journal of Medicine* 295 (1976): 1351–1355.

18. Starfield and Scheff, "Effectiveness of Pediatric Care," 547–552.

CHAPTER 2

National Approaches to Continuing Medical Education: Recurring Attempts, No Finality

It is almost impossible to determine when the idea of a national plan and philosophy for continuing medical education (CME) in the United States was first conceived. Chapter 1 of this book references the 1906 effort of the American Medical Association (AMA) to encourage county medical societies to offer weekly programs on basic medical science and therapy. Even though 350 county medical societies began sponsoring such programs, no concept of a national plan with any attempt at coordination evolved.

But interest seemed to exist. The AMA began to learn about and study other systems for postgraduate education (as it was then called) in Europe and identified several, including a system in Prussia that is described further in chapter 5. It seems clear that an interest in a national system for directing postgraduate medical education existed, but nothing happened for many years. Today, more than 100 years later, another call for a national approach is being heard but with a twist: a national institute that will focus on interprofessional medical education, a new emphasis that reflects current times.

Suggestions for a national approach are contained in the 1932 *Report of the Commission on Medical Education.*[1] The commission had been organized by the Association of American Medical Colleges (AAMC) in 1925 to review the entire field of medical education in the United States.

Chaired by A. Lawrence Lowell, LLB, PhD, president of Harvard University, its members were a virtual who's who of university leadership in the United States, including seven university presidents and five deans. Others included Olin West, MD, the secretary and general manager of the AMA, and Walter L. Bierring, MD, the secretary of the Federation of State Medical Boards of the United States. Staffing the committee were Fred C. Zapffe, MD, secretary of the AAMC, and Willard C. Rappleye, MD, the director of study.

It was a far-reaching report, covering the public health aspects of medicine, medical needs, supply and distribution of physicians, all aspects of medical education and training, and especially the relevance of having well-educated professionals who could provide adequate and effective medical services. One section was devoted exclusively to postgraduate medical education. It begins:

> In discussing the problems of an adequate program of medical care for a community and in visualizing the individual medical needs to be met, emphasis was placed upon the necessity of competent physicians who are familiar with current knowledge regarding the diagnosis, treatment, and prevention of disease, and upon the importance of every physician continuing to be a student throughout his professional life.[2]

And it goes on to state a truth as relevant today as it was then: "Many enthusiasts for the organization of medical services fail to appreciate fully that the successful development of adequate medical services in any community depends in the last analysis upon the training and ability of the professional personnel."

And where should the responsibility lie?

Every physician must continue to be a student throughout his professional life if he expects to be scientifically successful. The responsibility of providing opportunities for the continuing education of physicians must be shared by the medical profession and the medical schools if they are to work out this essential feature of public service, already recognized as a public responsibility in Germany, for example, where the state supports the instruction and all courses are free. . . . The educational sequence from pre-medical education to retirement from practice should be looked upon broadly as a single problem, not a succession of isolated and unrelated experiences. . . . No single phase of the educational program as a whole can be safely isolated. The university's endeavors in various aspects of medicine should be closely correlated under a unified program.

While the report generally avoided specifics, after considering the emerging role and in-depth training of specialists, it called for two types of short courses: one for the trained specialist and one for the general practitioner designed primarily to help the general practitioner improve his or her ability in diagnosis and nonspecialized treatment. It innovatively called for the use of extension education services to deliver medical education, citing the work of the Extension Division of the University of North Carolina in particular, and described circuit courses in North Carolina, Kansas, Minnesota, and Wisconsin, all different in their details but with courses that reached out to all physicians in the state. The expense of promoting the plan was to be borne by the university, usually in cooperation with the state board of health, but physicians would pay tuition to cover the salary and traveling expense of the instructor. Especially commended was the medical ex-

tension work in Wisconsin that linked a medical library service with the University of Wisconsin Medical Library in Madison.

The commission was also intrigued, as was the AMA in 1910, by the leadership roles in postgraduate education and training being played out in Europe, and commented on efforts in the United Kingdom, Germany, France, and the Netherlands, while admitting that all of these efforts were still in an embryonic stage. And so they concluded: "This outline may appear theoretical, but there is a public as well as a professional need for postgraduate and continuation education and a solution of the problems presented will be found."[3]

The next visible call for a national plan did not occur until 1955 when the Council on Medical Education of the AMA released a report titled "Postgraduate Medical Education in the United States." Based on a national survey of 5,000 physicians, the conclusions were dramatic; about a third of physicians did not participate in any formal education following their graduation. Many conclusions were reached, but a relevant one was the call for a permanent national advisory council to give guidance to the emerging field of postgraduate medical education. The Council was to have representatives from the AMA, the AAMC, the Federation of State Licensing Boards, the American College of Physicians, the American College of Surgeons (ACS), and the American Academy of Family Practice, among others.[4]

But it was never convened, for reasons lost to history. Instead the AMA proceeded alone to form the AMA Advisory Committee on Postgraduate Medical Education in 1957 (see chapter 5 for more detail about the committee).

In 1961, Ward Darley, MD, and Arthur Cain, MD, of the AAMC, published a brief paper in the *Journal of Medical Education* that called for the establishment of a national academy of medical education. It was in reality a response to other articles in that issue that examined issues that are encountered still today about the relationship between CME as a discipline and the pharmaceutical industry. Their opening paragraph summarizes it well:

If the preceding articles are read with the care they deserve, one cannot help but become aware of increasing turbulence between the medical profession and the pharmaceutical industry. Also, one cannot help but be made aware of the fact that the health and welfare of the nation are completely dependent upon harmony between these two groups—a harmony that unavoidably must come out of a situation in which the proper function of one depends on the other. If this dependency is to reflect the strength it should, both the profession and industry must pause, identify the denominators that are common to both sides of the problem, and then work together in shouldering their responsibilities and moving toward their goals.[5]

Darley and Cain's proposal was based on their observation that, due to advances in medical research, the amount of new information available to physicians is too great for existing CME sources to distribute. They noted that such an academy should not compete with or replace existing physician-controlled mechanisms for practitioner education but should fill a void. They noted that a problem had developed: "More and more, the physician is being asked to apply measures prescribed for him rather than those determined by him," a reference to their assertion that "industry had seized an opportunity and met a need."[6]

The national academy was proposed to be a separate organization run by a board of governors with appointees from at least the following sources: the AMA, the ACS, the American College of Physicians, the American Academy of General Practice (now the American Academy of Family Physicians), and the AAMC. They explicitly noted that financial support would have to be substantial and that in the early phases of development such funding should be supplied by the professional organizations represented "to guarantee maximum independence during the all important conceptual and planning period."[7]

With such funding in hand, the academy could apply to private foundations and voluntary health organizations and perhaps industry for support "if it came without strings." Support from grants-in-aid from governmental sources was also cited as another possible step.

They proposed that the focal point for the academy's efforts should be the hospital medical staff organization because staff meeting attendance was already required and usually the educational activities presented actual cases. The academy's graduate school philosophy could then provide "integration, continuity, and constant revision of basic scientific and professional concepts." For this purpose, the academy would provide media-based CME via radio, television, and film to hospitals across the country.

In summary, the goals of a national academy were to provide quality, pertinent, comprehensive educational programs; utilize delivery systems that were accessible and practical for the physician; and protect CME from exploitation. They concluded:

As far as continuing postgraduate medical education is concerned, we feel that the present gap between what is needed and what is being done is comparable to the situation that pertained in undergraduate medical education in the early 1900s. The sooner a forthright over-all approach to the problem is made, the better. Of course, the expense of such a proposed non-profit corporation would be considerable. But with the knowledge important to medicine increasing by leaps and bounds and with medicine's potential effectiveness increasing correspondingly, any program that will enhance the practicing physician's competence in the prevention and management of illness is a sound investment, no matter what the cost.[8]

Who responded in support of the challenge? The AMA took up the gauntlet, acting alone. As reported by Bernard Dryer, MD:

The AMA initiated a study of the nature and function of a national coordinating agency. After preliminary meetings of members of the AMA's Councils and staff, an invitation was issued to eight other organizations to attend a meeting "to consider the formation, under the sponsorship of major medical organizations, of a national agency to further continuing medical education." The meeting was held on March 29, 1961 with the following organizations represented: American Academy of General Practice, American Academy of Pediatrics, American College of Obstetricians and Gynecologists, American College of Physicians, American Medical Association, American Hospital Association, American College of Surgeons, American Psychiatric Association, Association of American Medical Colleges. As a result, a committee was appointed "to spell out the dimensions of a program of continuing medical education." The committee recommended that a careful study be conducted, with a full-time study director, in order that a detailed proposal might be submitted to the cooperating organizations for approval. . . . The report is expected to be both conceptual and practical in nature, and will include a plan or choice of plans for the activation of a national coordinating agency. It is of great significance to the success of the undertaking that the nine participating organizations have recognized the necessity for such a joint effort. With such a combined approach, there seems to be every reason to be optimistic about the possibility of a significant improvement in the status of continuing medical education.[9]

Dryer's full report appeared in 1962 in the *Journal of Medical Education* and summarized a joint study about CME titled "Lifetime Learning for Physicians: Principles, Practices, Proposals." Dryer's report, as published in the journal, was hardly a model of concise writing. The original 89-page report with its 28-page supplement is, however, exciting to read in its entirety. The bottom line of the report is a call for a nationwide "University without Walls." Dryer wrote:

The biochemistry of life requires two basic energy systems: the aerobic and the anaerobic. The metabolism of any vigorous plan for the continuing education means a minimum of four existing systems: the physi-

cian, the medical teaching center, the community hospital, and the medical organization. These four, in a nationwide "university without walls" coordinated for the benefit of the practitioner and his patient, can accomplish together what no one of them can accomplish alone.[10]

The working agenda to create a nationwide university without walls for CME is preceded by this commentary: "The liberal use of analogies throughout this document leads to the comparison of this portion of the report with a prescription. Like any prescription, it needs to be as short as possible, to the point, and accompanied by the explanation that a therapeutic trial with appropriate adjustments may improve its value."[11]

And then Dryer outlines his ideas and thoughts:

The prescient ideas for the *University of Continuing Medical Education* are so good as to repeat them here, since most readers have never had access to the concept or the document. Much as a new medical school is conceived, planned, designed, built, and staffed, so can this Report be put into action. Such an organization should meet these community, professional, and personal criteria:
A. Focus should be on the patient, through the physician.
    1. Goals are improved patient care and health maintenance, and enrichment of medical careers.
    2. Goals will be achieved—insofar as the doctor-patient and doctor-community relationship can contribute to them—by maintaining lifelong competence of physicians and by increasing "health competence" of patients.
B. All physicians should have equal opportunity to continue their medical education, in order that all physicians may be lifelong students. Local inadequacies in CME opportunities should be minimized or eliminated by new educational patterns and technology.

C. Opportunity for continuing education should be available at a time, place, and pace convenient to each physician:
    1. Individual learning opportunities, at home or office, should be reinforced by interrelated self-instructional devices.
    2. Group learning opportunities, with an active, individual, doctor-patient, "bedside" orientation, should probably be centered in the community hospital and the medical center.
    3. Additional opportunities, with the foundation materials available under the two preceding paragraphs, should be made available through the county medical society, general or specialty society, voluntary or governmental health agency.
D. The continuing education program should take the form of an organized, sequential curriculum comprehensive in scope.
E. The curriculum should be continuously available.
F. The physician should have the right to chose any or all of the curriculum.
G. The physician-learner should participate actively in the program and not be only a passive recipient.
H. Some means of evaluation should be built into the program, both for the physician-learner and the educators.
I. There should be a variety of voluntary examinations designed primarily as a part of the learning procedure, and kept separate from any other purpose.
    1. The physician may elect to take examinations.
    2. The physician may take examinations for self-appraisal purposes and remain anonymous if he chooses.
    3. The physician may receive credit for passing examinations if he chooses.
J. The curriculum should be designed and produced by a national "faculty," made up of expert and scholarly teachers in the subject

matter of the life sciences, and such neighboring fields as the physical sciences, the many disciplines convergent on our educational processes, the arts, and the humanities.
K. The curriculum should be nationally organized and developed, but made available on a regional and local selective basis.
L. Existing institutional programs should be reinforced and augmented and not disturbed or displaced by the national educational program.
M. Administrative and technical methods, to satisfy the above criteria, are:
    1. There should be developed, with the guidance of individual specialty groups, "core curricula" for each of the specialty areas.
    2. Using "core curricula" as a base, the national agency would develop teaching materials and methods of delivery to be used in curriculum presentations made by a faulty of national experts. These would be indexed and codified for repeated library accessibility and would include: (*a*) syllabi and books, (*b*) motion picture films, (*c*) videotapes, (*d*) programmed instruction ("teaching machines"),[12] (*e*) slides and film strips of pathology, including X-ray film materials, and (*f*) other modalities of instruction.
    3. The organized sequential curriculum for each would be presented over nationwide distribution systems on a continuous basis, i.e. the curriculum would be rotated sequentially and continuously, with the pattern starting over again as soon as it had been completed. Modifications should be made whenever required by advancing knowledge.
    4. National presentations would be focused by medical centers, individual hospitals, or other group arrangements which would make use of direct bedside teaching, group clinics, discussion groups, question

and answer sessions, clinical-pathological conferences, seminars, and other modalities for patient-centered, active, physician participation.

5. Teaching materials for the local programs would be furnished by the national agency, in time to permit their correlation with the national presentations, which would be scheduled far in advance. Teaching program guides, syllabi, and other instructional materials, would be sent to the community hospital education director well in advance of the national programs.

6. Each regional or local distribution center could decide to receive and distribute all or any part of the national presentations, depending on regional needs.

7. Each individual physician could elect to participate in any part of the program, or to take the entire program.

8. Since the national presentations would be organized, sequential and continuous, the physician who was unable (or did not choose) to participate at the first rotation, could join at the second or third, or could elect to take part of the program the first time around and pick up the rest at a later time.

9. A series of self-appraisal examinations would be designed along with each "core curriculum," with the partnership of self-test design specialists.

   a. The physician-learner could elect to take self-examinations on any given segment of a program, to determine only for himself whether his progress was satisfactory.

   b. If the physician wished to receive formal recognition, or credit, for what he had done, he could choose more formal examinations.[13]

Dryer reflects on the costs of such a national plan and likens them to the cost of starting a new medical school: "an approximate working figure is twenty-five million dollars during the tooling up period before the school opens its doors to student. A somewhat similar expenditure would be required for the first of three components—the educational—of a continuing medical education system with nationwide university-like functions."[14]

The costs of such an initiative today would be staggering, as they were at the time of Dryer's report; but Dryer writes:

> A number of national-level medical, health, welfare and commercial organizations currently spend sums reasonably estimated above one hundred million dollars per year in postgraduate medical educational opportunities. Many of these organizations might prefer to achieve their educational objectives more efficiently—albeit indirectly—by contributing portions of their instructional budgets to a national body of major university status.[15]

And he cautions that "medicine will do well to resist the temptation to compare the magnitude of the above estimates with the billions spent annually in the United States on cosmetics or liquor, or bowling or bombers." He backtracks a bit when he states that "more aptly we may recall the 5.2 billion dollars spent in 1960 on hospital services, plus the 5.0 billion for physician services." To put it into perspective, merely reflect on the amounts spent on these items in 2011.

A corollary recommendation of the Joint Study Group was that a national academy of CME similar to the proposal of Darley and Cain be established. Again, the resources for this were not forthcoming, but the idea of a national plan was kept alive in the Department of Postgraduate Programs at the AMA. Pulmonologist Patrick Storey, MD, was recruited from the University of Pennsylvania and appointed to lead the effort. Over time, he and others developed a new concept titled a New Emphasis for CME. Eventually the AMA provided funding to an ambitious project that included a pilot program focused on practicing physicians in Utah (see chapter 5 for more detail). In the preface of his book *Continuing Medical Education: A New Emphasis,* Storey wrote,

"There were certain problems involved in the further development of the idea, not the least of which were those of a philosophical and methodological nature. These appeared to be fundamental to all the rest. The attempt to resolve these problems is recorded here."[16]

Forty-eight years later, we must face the fact that as a profession we messed up by collectively failing to consider the ideas of Darley, Cain, Dryer, and Storey. I believe that the CME field has been wandering randomly, to my mind, in a manner analogous to a continuing Brownian movement. Other chapters in this book will offer in-depth perspectives on what happened; this chapter introduces an awareness of the former (and often well formulated) plans to bring CME into the mainstream of medical education and into the prominent position it must have in the medical educational continuum.

The Regional Medical Program (RMP) established by the federal government in 1967 to close the gap between "bench to bedside" had the possibility of becoming a national plan though the RMP by legislation focused on only three disease areas: heart disease, cancer, and stroke.[17] Under the program, medical schools would take responsibility for a continuum of medical education, including CME serving practitioners in their geographic area. The RMP program was funded federally between 1967 and 1973, and many good things came out of it, including the University of Alabama's popular Medical Information via Telephone (MIST) consultation system, which was developed under the leadership of Margaret Klapper, MD. A critical decision was made in Alabama: from the beginning, only faculty clinicians answered the telephone calls from practicing physicians with patient management problems, and they were scheduled on-call for 24-hour periods. MIST was further refined by George Smith, MD, and became so essential to Alabama physicians that it received line-item funding in the state budget separate from the university. To my knowledge, it is the only RMP effort that has lasted. MIST continues today and has expanded

gradually to become regional, national, and now international in scope. But federal funding for the RMP program would end. Manning and De-Bakey in chapter 1 sum up the demise of the RMP program, writing that it "became diffuse and unwieldy and prompted complaints that tax dollars should not be used for physicians' CME"—a theme and an unfortunate thought that has continued throughout the years.

Another attempt to create a national think-tank for CME came about in 1974 at a New York meeting of 36 individuals interested in CME. As highlighted in chapter 13 of this book, the meeting was hosted by Lewis Miller and brought together thought-leaders from academia, industry, medical practice, government, and organized medicine to discuss CME's future. The group developed this charge for themselves: "To identify, and promote the implementation of, a rational, pluralistic, and coordinated system of CME, for the purpose of enabling practicing physicians to be optimally effective in the delivery of patient care."[18]

In 1978, however, a decision was made to convert this informal think-tank invitational organization into a formal dues-paying membership organization with a major philosophic change in its goals. Thus emerged the Alliance for Continuing Medical Education.

The last and, in retrospect, weakest attempt at creating a national institute for continuing physician education was announced by the AMA in 1992 (see chapter 5). Although input had been solicited from several organizations, the AMA's unilateral announcement of a new national approach to bring coordination to the field of CME was not well received. The AMA Board of Trustees organized and chartered a new not-for-profit organization that would in many ways try to replicate the ideas of Darley, Cain, and Dryer.[19] In retrospect, all of the organizations who were substantial stakeholders in CME should have been involved in the planning and chartering of such an institute; many believed the AMA was attempting to dominate and control the field of

CME. When funding could not be developed and overt hostility became rampant, the AMA eventually and quietly abandoned the effort.

But history repeats itself. Yet another call for a national effort has been issued. In November 2007, the Josiah Macy, Jr. Foundation convened an invitational conference on continuing education in the health professions.[20] It should be noted that *all* health professional continuing education is under consideration by the Macy group. While most of the attention received by the report focuses on recommendations regarding industry support of continuing education, including a phasing out of all commercial support over a five-year period, a final recommendation calls for the creation of a national interprofessional continuing education institute. As outlined at the time, such an institute would have several functions, including the need to:

- Promote the discovery and dissemination of more effective methods of educating health professionals over their professional lifetimes and foster the most effective and efficient ways to improve knowledge, skills, attitudes, practice, and teamwork
- Be independent and composed of individuals from the various health professions
- Develop and run a research enterprise that encourages increased and improved scientific study of continuing education
- Promote and fund the evaluation of policies and standards for continuing education
- Identify gaps in the content and processes of continuing education activities
- Develop mechanisms needed to assess and fund research applications from health professional groups and individuals
- Stimulate development and evaluation of new approaches to both intra- and interprofessional continuing education and determine how best to disseminate those found to be effective and efficient
- Direct attention to the wide diversity and scope of practices with special continuing education needs, ranging from highly technical specialties on the one hand to solo and small group practices in remote locations, on the other
- Acquire financial resources to support its work and provide funding for research, with possible funding sources including the federal government, foundations, professional groups, and corporations

In conclusion, the Macy report calls for a concerted effort to make the concept of a national continuing education institute a reality, recommending that the Institute of Medicine (IOM) convene a group to bring together interested parties to propose detailed steps for developing such an institute. To ensure that such is considered, the Macy Foundation provided funds to the IOM to convene a Committee on Planning a Continuing Health Care Professional Education Institute. Its report was issued in late 2009 and the Statement of Task reads:

An ad hoc IOM committee will undertake a review of issues in continuing education (CE) of health care professionals that are identified from the literature and from data-gathering meetings with involved parties to improve the quality of care. Based on this review, the committee will consider the establishment of a national interprofessional CE Institute to advance the science of CE by promoting the discovery and dissemination of more effective methods of educating health professionals over their professional lifetimes, by developing a research enterprise that encourages increased scientific study of CE, by developing mechanisms to assess research applications, by stimulating new approaches to both intra- and interprofessional CE, by being independent and composed of individuals from the various health professions, and by considering financing (both short and long term).[21]

The report has seven detailed recommendations to create a new public-private institute: the Continuing Professional Development Institute (CPDI). It calls on (1) the secretary of the Department of Health and Human Services to commission a planning committee to develop the institute, (2) the committee to design a new vision of a CPD system, and (3) the committee to design the CPDI to work with other entities whose purpose is to improve quality and patient safety by:

(a) Collaborating with the Agency for Healthcare Research and Quality, the Centers for Medicare and Medicaid Services, the Joint Commission, the National Committee for Quality Assurance, the National Quality Forum, and other data measurement, collection, cataloging, and reporting agencies to evaluate changes in the performance of health professionals and the need for CPD in the improvement of patient care and safety; and (b) involving patients and consumers in CPD by using patient-reported measures and encouraging transparency to the public about performance of health care professionals.[22]

The report recognized that adequate and ensured long-term financial support for the CPDI would be necessary, acknowledging that no data existed to project whether the costs of a comprehensive CPD system would be greater or less than the costs of the current system. Report recommendation no. 7 reads: "The Continuing Professional Development Institute should analyze the sources and adequacy of funding for CPD, develop a sustainable business model free from conflicts of interest, and promote the use of CPD to improve quality and patient safety."[23]

At this writing, nothing more is known about the progress of the CPDI. However, I am concerned that the report fails to mention the activities undertaken by the medical or other professions over the years and of the role professional associations play in the continuing education of doctors and other health-care professionals. The report barely mentions the role of professional societies and the major efforts of the AMA. Although mention is made of the 1955 AMA Vollan report, it is unattributed, and the AMA's role is defined in one sentence: "Regulation of CME began largely as a method for the American Medical Association, and eventually state medical socie-

ties, to monitor pharmaceutical influence on physician education."[24]

Perhaps this will change as the CPDI comes into being. What is especially important in the report is the call for a continuing education research imperative. In commenting on the new initiative, Paul Mazmanian called for the health professions continuing education community (i.e., continuing education providers and practitioners, regulatory and accrediting agencies, and the health professions) to rise to the challenge:

Without a sound evidence base, CE may continue to be played out and practiced in the flawed and fragmented world revealed by the IOM report, but with good science, the CE community shares a reasonable chance of advancing the development of practitioners, enhancing the discipline of CPD, and improving health outcomes for patients.[25]

I have traced the evolution of the thinking of organized medicine and serious scholars about the need to bring national formal organization to the field of CME, now within the broader scope of continuing professional development and continuing interprofessional education. But I also believe that the chances of doing anything are few, and the possibility may be as remote as it always has been.

Notes

1. A. Lawrence Lowell, *Final Report of the Commission on Medical Education* (New York: Office of the Director of Study, 1932).

2. Lowell, *Final Report*, 122–140.

3. Ibid., 144.

4. Report of the Council on Medical Education, "Postgraduate Medical Education in the United States," *Journal of the American Medical Association* 157 (1955): 701–707.

5. W. Darley and A. S. Cain, "A Proposal for a National Academy on Continuing Medical Education," *Journal of Medical Education* 36 (1961): 33–37.

6. Darley and Cain, "A Proposal," 35.

7. Ibid., 36.

8. Ibid., 37.

9. B. V. Dryer, "Lifetime Learning for Physicians:

Principles, Practices, Proposals," *Journal of Medical Education* 37 (1962): 1–89.

10. Dryer, "Lifetime Learning," 90–134.

11. Ibid.

12. Leo L. Leveridge, "Experience in Educational Design for Interactive Videodisc and Quadrasync Presentations," *Journal of Educational and Technology Systems* 8 (1979): 221–230.

13. Dryer, "Lifetime Learning."

14. Ibid.

15. Ibid.

16. P. B. Storey and others, *Continuing Medical Education: A New Emphasis* (Chicago: American Medical Association, 1968), iii.

17. *The President's Commission on Heart Disease, Cancer and Stroke: A National Program to Conquer Heart Disease, Cancer and Stroke. Report to the President* (Washington, DC: Government Printing Office, 1964).

18. W. C. Felch, *The Alliance for Continuing Medical Education: The First Twenty Years* (Dubuque, Iowa: Kendall/Hunt Publishing Company, 1996), 3–7.

19. Dennis K.Wentz, "The National Institute for Continuing Physician Education" (presentation, Society of Medical College Directors of CME, Washington, DC, November 6, 1993).

20. *Continuing Education in the Health Professions: Improving Healthcare through Lifelong Learning* (New York: Josiah Macy, Jr. Foundation, 2008).

21. Institute of Medicine, *Redesigning Continuing Education in the Health Professions* (Washington, DC: National Academies Press, 2009).

22. IOM, *Redesigning*, 6.

23. Ibid., 8.

24. Ibid., 14.

25. Paul E. Mazmanian, "Institute of Medicine Recommends a Continuing Professional Development Institute for US Health Professionals," *Journal of Continuing Education in the Health Professionals* 30 (2010): 1–2.

M. Roy Schwarz

CHAPTER 3

Is There a Continuum of Medical Education? Fact versus Fiction

Over the past decade, it has become increasingly clear that we live in an era of global health. In late 2008, a joint Sino-US conference was held at Johns Hopkins University that focused largely on the components of global health. Many themes emerged from this conference, with the most important being that for the world to effectively face the global health challenges of the future, there must be a seamless continuum from the laboratory benches of biomedical science to the bedsides of patients and populations of people. Many examples were given, but the most compelling was the natural history of vaccines. Vaccines begin with breakthroughs in the laboratory and continue until patients are immunized and the threat of the infectious disease has been significantly attenuated at both the individual patient and the population of people levels.

In light of the emergence of global health and the global village of which it is a part, the question of whether a continuum of medical education covering medical school, residency training, and continuing medical education (CME) exists takes on new meaning and is both timely and important. The short answer to this question is no, a continuum *does not exist* at this point in history. While lip service is paid to such a continuum, scant evidence supports its existence. To understand why it does not exist, one must begin with a brief history of medical education in the United States.

History of Medical Education

In the early 1900s, medical education leading to the MD degree was largely in disarray. Many medical schools served as nothing more than for-profit diploma mills. There was little or no planning for medical education, poorly defined and non-uniform curricula, limited buildings, and the core needs of medical education were wanting at best. In addition, the faculty varied greatly in their quality and credentials, and admissions to medical school, the educational experience, and the requirements for graduation lacked quality control. Not surprisingly, educational programs received little, if any, evaluation. In short, educational chaos reigned largely unchallenged in the medical education system. Exploited for profit and personal gain and not for improving patients' welfare, medical education was, to a large extent, a national disgrace.

Change came about because the Flexner Report of 1910 challenged the status quo. It established new quality standards to define proper medical education. The report created a revolution that purified medical school education (undergraduate medical education or UGME), which in turn spawned residency education programs (graduate medical education or GME) using, to a large degree, the same standards as used in UGME.

After the closure of many, if not all, poor-quality schools, the remaining medical schools and the American Medical Association (AMA) became responsible for advancing and applying the Flexnerian standards. From the moment of its original formation in 1876 to its closing in 1880 and then after its second initiation in 1890, the Association of American Medical Colleges (AAMC) joined the fray. With the establishment of these quality standards came public acceptance of medical education, prestige, money, buildings, highly trained faculty, schools, prizes, promotions in academia based upon effectiveness as educators, reviews, reforms, research in medical education, journals containing scholarly research articles, conferences, professional societies, and great pride in the educational institutions. As a result, in the century since publication of the Flexner Report, American UGME and GME have become world standards for developing countries and have been in total, or in large part, reproduced around the globe.

Pre-Flexner State of Continuing Medical Education

Comparing the status of CME to UGME and GME brings the realization that the difference between (1) medical school and residency training and (2) CME is vast. CME is largely fragmented and lacking an integrated structure. Some have observed that "there is a CME enterprise on every street corner." Continuity of CME planning and experiences is limited. The definition of educational needs lags behind UGME and GME. CME contains a large, for-profit element to the enterprise. CME has no dedicated faculty, i.e., those whose primary educational job is CME. CME has limited funds except what it can raise. Except at Meharry Medical College, no CME buildings or schools exist. CME has limited prestige in the public eye, and no CME prizes for excellence are widely applauded. Academic promotions for creativity and excellent achievement in CME are rare. CME has not been the subject of major national reviews that would result in recommenda-

tions that professionals and policymakers would embrace strongly. The number of CME research projects, scholarly papers, journals, and conferences pale in comparison to those of UGME and GME.

The biggest and most critical difference, however, is that CME has never been adopted by medical schools, universities, and professional societies as a highly important, integral, and legitimate part of their missions. In short, CME has never been baptized with academic holy water and, hence, has never been accepted as being equal to UGME and/or GME. It has always been a not-too-important outsider that must raise its own funds and pay faculty members to participate. CME, therefore, differs greatly from UGME and GME, and the lack of acknowledgment that CME is equal to UGME and GME prevents a continuum of medical education from becoming a functioning reality.

Looking over the weaknesses in the CME effort, it is not a stretch to conclude that CME is in a pre-Flexnerian stage of evolution similar to where UGME and GME were in 1910. Until CME matures as UGME and GME did after release of the Flexner Report, it is safe to say that a continuum of medical education that incorporates CME will exist in word only.

Implications

Given that a continuum does not exist at this time, a legitimate question must be raised as to whether medical education needs a continuum. The answer to this question is most assuredly yes. Reasons for this answer involve time and globalization.

Time

For most educators, the time in the educational process to impact the learner is thought to bear a near straight line relationship to changes in behavior and the acquisition of knowledge and skills. If this is true—and most educators would agree that it has great merit—then CME is infinitely more important than UGME and GME. This reflects the fact that the CME portion of medical education covers the entire practicing life of a medical professional or usually a period of up to 40 years. In contrast, UGME covers four years and GME usually lasts from three to seven years. At a minimum, CME should be of equal importance to UGME and GME. Such importance for CME should be reflected in the time, energy, and creative thought educators put into it, and CME should adhere to the same Flexnerian standards as UGME and GME.

Globalization

The four forces of globalization are rapidly producing a single global village of which all human beings are a part. These forces are (1) a global economy linking all national economies together, (2) a global language of English, (3) a global communication system involving communication satellites and cables, and (4) a global transportation system. These four forces pull all members of the human race closer together and make us increasingly dependent on one another. Additionally, as time and distance shrink, a new world unlike anything mankind has known is emerging.

Given the magnitude of change brought about by the four forces that are creating the global village, it is not surprising that the four cornerstones of the profession—biomedical science, medical education, patient care, and ethics—are in the process of becoming globalized as well.

Biomedical Science
Biomedical science has become a global enterprise. An unprecedented number of multinational projects have occurred or are underway. Examples include mapping the genome, exploring RNA biology, searching for genetic predisposition to many diseases, and the search for stem cells with regenerative capacities. In addition, clinical trials are being globalized as indicated by the fact that in 2008, 956 companies conducted

clinical trials in 70 different countries. Furthermore, globalized regulation of scientific products is evidenced by the opening of three US Food and Drug Administration (FDA) offices in China and FDA plans to open more foreign offices. These FDA offices are designed to protect the quality of products imported into the United States.

These developments have profound implications for CME. The instructional challenge that comes with globalized biomedical science is to educate all practicing physicians throughout the world as to these developments and their effects on public and patient health. Hence, the importance of CME will increase in the future.

Medical Education
Motivated, in part, by the fact that most US universities have or are developing global education programs, medical schools have slowly entered the new world of the global village. For example, the University of Colorado assisted in the formation of the University of Riyadh medical school, the Weill Cornell Medical School established a branch campus in Qatar, and Duke University assisted in starting a new medical school in Singapore. In addition, some medical schools, including those in Nepal and China, offer medical education to students from around the globe. Some universities, such as the University of Michigan, also offer a portion of their UGME experience in an online or virtual form to anyone in the global village. Given these activities, it seems safe to predict that this process will sweep across all three segments of the educational continuum and boost the importance of CME in medical education in the future.

Patient Care
Patient care is also becoming globalized as evidenced by three movements: patient travel, physician relocation, and animal transport. First, many employees of multinational businesses work and live outside of their home countries. In addition, in a process called *medical tourism*, patients leave their home countries to seek medial care in

foreign countries for reasons of cost and quality of health care. Furthermore, this movement of potential patients is compounded by recreational tourism, which has reached historic global levels. Each of these tourists represents a potential patient.

Second, an increasing number of physicians are leaving their home countries and settling in foreign settings to practice medicine. While this is not a new phenomenon, what is new is the magnitude of the migration.

Third, animals that will become pets are transported around the globe and, in the process, act as mobile reservoirs of disease. One example is the spread of the Hanta virus by rodents.

Through these three patterns of movement, any disease *anywhere* in the world may emerge *everywhere* in the world. This poses an enormous challenge for medical educators. Nowhere is this challenge larger than in the CME portion of the continuum.

Ethics

Ethics, reflecting the cultural traditions of different countries, is the most complex and difficult of the four cornerstones when it comes to globalization. It is also the least globalized, lagging far behind biomedical science, medical education, and patient care. For decades, the World Medical Association (WMA) has, through its representatives of national medical associations, issued ethical opinions that it has hoped would become standards for the global village. Unfortunately, these "standards" have been adopted to only a limited degree by individual professional societies around the globe.

Additionally, all would acknowledge that for a profession to exist, it must have a set of core values that clearly define that profession. Sometimes, these core values are expressed in the form of oaths (e.g., Hippocratic), sometimes as prayers (e.g., Prayer of Maimonides), or through professional and/or government pronouncements. These core values become the standards by which all members of a profession are expected to aspire

and live. Unfortunately, to date no such uniform core value standards have been enunciated and accepted by physicians around the globe. Hence, a global profession of medicine has not emerged.

In 1999, an attempt was made to determine whether it is possible to achieve a global consensus on what constitutes the core values of a global medical profession. A conference was held in Beijing, China, to compare the core values of the medical profession in China with those in the United States.[1] The planners reasoned that if the core values of these two widely different cultures were the same, then it would be reasonable to envision, at least, that a global profession of medicine is possible. Interestingly, after 11 major presentations, divided equally between Chinese and US speakers, a general consensus emerged that the core values of the United States, which emerged from Judeo-Christian ethics, and the core values of China, which emerged from Confucianism, are the same.

A second US-China conference sought to determine whether the application of these common core values to the use of humans in experimental research would be equally compatible.[2] Fourteen papers representing 18 individuals from both countries concluded that the answer to the question was yes. Not surprising, vast differences of opinions remained on what actions should be taken on the technical aspects of this issue. Such differences existed within the US delegation and among the Chinese attendees as well as between the two countries. All participants agreed on the need to harmonize the guidelines so that they could be applied around the globe.

The growing focus on values underlying the profession of medicine at a global level is saturated with educational needs in all three portions of medical education. As such, these needs are pushing the creation of a continuum of medical education.

Clearly, the process of globalization and its impact on the four cornerstones of medicine usher in a world of opportunities for CME. If global standards are demanded for financial management and trade in the global economy, along with global standards for the quality of food, drugs, devices, toys, and other products traded around the globe, how can the four cornerstones of medicine expect to be exempt from this standard-setting tsunami? The answer is they cannot and, hence, it will fall to CME to educate all practicing physicians on these global standards when these standards appear.

Outcomes and Competency-Based Medical Education

Outcome-oriented education is relatively new to the educational scene. Under this philosophy, educators must define, in the form of competencies, what they want the products of their educational programs to know, what they want them to be able to do, and how they want them to think and act. For medicine, this would include the knowledge, skills, clinical reasoning abilities, and the professional behaviors that medical educators expect their graduates to possess.

Outcomes-based education is a revolutionary idea because it sets achievement as the constant (outcome competencies) and time (length of educational process) and methods of instruction as the variables. Currently, our educational efforts focus on time and, to a large extent, methods as being the constants and on outcomes as being the variable. In fact, little creative thought has been given in the global educational system to outcomes in medical education.

Outcomes-based education provides the basis for research studies to compare different lengths of educational programs as to their effectiveness. In the same vein, it provides the framework for determining which methods of instruction are the most effective in achieving the desired competencies. It also allows for the study of the different learning styles of individual students as well as the impact of different preparatory experiences before medical school and in competency acquisition during the medical education process. A recent article even proposed establishing

outcome competencies for teachers across the continuum of medical education.[3]

For UGME or medical school education, the Global Minimum Essential Requirements (GMER) Project defined not only the 60 outcome competencies that every graduating medical student of any medical school in the world should possess,[4] but it also developed ways to test for the presence of these competencies. In addition, it conducted an implementation trial involving the soon-to-graduate medical students of eight of China's best medical schools. It also established performance standards for students, individual schools, and all eight schools combined, and it developed quantitative report cards for each student, for each school, and for all schools together.

Individual student report cards showed where each student stood compared to all students in their class, how they compared to all students who took the exam, and how their individual performance measured up to the global performance standards that had been set for the exam. The report cards delineated student strengths and weaknesses as well as borderline performance. In short, it gave the students a quantitative menu for further education focused on their individual educational needs.

The report cards for individual schools showed how the performance of each school's students as a group compared with all students who took the exam and how they compared to the global performance standards. The quantitative reports showed the school's strengths, weaknesses, and borderline areas, thereby providing a blueprint for educational reform based upon the needs of each school as defined by the GMER competencies and their students' performance. It should also be emphasized that strict security was maintained so that the names of the schools and/or the students never became public. Hence, there was no competition between individuals or schools, only competition against the GMER competencies.

As with the two previously described report cards for students and individual schools, the quantitative report cards given to the ministers of education and health documented the aggregate performances of all eight schools and compared it them to the global performance standards for schools.[5] The report also indicated the strengths, weaknesses, and borderline areas that in turn presented a checklist for medical educational reform in the People's Republic of China.

At the residency level of medical education, the Accreditation Council for Graduate Medical Education has also established six broadly defined competencies that every person who completes a residency training program must possess regardless of the subdiscipline of medicine in which the training occurs. The definition of how these general competency requirements are defined in specific terms for any given residency and how to evaluate if the graduates possess these competencies has been left to the individual training programs. If these competencies could be defined in more detail for both the core requirements of all residency training programs and for each specialty area, they would, in essence, become the basis for defining the competency requirements for each physician practicing in every specialty. When this happens, the competencies required of residency graduates will become critically important to CME educators as the core competencies for medical school graduates will become of great interest to residency educators. As such, outcomes-based education will demand a continuum of medical education. That this will become global in scope may be seen from developments in Europe.

In Europe, the European Union (EU) has adopted an educational philosophy that is captured in the Bologna Accord. In its simplest form, this accord sets as a goal to have no national boundaries in Europe for education. This means that there would be uniform educational standards in all universities in Europe with a free flow of faculty, students, and graduates across national borders. For medicine, this accord has resulted in the establishment of the Tuning Project, which is attempting to define the core requirements for graduation at all medical schools in the EU. Competencies are playing a major role in their deliberations.

Given the emergence of outcome-competency–based education, it is easy to see how this approach can be readily incorporated into the accreditation process of UGME, GME, and CME. This will, when implemented, push the emergence of CME as an integral and equal partner of UGME and GME and initiate the emergence of a true medical education continuum.

Physician Performance Assessment

While educators can instill the desired competencies into their trainees, they cannot ensure that the trainees will perform according to their competencies when they practice medicine. For this and many other reasons, assessing physician performance has become an increasingly important area of study. However, for this type of assessment to become widely accepted and implemented, two developments must occur: (1) the implementation of a standardized, computerized patient health record and (2) the definition and acceptance of surrogate end points for quality of care. The latter will serve the same role as competencies play in an outcomes-based educational process.

When these two requirements are satisfied, it will be possible for the individual physician to profile his or her practice and to compare his or her performance to others in the group, community, or state and to national or global standards established by the specialty group. Such an analysis should define each physician's weaknesses such that a tailored CME program can be designed to correct those weaknesses. It may also be possible to include experts' input into the design of the educational effort through a process known as *academic detailing*. After the physician completes this tailored education program, he or she can return to practice and reprofile his or her effort to see if the CME program corrected the weakness. When this process is implemented, CME will immediately become equal to—if not more important than—UGME and GME, and a functioning continuum of medical education will finally become a reality. It will also usher in the dawn of the golden age of CME.

Genomic Century

Medicine has entered the new world of genomic medicine with its personalized health care based upon one's own genetic profile and predispositions to disease. In this new world, some believe that science will finally be able to settle the age old question of whether a disease is nature or nurture based in its genesis; others believe a genetic basis for many diseases may be found, though this may be a complex interaction between many different genes.

Especially exciting is the use of stem cells, which is thought to be building toward regenerative medicine in which newly developed organs or parts of organs can be grown by engineering stem cells to follow certain pathways of development. For the visionaries, nanomedicine, which will involve medicine at the molecular level, also beckons on the horizons of science.

Whether these scenarios play out as envisioned, enough new developments will occur in medicine to pose an enormous challenge for medical educators. This challenge emanates from the fact that only a small part of what a physician will encounter in his or her 30 to 40 years of practice will be taught in medical school and residency training. The reason is that the majority of new information will be discovered after physicians finish their formal training. Hence, the burden of seeing to this transfer of information will be, as it always has been, on the backs of CME providers. It follows that as scientific discoveries accelerate so will the CME burden. To maximize both the effectiveness and efficiency of the CME efforts, the prior knowledge of the learner, including medical school and residency training, will be increasingly critical. It will also not be possible to assume that the information base of all physicians will be the same and, therefore, individualized educational efforts will have to be pursued. This sequence will make CME increasingly more important and at least equal to UGME and GME.

Information Technology

The information technology revolution is reshaping the landscape of how, where, and when people learn. Widespread utilization of technology such as online (distant) education, computer-assisted instruction, messaging, texting, etc., affects all three segments of medical education and forces revisions of educational pedagogy and methods of instruction and evaluation. This is especially important to CME where educational materials must be available when a physician is available and recognizes that he or she has an educational need. The preparation of electronic information should always raise the following questions: (1) what has the physician been taught in medical school and residency training? and (2) how do the electronic materials build upon this information base? Hence, the continuum emerges.

Health Care Reform

The need for health care reform spurs a great deal of discussion. Some educators believe CME can play a major role in educating physicians on evidence-based medical practice, on how to improve the efficiency and effectiveness of health care, and on changes in the system of care that lead to improved patient outcomes. Some even believe that by doing this, the costs of health care will be reduced. Achieving these goals will require an enormous CME effort. For greatest cost effectiveness, this effort again must build upon the prior experiences of one's educational sequence, therefore allowing the continuum to emerge further.

Epidemic of Ethical Misconduct

Even the casual reader of newspapers, professional journals, and/or special interest publications comes to the conclusion that the medical profession has a serious problem of ethical violations and perhaps even an epidemic of ethical misconduct in many, if not all, countries. Among the adverse behaviors seen in these publications are such things as cheating and drug abuse by medical students; inappropriate contact between residents and patients and between residents and trainees during the educational years; and conflicts of interest, fraud, lying, and inappropriate physician-patient relationships during the practice years. Of these, it could be argued that the most serious transgressions occur in the CME part of a physician's life.

Simultaneous with the appearance of this epidemic has come an increasing emphasis on medical professionalism and the importance, if not the sacredness, of the physician-patient relationship. Many believe this relationship forms the foundation for the unwritten contract or covenant that exists between the profession of medicine and society. Clearly, courses on professionalism and standards of ethical behavior during medical school and residency training have not stemmed the tide of this epidemic. Neither have pronouncements and regulations emanating from professional societies and government agencies. What is needed, among other things, is a declaration that unethical behavior is a syndrome that expresses itself at least as early as medical school and achieves full blossom during the practice years. Such a declaration would lead to studies about the causes of the disorder, how it can be prevented, the natural history of the disease, and what therapies may help cure or mitigate its expression.

In addition, in medical education, a mandatory longitudinal ethics curriculum covering the three segments of the educational continuum must be developed. In such a longitudinal endeavor, course content must build on what came before and it should make extensive use of actual cases of misconduct to repeatedly demonstrate the ethical principle involved. These cases must also be made appropriate to where the learner is in the continuum. CME, being the longest segment of the continuum, is critical to this prevention strategy. To be successful or to have any hope of success, it must build upon what has been taught in the previous two segments of medical education and, if nothing has been presented in medical school and/or residency training, CME must correct this shortfall in the educational experience it provides.

Leadership

As previously mentioned, the United States and its medical education programs have been looked upon by people outside of the United States as one of the leaders, if not *the* leader, in global medical education. Trainees have come to the United States from around the globe for educational experiences. Some have remained to continue their education or to practice medicine in this country; many others have returned home to create training programs resembling US programs. Clearly, the developing world has watched, with great interest, the educational developments in the United States and other developed countries. At this moment in time, as the developing countries labor to build their first two phases of the continuum, they show growing interest in what the United States is doing in the CME realm and how this relates to UGME and GME. Hence, if the United States wishes to continue to be a world leader, the US CME system must emerge as a part of a functioning medical education continuum.

For these and many other reasons, it is imperative that educators shift their thinking, creativity, and programs to be continuum oriented. When such is done, a number of issues come clearly into focus. For example, why do some physicians who are fully competent, and have the knowledge, skills, and know-how to think and behave professionally, fail to perform properly? To pursue an answer to this question will require a study of behavior across the continuum.

Another example is the life-long learner. At a 1989 international meeting on CME at the Annenberg Center on the Eisenhower Medical Center campus in California, professor Andre Wynen stated, *"CME begins the first day of medical school* [emphasis added]." For this to happen, learning must become a habit that brings joy and satisfaction to the learner. When this is achieved, the individual becomes a life-long learner. This process must begin at least on the first day of medical school, if not long before formal medical education begins. It is likely that if medical educators view the creation of life-long learners as one of their major educational responsibilities, then carrying out this sacred duty will require that they approach the issue over the continuum of medical education and not just in one of the three segments.

Where Do We Start?

If a functioning continuum does not exist and if the developments discussed in this chapter convince the reader that such a continuum will be essential in the future, then where do we start to make such a continuum a reality? It is encouraging that the president of the Association of American Medical Colleges (AAMC), Darrell G. Kirch, MD, has recognized the importance of CME and has hired a premier member of the CME club, David Davis, MD, to create a CME focus within that organization. This could be a first but gigantic step to baptize CME in the holy water of medical academia. If so, it may lead to the ultimate acceptance of CME as an equal to UGME and GME. In addition, if the AAMC can now cooperate fully with the American Medical Association (AMA), which has held CME as an important mission since its founding in 1847, significant progress toward making the continuum a functioning reality is possible.

Looking beyond organizations, if the analogy is correct of CME being at a pre-Flexnerian stage in its development and if a CME Flexner-like report could have the same transforming effect on CME that the 1910 Flexner Report had on UGME (and secondarily on GME), it is imperative that such a study be undertaken. To be maximally effective, this study would have to be undertaken through the eyes of a medical education continuum and not through CME eyes. The latter, while valuable in defining the status of CME, would likely miss the forces that are causing the emergence of the continuum. Among other things, it would fail to ask questions of how the three components of the continuum are related, where the key research questions exist in the continuum, and how to change the perception of CME from an independent entity to an equal part of the continuum. Most importantly, it would fail to wrestle with the issues of how to leverage what has gone on before in the continuum to maximize the effectiveness of CME in changing knowledge, behavior, and thinking and how to make all physicians life-long learners.

If the study were conducted on a global basis, it would be even more useful given that a global system of medical education is beginning to appear in the minds of the world's educators. Evidence for this are the global accreditation programs for UGME, GME, and CME that the World Federation for Medical Education has developed and the GMER Project of global outcome-competency for medical schools, which was discussed previously. Eventually, competency-based (outcomes-based) education will become a cornerstone of accreditation activities. In addition, the increased migration of physicians from the countries where they received their medical education brings the issue of equivalency of learning sharply into focus. Although a global focus for a CME Flexner study would be considerably more challenging than a national focus, the findings and recommendations would be infinitely more useful in the global community of which we are all a part.

Regardless of whether national or global in its focus, if a CME Flexner study is commissioned by a prestigious organization or organizations and if the members on the study committee are highly respected professionals, the likelihood of the study having a transforming and lasting effect would be markedly enhanced. In such a circumstance, a true continuum of medical education should emerge.

Thinking about where the world is and where it seems to be going, one cannot escape the conclusion that CME will become, if it is not already there, the endless frontier of medical education. Such a dream beckons all medical educators from the mists of the future, and it will have to be built on a continuum of medical education that is in the realm of fiction today.

Notes

1. A Global Profession—Medical Values in China and the United States. July–August 2000; A Hastings Center Report Special Supplement, 1–48.

2. M. R. Schwarz and D. T. Stern, eds., "Special Issue: The Human Subjects in Research: Comparing Core Values in the People's Republic of China and the United States," *Journal of Clinical Ethics* 15, no. 1 (2004): 1–96.

3. Yvonne Steinert, "Mapping the Teacher's Role: The Value of Defining Core Competencies for Teaching," *Medical Teacher* 31, no. 5 (2009): 371–372.

4. Core Committee of the Institute for International Medical Education, "Global Minimum Essential Requirements in Medical Education," *Medical Teacher* 24, no. 2 (2002): 130–135.

5. M. R. Schwarz and others, "The Outcomes of Global Minimum Essential Requirements (GMER) Pilot Implementation in China," *Medical Teacher* 29, no. 7 (2007): 699–705.

PART II

Organizations in the Early Development of Continuing Medical Education in the United States

Daniel J. Ostergaard, Mindi K. McKenna,
Elaine Kierl Gangel, and Penelope L. LaRocque

CHAPTER 4

The American Academy of Family Physicians Contribution to Continuing Medical Education

The American Academy of Family Physicians (AAFP), founded in 1947, is one of the largest national medical specialty societies, representing more than 94,000 family physicians, family medicine residents, and medical students. Its vision is to transform health care to achieve optimal health for everyone, and its mission is to improve the health of patients, families, and communities by serving the needs of members with professionalism and creativity.

The Influence of CME on the AAFP Vision and Mission

The importance of continuing medical education (CME) was clear and embedded in the very origin of the AAFP. CME remains central to its organizational framework today.

The AAFP, then known as the American Academy of General Practice (AAGP), was founded in 1947 to establish an organization of general practitioners of medicine and surgery to promote and maintain high standards of general practice and to promote the betterment of the public health. Its founders were committed to the concept of CME and its mandatory completion to better ensure the competence of its members and their ability to provide care for patients.

One of the values of the AAFP and its members is a commitment to care that is supported by lifelong professional learning. Its original bylaws included a committee on education and, as of 2009, the AAFP bylaws contain a requirement for only three standing committees, one of which is a committee on education. Although other medical organizations have had similar initial goals, the AAGP was the first to require, as recorded in its original constitution and bylaws, that "a member each three years must complete 150 hours in postgraduate study of a nature acceptable to the board of directors."

At the time of the AAFP's founding, some observers said the requirement for postgraduate medical education would prevent the AAFP from thriving because it represented a standard to which no other medical society aspired at that time. History has proved those naysayers wrong as the AAFP has flourished.

Following World War II, the practice of medicine in the United States focused on technological advances gained during wartime, and far greater emphasis was placed on medical subspecialties devoted to the care of specific organs and organ systems.[1] General practitioners returning from the war faced daunting professional challenges; specialists received hospital privileges, higher incomes, and greater prestige that general practitioners did not. The change in both

American medicine and societal interest in technology caused student enrollment in general practice to decline. That decline was part of the impetus for the creation of the AAFP. Its tenacious pursuit of, commitment to, and reliance upon CME served as a means to maintain quality among general practitioners for the benefit of their patients.

The Specialty of Family Medicine

The 1960s saw a movement that gravitated away from general practice toward development of a new specialty: family practice. Nicholas Pisacano, MD, was the leader of this movement, and some vilified him for taking a position they thought would result in the creation of boundaries for the specialty. At that time, a certifying board for general practice did not exist, which was perceived as a hindrance to general practice training and residency programs.[2] After years of negotiations, the American Board of Family Practice (ABFP) gained approval in 1969 and joined other formal certifying boards that granted diplomate status.

The formation of the ABFP (renamed the American Board of Family Medicine [ABFM] in 2005) was another demonstration of family practice leadership in CME. When the ABFP was chartered, its eligibility requirement of 150 CME hours every three years for family practice certification was unique. Additionally, the ABFP structure was singular among medical specialties in that it offered a time-limited certificate rather than "a specialist for life" recognition. Again, the educational requirements for family physicians were greater than those required for other specialties. In addition to the required 150 hours every three years, diplomates of the ABFP were also required to pass a secure examination every seven years in order to retain diplomate status; family practice was first in this requirement, but all other specialties have since followed.

The AAFP Dual Role as CME Provider and Accreditor

Family medicine has a demonstrated legacy of commitment to CME. In keeping with that tradition, the AAFP has been and continues to be a leader and innovator in both providing and accrediting CME. Today, it is one of only three national CME-credit-granting entities in the United States, along with the American Osteopathic Association (AOA) and the American Medical Association (AMA), which delegated accreditation authority for its AMA Physician's Recognition Award (PRA) Category 1 CME credit to the Accreditation Council on CME (ACCME) in 1980. The AAFP accredits CME activities whether live, enduring, or online; the AOA accredits organizations and activities; and the ACCME accredits CME provider organizations, including the AAFP, which offer independent certified CME activities.

Over the years, the AAFP has maintained a dual role in the CME community: it functions as both a standard-setting, credit-granting entity and a CME provider. As an accreditor, the AAFP acts as a quality agent for CME activities intended for family physicians, as well as for the outcomes of the activities it accredits. In its role as a CME provider, the AAFP recognizes that family-physician educators and faculty—from planners and developers to authors, editors, and reviewers—have unique and important insights into and knowledge about the CME needs of family physicians. These insights result in the creation of relevant, high-quality CME designed for family physicians.

To better understand AAFP accreditation, an explanation of its credit system and the types of AAFP CME credit granted is necessary. Until 1955, the AAFP described its educational training as *formal* and *informal*; those terms were later replaced by the terms *Category I* and *Category II*. Category I refers to training delivered by medical schools and the AAFP; Category II refers to training delivered by any other organization.

In 1958, the AAFP Commission on Education (which later was refocused and renamed the Commission on Continuing Professional Education) published criteria by which external organizations could develop CME for family physicians. The criteria for an activity to be considered for Category I credit required that an advance copy of the activity program, along with documentation of compliance with AAFP established policies, be submitted through an AAFP advisor. This action, which formed the construct of what would become the AAFP accreditation system, made a clear distinction between the two types of credit.

In 1963, in an effort to better regulate the quality of courses and scientific programs in which AAFP members participated to fulfill their credit requirements, the AAFP Commission on Education recommended that the terms *Category I* and *Category II* be dropped, stating that "the concept is misunderstood, misinterpreted, and misused." Under the new system, members would complete one-third of the required 150 hours by attending accredited AAFP or medical school courses.[3]

In 1966, the AAFP instituted new terms— *Prescribed* and *Elective*—that aimed to more effectively distinguish courses that would meet the 150-hour requirement. In order for a CME activity to be granted Prescribed credit, it must have a direct bearing on patient care or a physician's ability to deliver patient care, or it must relate to select nonclinical topics. Additionally, any activity granted Prescribed credit must be developed with direct involvement by a family physician who is an AAFP member. This last requirement ensures relevancy of CME to family physicians.

In contrast, Elective credit can be granted to those activities designed for other health-care professionals, not specifically family physicians. Elective-credit activities must enhance the physician's professional ability, though not directly influence patient care or delivery.

Early CME Programs and CME Credit

The terminology used to describe types of credit has changed and so too have the types of CME activities for which credit is sought. Traditional CME, primarily the didactic lecture and repurposed materials from those lectures, has evolved over the years to include computer- and Web-based activities. The dynamic nature of CME activities has required nimbleness as well as diligence on the part of the AAFP as a credit-granting entity *and* as a CME-producing entity in order to provide the most relevant and user-friendly learning experience possible for its members.

The AAFP's earliest educational offering was its annual Scientific Assembly, a national conference for thousands of family physicians covering a broad spectrum of education relevant to their scope of practice. Even in its nascent form, this valuable forum allowed practicing physicians to acquire and share advances in medicine to improve patient health. The first Scientific Assembly, held in Cincinnati, Ohio, in 1949, included programs on cancer, heart disease, industrial and rural medicine, malnutrition, and obstetrics. Just as they are today, most of the first Assembly CME sessions were approved for AAFP CME credit.

While the Scientific Assembly provided a venue for members to become immersed in educational opportunities and make personal and professional contacts, the AAFP recognized the need for, and potential of, CME that integrated the emerging technologies of the post-war era. In 1955, with sponsorship from Wyeth Laboratories, the AAFP presented what was, at the time, the largest-ever, closed-circuit television program for postgraduates. On February 24, CBS broadcast *Management of Streptococcal Infections and its Complications*, a five-person panel-discussion program, to television stations in 60 US and five Canadian cities. In each city, a leading AAFP member acted as a moderator for groups of physicians attending the event on-site in local television stations.[4] This innovative program was approved for CME credit.

In another effort to make accredited education available to family physicians in a variety of formats, the AAFP began collaborating in 1963 with the Public Health Service to produce "Shop Talk," a forum for small-group discussion of medical problems on preselected topics. The first program, on cancer detection and control, resulted in a library of four filmstrips and coordinated audiotapes; by 1965, AAFP chapters could access 14 "Shop Talk" programs when developing discussion programs.[5]

In 1967, the AAFP introduced interactive educational technology in the form of *teaching machines*. Teaching machines were simple computers that presented programmed instruction and provided feedback on learners' responses to the questions posed by the machines; these proved popular and were used heavily.

Evaluation of Educational Impact on Physician Practice Performance

In 1967, in an effort to fulfill the AAFP commitment and responsibility to providing CME, the AAFP Commission on Education adopted plans for the first "significant and objective project in the evaluation of continuing education." The goal was to measure physician performance in a particular portion of practice before and after educational experiences.[6]

This appears to be the earliest example that invokes the transition from CME to continuing professional development (CPD). While CME describes the formal educational activities, CPD refers to the continuous enhancement of clinicians' proficiency in providing patient care. Fortunately, pre– and post–self-assessment are now typical components of continuing education, but in the 1960s, that commitment was uniquely innovative.

In addition to its efforts to lead and innovate in the area of CME, the AAFP has remained mindful of members' needs, not only with respect to content but also in considering the manner in which educational activities are provided. In 1970, in response to a survey that asked members about preferred learning environments at the annual assembly, the AAFP offered small-group (up to 15 attendees) seminars as well as traditional large-group lectures.[7]

The most significant action the AAFP took on behalf of its members during this period was in 1971 when it changed its name from the American Academy of General Practice to the American Academy of Family Physicians. This change was undertaken in an effort to be consistent with the ABFP and to "eliminate any semantic distinction between 'general' and 'family' practice, make the [AAFP's] work in establishing family practice programs more effective, and help eliminate misunderstanding among the public and medical community."[8] By 1972, in a related action to support this distinction, the AAFP officially adopted the term *continuing education*, which had first been proposed in 1961, as a replacement for *postgraduate education*.

While the minimum number of 150 credits for membership was maintained, in 1973 the AAFP increased the number of required Prescribed credits from 50 to 75 of the 150 and broadened the options for earning Prescribed credit. The new requirements allowed up to 30 of the 150 hours of credit to be earned via multimedia programs.[9]

In 1974, the AAFP premiered its subscription professional-study program and once again turned to closed-circuit television technology to produce videocassette tapes with the assistance of a communication service company. The project was short-lived, but the AAFP continued to research methods for offering CME to members via video technology and, ultimately, developed other options.[10]

In 1976, the AAFP Commission on Education proposed the creation of a freestanding Committee on Continuing Medical Education (COCME), the forerunner of the current Commission on Continuing Professional Development. The purpose of the committee was to "assist AAFP members by providing the fullest possible access to continuing medical education programs of quality, relevance, structure and involvement."[11] The COCME held its first meeting in February 1977; in 1981, the committee became a commission. The AAFP now has a Commission on Education for student interest and residency as well as a Commission on Continuing Professional Development for CME.

Further Advances in Physician Self-Assessment and Lifelong Learning

In 1976, a plan was approved for an AAFP core curriculum self-assessment program as a means to provide targeted educational opportunities for lifelong learning and professional recertification; in 1978, this became the Home Study Self-Assessment (HSSA) program.[12] Now known by the product names *FP Essentials* and *FP Audio*, the monthly self-study programs follow a nine-year curriculum, divided into three three-year curriculum cycles, and include printed and PDF versions of the monographs and written outlines, CDs and MP3s, and testing materials with pre- and post-tests. The curriculum cycle covers the topics on the ABFM recertification examination that diplomates must take every seven or 10 years and provides a comprehensive review of specific clinical and practice-related topics. Each *FP Essentials* edition is granted five to eight Prescribed credits and each *FP Audio* edition is granted two Prescribed credits.[13]

Record Keeping as Part of CPD

The AAFP recognized that the ability to report credits earned as a result of participating in a CME activity was, from the physician's perspective, a critical element in the CME process. In 1976, five AAFP chapters participated in a pilot project to test a system in which members could submit personalized computer cards each time they attended an approved course. These cards were sent to the AAFP headquarters in Kansas City where the credits were added to each member's computer record. By early 1977, the AAFP had created a computerized records department capable of managing the CME records of more than 16,000 members in 37 participating state chapters; by 1978, the number of participating chapters increased to 47.[14] By April 2003, the AAFP began using scannable answer sheets to more rapidly and accurately record CME credit for members and nonmembers.[15] Today, much of the AAFP CME is accessible online, and quiz results are automatically recorded for members; nonmembers also use the online system and can easily request statements of credit.

Further Enhancements to AAFP CME Programming

Continuing in its commitment to provide CME activities in a variety of formats and media, the AAFP launched its video CME program in September 1983. Early video programs included *Sports Injuries of the Knee and Ankle*, *Medical Management of Arthritis*, and *Suturing Techniques*. While the delivery formats have evolved over the decades from VHS to DVD to Web access, the commitment to quality and relevant CME remains constant.

Between 1986 and 1993, the AAFP produced a monthly program called *Family Practice Update* that aired on the Lifetime Medical Television network. The program's talk-show format featured a host who interviewed expert guests about the most recent diagnostic and treatment techniques in family medicine.

Collaborations with Other Organizations

In its efforts to develop the most up-to-date and valuable educational programs for family physicians, the AAFP has often collaborated with other CME provider organizations, including other medical specialty societies. For instance, in 1977 alone, the AAFP developed and participated in an obstetrics conference with the American College of Obstetricians and Gynecologists, developed a program titled "Contemporary Management of Acute Myocardial Infarction" with the American College of Cardiology, and cosponsored programs with the American Academy of Dermatology and the Society of Teachers of Family Medicine. The AAFP also developed the CME section of the AMA 31st National Conference on Rural Health.[16] The value of collaboration is explicitly reflected in current ACCME criteria for Accreditation with Commendation, an esteemed designation that AAFP consistently earns in its ACCME accreditation review cycles.

To serve educational needs beyond those of allopathic family physicians, in 1995, the AAFP sought and was granted accreditation from the American Osteopathic Association for its self-study subscription program. This AAFP effort ensures that osteopathic physicians practicing in primary care settings continue to receive educational access to and earn CME credit from this important educational program.[17]

AAFP's Relationships with Industry in Support of Patient Care

Consistent with the AAFP's more than 60-year heritage of commitment to optimal patient care, the AAFP has long understood the benefit to patients of collaboration with government and industry. Such interactions, when appropriately managed, can facilitate and accelerate the appropriate translation of research into education and patient care. And yet, such relationships can be susceptible to potential conflicts of interest that must be identified and addressed. This requires purposeful deliberation and an unwavering commitment to the highest standards of ethics and professionalism. Since its inception, the AAFP has recognized its responsibilities to establish and uphold policies and practices that are above reproach.[18]

The AAFP approach makes a thorough and unrestricted analysis of its present and potential relationships with commercial companies to en-sure such relationships are designed to improve patient health. For example, in order to demonstrate its commitment to science by applying rigor to the CME activities that it produced and accredited, the AAFP formed, in 1991, an ad hoc committee on proprietary practices.[19] Of the two issues studied by that 1991 committee—(1) the relationships between the pharmaceutical industry and physicians and (2) direct-to-consumer advertising in medical journals—the first issue would have direct and significant bearing on CME.

The committee utilized two reference reports to formulate its policies on the role of commercial support: the ACCME Standards for Commercial Support of Continuing Medical Education and the AMA Ethical Guidelines for Gifts to Physicians from Industry. While the AAFP supports the current (2004) version of the ACCME Standards for Commercial Support, the AAFP has taken a more rigorous stance than required by such guidelines that defined *industry* as being related only to pharmaceuticals, medical devices, and equipment. For example, AAFP policies ensure independence from inappropriate influence by "all proprietary health-related entities that might create a conflict of interest."[20] The AAFP holds to a high standard the actions of all involved in AAFP-accredited or AAFP-produced CME, including external supporters and faculty responsible for planning, producing, delivering, or influencing AAFP-accredited CME to ensure such activities are not biased by conflicting interests.

A key mechanism used to ensure content validity was, and remains, the editorial control exercised in the creation and review of educational content; in effect, the entity producing the CME activity would retain *complete* editorial control.

As to the CME content directly produced by the AAFP, a policy was adopted requiring all faculty to report any funding received from external supporters of activities with which they have involvement. Furthermore, this information was made available prior to participation in the CME activity. In current times, such funding does not flow directly to physician faculty for independent accredited CME.[21] But at that point in history, the AAFP Conflict of Interest Declaration was rather revolutionary. The organization continues to require all faculty (speakers, authors, advisors, or planners) of AAFP-produced CME activities to comply with all relevant laws, regulations, policies, and standards to ensure the highest level of ethics and professionalism. As a result, all involved parties are diligently conscientious about disclosure of relationships and mitigation of real or perceived conflicts of interest in order to ensure the independence of professional education.

In 2000, the AAFP acted once more to ensure its programs' integrity and independence from commercial influence. Its Commission on Continuing Medical Education explicitly conveyed that certain activities produced by proprietary entities such as pharmaceutical companies, medical device manufacturers, or health-care communications companies acting on behalf of proprietary entities, would be deemed ineligible for credit. The AAFP granted an exception for CME activities produced by private foundations established by proprietary entities if the focus was "on non-clinical topics that are eligible for review under established Academy policies." Such activities included medico-legal and ethical issues, faculty development, physician-patient relations, practice management and quality assurance, among others.[22]

In 2005, the AAFP adopted the ACCME Updated Standards for Commercial Support, which had been revised in 2004 to be more stringent. Strict adherence to the revised standards reduced the risk of inappropriate commercial influence or content bias in CME.[23]

The Advanced Life Support in Obstetrics Program

Whether through policies intended to eliminate bias in CME content or policies intended to increase relevancy of content, the AAFP has always had an unwavering commitment to professional education that improves public health. This commitment is exemplified in the AAFP Advanced Life Support in Obstetrics (ALSO®) program.

The ALSO program, initially developed by the University of Wisconsin Department of Family Medicine, teaches all members of a health-care team to provide nonsurgical emergency maternity care.[24] In addition to providing the needed and desired continuing education courses in obstetric emergencies, the acquisition of the ALSO program was initiated as a proactive step to bolster family physicians' waning interest in obstetric practice, as well as to provide a refresher course for family physicians who wished to return to obstetric care.[25]

In the years since 1993, when AAFP acquired the program and its copyright, the course has been administered in 50 countries and has trained more than 100,000 maternity care providers worldwide. ALSO courses are highly structured, interactive, and rely on evidence-based content. High-quality skills are developed through the use of mnemonics, supervised practice, and case-based discussions. In addition to the curriculum, the program includes pre-course self-assessment tools and concludes with a written exam and the requirement that learners demonstrate acquired skills at a "megadelivery testing station." Along with courses on nonemergency and emergency maternity care, the ALSO program offers an instructor course for physicians, obstetricians, registered nurses, and certified nurse midwives who wish to teach ALSO skills to other caregivers in their communities.[26]

Expansion of Educational Opportunities

In another effort to expand educational opportunities, the AAFP grants CME credit to physicians who complete quiz cards after reading select professional, peer-reviewed journal articles, including the AAFP premier clinical journal *American Family Physician* and some publications produced by other entities for which AAFP CME credit is sought. In keeping with its ongoing commitment to educational and editorial rigor, the AAFP established mechanisms to ensure the CME articles would meet appropriate standards of content validity and scientific objectivity and that there was a clear distinction between journal advertisements and educational content. To monitor this distinction, AAFP accreditation advisors and staff preview the journals before credit is granted and conduct post-publication reviews as an additional oversight mechanism.

Annual Clinical Focus

Recognizing the value of focusing educational efforts on conditions that affect wide ranges of the patient population, the AAFP launched the innovative Annual Clinical Focus program in 1998. This program was "an education initiative designed to bring members state-of-the-art information and resources in a specific clinical area each year."[27] The clinical focus for 1998 was cardiovascular disease management.[28] Subsequent years brought educational focus to other important health concerns addressed by family physicians, such as cancer, genetic diseases and risk factors, infectious disease, and chronic illness. The AAFP has since redesigned the program to provide educational support for closing gaps in knowledge or practice performance in a manner that is consistent with current best practices in patient-centered, learner-directed, needs-driven, outcomes-oriented CPD.

The AAFP Commitment to Scientific Advances: Evidence-Based CME

In 1999, the AAFP undertook another endeavor to protect the integrity of AAFP CME activities and to demonstrate its unwavering commitment to science. The AAFP recognized that topics pertaining to complementary and alternative medicine (CAM) were becoming more prevalent in CME activities as a result of increased use of CAM therapies by patients. Furthermore, it was recognized that such CME activities were being awarded Prescribed credit.

The AAFP invited the ACCME, the ABFM, the AMA, the AOA, and the Federation of State Medical Boards to a forum to discuss controversies related to CAM and to devise a strategy for addressing them in the context of CME. Those deliberations triggered a broader advancement: the AAFP's advocacy of evidence-based CME (EBCME). EBCME was introduced as a unique category of AAFP CME because it met certain unique criteria. Specifically, to be designated as EBCME, the live activity or online or enduring material had to include key practice recommendations (points intended to change physician behaviors) that were substantiated by AAFP-approved evidence-based sources.

Evidence-based sources, such as the Cochrane Collaboration, the Agency for Healthcare Research and Quality (AHRQ), and the US Preventive Services Task Force (USPSTF), contain medical information derived from the best currently available research, ideally double-blind, placebo-controlled, randomized clinical trials or comparably rigorous peer-reviewed, methodologically sound meta-analyses. The topics must be systematically identified, appraised, and summarized according to predetermined criteria. This is meant to assure clinician learners that practice recommendations are the result of a systematic review of all available best evidence.

At the same time that EBCME was introduced, the AAFP changed its designation of Prescribed credit to refer to AAFP CME credit approved for customary and generally accepted medical practice, if an AAFP member was involved in developing the activity. Elective credit would be granted to topics for which the evidence base was not yet as rigorous but that were customary and generally accepted medical practice and that were not dangerous to patients; this included most CAM therapies.[29]

In May 2000, the AAFP HSSA program was included in the AAFP pilot revision of accreditation toward an evidence-based approach with a monograph on hypertension.[30] By 2002, the AAFP established the evidence-based designation for CME credit and instituted a new process for awarding EBCME credit.

Later, the AAFP updated its definition of EBCME to include practice recommendations from other sources, so long as they met certain rigorous criteria. The AAFP continues to provide an evidence-based resources list to anyone involved in planning, producing, or reviewing CME.

Many different classifications were and still are used to stratify the quality of studies as well as the strength of recommendations related to evidence-based recommendations. In an effort to present evidence in a unified way for publications focused on family medicine, a unique classification or taxonomy was developed.[31]

The Strength of Recommendation Taxonomy (SORT) system addresses the quality, quantity, and consistency of evidence and allows authors and readers of journal articles to rate individual studies or bodies of evidence. SORT emphasizes the use of patient-oriented outcomes that measure changes in morbidity or mortality.[32]

In the SORT ABC scale, a rating of A is the highest level of recommendation based on "consistent and good-quality patient-oriented evidence." B-level recommendations are based on inconsistent or limited-quality evidence. C-level recommendations are based primarily on consensus, usual practice, or expert opinion.[33] This taxonomy remains in use today.

An outgrowth of EBCME was the AAFP decision in 2004 to grant double credit for any portion of a CME activity granted the evidence-based designation. The AAFP saw this as a means to build awareness of the importance and value of CME based upon best available evidence. Over the years, awareness has grown of the importance of evidence-based content and evidence-based practice in the design of all CME. Thus, the AAFP eliminated the transitional mechanism of double credit in 2010 and now expects that all AAFP-accredited Prescribed CME should be developed and provided by using best available evidence in educational design and medical science.[34]

Point-of-Care CME

In 2006, the AAFP, in a collaborative initiative with the AMA, launched a new category of CME credit for point-of-care CME activities. Point-of-care CME is practice-based learning that takes place in the clinical setting when the physician uses one or more computer-based clinical decision-making reference tools to search for an answer to a clinical question and then, if appropriate, applies the knowledge to care for the patient.[35] Current available reference tools feature regularly updated, searchable databases that include synthesized evidence on thousands of medical topics and terms; practice recommendations; disease descriptions, diagnoses, and treatments; drugs and dosing recommendations, contraindications, adverse reactions, and pregnancy categories; laboratory manuals and medical calculators.[36] A 2005 study of one major database showed that, while search times (averaging approximately 4.8 to 5.2 minutes) remained the same whether physicians used the database or more traditional search sites such as MEDLINE, searchers were able to answer more of their questions and find answers that changed clinical decision making when using the database because of the centralization of a broad range of information.[37]

Up to half of a CME credit is granted for each search, and up to 20 Prescribed credits per year can be claimed for these activities. In order to be eligible for credit, the AAFP requires that point-of-care activities—even those that do not result in a change in clinical decision making—be delivered by an ACCME-accredited CME provider and meet the following criteria:

- Provide consistent, reproducible search of evidence by including the learner's question and the citation for the AAFP-approved source

- Document how evidence is reviewed, updated, and applied in practice
- Describe how the strength of the evidence is evaluated
- Emphasize patient-oriented evidence over disease-oriented evidence
- Involve family physicians and the family medicine perspective in the generation of the content
- Rate explicitly the strength of evidence

Interestingly, point-of-care CME has not yielded as much practical application as originally expected. For example, during 2008, only 1.4 percent of CME reported to the AAFP was for point-of-care activities.[38] It seems that point-of-care CME is not a natural extension of point-of-care learning. In a practical sense, so long as physicians are engaged in practice-based learning and improvement, they will be experiencing CPD, which is ultimately what matters for optimal patient care.

Performance-Improvement CME and Maintenance of Certification and Licensure

The AAFP has always understood that physicians must continually assess and improve their performance. In recent years, growing synergy among quality-improvement experts and educators has resulted in quality-improvement (QI) and performance-improvement (PI) initiatives involving CME. The AAFP first proposed such a program in 1997. At that early stage in the development of the QI movement, this proposal was determined to be impractical because of the cost to develop such an innovative program as well as the small number of physicians who were likely to participate.

In 1999, the American Board of Medical Specialties imposed new requirements for maintenance of certification for all medical specialty organizations.[39] One important difference was the requirement for measuring practice performance. Consequently, the ABFM diplomates were required to demonstrate performance improvement in practice. This new requirement, which addressed practice performance, would become known as MC-FP Part IV.

In 2000, the AAFP considered another QI program but with a different development approach. The Family Physicians–Improving Quality (FP–IQ) program was developed in collaboration with the American Academy of Neurology, which made its development affordable. This was the first PI activity for which AAFP Prescribed credit was available.[40]

FP-IQ was a self-assessment program, which, by 2002, included one module on the topic of migraine headache. The module contained a baseline practice questionnaire and a confidential report of peer- and evidence-based data from which to make comparisons. Following the comparisons, the learner was presented with clinical guidelines, interventions, and various tools or strategies for use in implementing change in practice. A follow-up questionnaire was generated, after which comparison feedback was available. Additionally, peer and expert interaction was available via an e-mail group.[41] Participants included 16 family physicians and neurologists. In March 2003, the program was discontinued after it was recognized that a different strategy would be necessary to meet the newly emerging requirements for the ABFM MC-FP Part IV program.

In 2003, the ABFM accepted a proposal from the AAFP to be the sole provider for the MC-FP Part IV program. This arrangement, however, was subsequently determined to be impractical, and the AAFP set about developing its own program that would be acceptable to ABFM as satisfying Part IV.

In 2004, in the absence of definitive language from the ABFM regarding specific requirements and while recognizing the urgency for family physicians to have a means for meeting recertification requirements, the AAFP began developing and testing an MC-FP Part IV program in order to meet the ABFM goal of having a program available in 2005. The new AAFP Measuring, Evaluating, and Translating Research into Care (METRIC) program was designed to contain modules on specific disease states with each module composed of five elements. The first element was a chart audit based on specified performance measures; the second, a feedback report with data comparisons between participants, peers, and national benchmarks; the third, support for developing and implementing a QI plan; the fourth, a subsequent chart audit to determine whether improvements were made; and finally, a report comparing performance at the beginning and the end of the program.

The first AAFP METRIC module focused on diabetes and the second focused on hypertension. Currently, seven modules are available, including METRIC modules on coronary artery disease, chronic obstructive pulmonary disease, depression, diabetes, and geriatric care. The modules are available to AAFP members and other health-care professionals, including the 450 family medicine residency programs that can use METRIC to help residents meet the Accreditation Council for Graduate Medical Education QI competency requirements.

Future of CME

The AAFP uses increasingly rigorous standards to design accredited teaching and learning activities that are needs-driven, outcome-oriented, evidence-based, and active or interactive for maximum improvement of professional competence, practice performance, and patient outcomes.

As an ACCME-accredited CME provider, the AAFP continues to refine its needs-driven practice-relevant-CME curricular framework and to incorporate that core curriculum into all AAFP-produced CME activities through application of current best practices in adult learning. The AAFP is exploring new approaches to facilitate CPD for all core competencies needed by family physicians and patient-care teams, in-

cluding medical knowledge and patient care, of course, but also including communication and interpersonal skills, professionalism, system-based care, and practice-based learning and improvement.

The AAFP is investing in greater enhanced educational technologies for content/data management and learning management systems to provide state-of-the-art tools for physician learners to assess their educational gaps, establish and implement lifelong learning plans, and conveniently track educational impact and clinical outcomes of that lifelong learning based on systematic measurement of practice data. The AAFP is also investing in various innovative approaches to faculty development in order to ensure independence, identify and address potential conflicts of interest, and equip faculty to provide CME and facilitate CPD using current best practices in adult learning.

As a credit-granting entity, the AAFP is proud to have established the country's first national CME accreditation system and to have done so through a system that involves activity-level oversight. The AAFP recently introduced technology to allow for online applications for AAFP CME credit by provider organizations, and it continues to explore ways of ensuring that AAFP-accredited CME meets the highest possible standards of quality, relevance, educational rigor, and freedom from inappropriate influence such as commercial bias or other potential conflicts of interest.

In some respects, the future of CME is much like the past: expectations and needs continue to change. At the time of this writing, significant turbulence is evident in the US system of continuing education for physicians and other health-care professionals. Significant concerns exist regarding the educational impact, funding models, accreditation mechanisms, and societal benefit of CME and CPD. The AAFP is eager to continue its decades-long legacy of leadership in medical education by having a voice in these matters. As a CME provider and accreditor, the AAFP is a uniquely positioned medical specialty society. It is an organization that exists to advance public health by advocating for and meeting its members' educational and practice enhancement needs. Leadership in CME and CPD will continue to be an important aspect of the AAFP mission.

Notes

1. R. B. Taylor, "The Promise of Family Medicine: History, Leadership, and the Age of Aquarius," *Journal of the American Board of Family Medicine* 19, no. 2 (2006): 183–190.

2. American Academy of Family Physicians, "FP Report: 50th Anniversary Edition, A Celebration of the Academy, 1947–1997," AAFP Web site, http://www.aafp.org/ fpr/970100fr/4.html (accessed July 13, 2010).

3. American Academy of Family Physicians, *Annual Report* (Kansas City, Mo.: AAFP, 1963).

4. American Academy of Family Physicians, *Transactions of the Congress of Delegates* (Kansas City, Mo.: AAFP, 1955), 41.

5. American Academy of Family Physicians, *Annual Report* (Kansas City, Mo.: AAFP, 1965).

6. American Academy of Family Physicians, *Annual Report* (Kansas City, Mo.: AAFP, 1967).

7. American Academy of Family Physicians, *Annual Report* (Kansas City, Mo.: AAFP, 1970).

8. American Academy of Family Physicians, *Annual Report* (Kansas City, Mo.: AAFP, 1971); American Academy of Family Physicians, *AAFP Daily News* (Kansas City, Mo.: AAFP, 1971).

9. American Academy of Family Physicians, *Annual Report* (Kansas City, Mo.: AAFP, 1973).

10. American Academy of Family Physicians, *Annual Report* (Kansas City, Mo.: AAFP, 1974).

11. American Academy of Family Physicians, *Transactions of the Congress of Delegates* (Kansas City, Mo.: AAFP, 1976).

12. American Academy of Family Physicians, *CME Historical Perspective* (Leawood, Kans.: AAFP, 2008), 16.

13. American Academy of Family Physicians, *Transactions of the Congress* (1976).

14. American Academy of Family Physicians, *Annual Report* (Kansas City, Mo.: AAFP, 1977).

15. American Academy of Family Physicians, *CME Historical Perspective*, 16.

16. American Academy of Family Physicians, *Annual Report* (1977).

17. American Academy of Family Physicians. *Transactions of the Congress of Delegates* (Kansas City, Mo.: AAFP, 1995), 161.

18. Daniel J. Ostergaard, "Relationships between Family Physicians and the Pharmaceutical Industry," *Journal of Family Practice* 34, no. 1 (1992): 29–31.

19. American Academy of Family Physicians, "Board of Directors Report, Attachment A, Board Report J: White Paper on Proprietary Practices," *Transactions of the Congress of Delegates* (Kansas City, Mo.: AAFP, 1991), 39–50.

20. Ibid.

21. Ibid.

22. American Academy of Family Physicians, *Board of Directors Minutes* (Kansas City, Mo., March 15–19, 2000), 8–9.

23. American Academy of Family Physicians, *COCPD Decisions on Accreditation* (Leawood, Kans., November 3, 2008).

24. American Academy of Family Physicians, "ALSO," AAFP Web site, http://www.aafp.org/online/ en/home/ cme/aafpcourses/clinicalcourses/also/ aboutalso.html (accessed July 13, 2010).

25. American Academy of Family Physicians Task Force on Obstetrics, *Transactions of the Congress of Delegates* (Kansas City, Mo.: AAFP, 1992), 26.

26. H. W. Beasley and others, "The Advanced Life Support in Obstetrics (ALSO) Program: Fourteen Years of Progress," *Prehospital and Disaster Medicine* 20, no. 4 (2005): 271–275.

27. American Academy of Family Physicians, American Cancer Society, American Diabetes Association, and American Heart Association, *Annual Clinical Focus Report*, December 12, 2005.

28. American Academy of Family Physicians, *CME Historical Perspective* (Leawood, Kans.: AAFP, 2008), 27.

29. T. Komoto and N. Davis, eds., "Evidence-Based CME," *American Family Physician* 66, no. 2 (2002): 200–202.

30. American Academy of Family Physicians, *CME Historical Perspective* (Leawood, Kans.: AAFP, 2008), 44.

31. M. H. Ebell and others, "Strength of Recommendation Taxonomy (SORT): A Patient-Centered Approach to Grading Evidence in the Medical Literature," *Journal of the American Board of Family Practioners* 17, no. 1 (2004): 59–67.

32. Ibid.

33. B. Weiss, "SORT: Strength of Recommendation Taxonomy," *Family Medicine* 36, no. 2 (2004): 141–143.

34. American Academy of Family Physicians, *Board of Directors Minutes* (Leawood, Kans., April 20–24, 2009).

35. American Academy of Family Physicians, "Point of Care CME," AAFP Web site, http://www.aafp.org/ online/en/home/cme/cmea/cmeapplying/point ofcare.html (accessed July 14, 2010).

36. "About DynaMed," DynaMed Web site, http:// www .ebscohost.com/dynamed/what.php (accessed

April 13, 2009); PEPID Online Web site, http://www.pepidonline .com (accessed April 13, 2009).

37. B. S. Alper and others, "Physicians Answer More Clinical Questions and Change Clinical Decisions More Often with Synthesized Evidence: A Randomized Trial in Primary Care," *Annals of Family Medicine* 3, no. 6 (2005): 507–513.

38. American Academy of Family Physicians, *2008 AAFP Reported CME Analysis* (Leawood, Kans., January 2009).

39. K. B. Weiss, "ABMS Maintenance of Certification: Raising the Bar in Measuring Physician Competency," *Synergy* 2009, no. 1: 20–22.

40. American Academy of Family Physicians, "FP Report," AAFP Web site, http://www.aafp.org/fpr/2002 0300/new.html (accessed July 15, 2010).

41. American Academy of Family Physicians, *CME Historical Perspective* (Leawood, Kans.: AAFP, 2008), 54.

CHAPTER 5

Continuing Medical Education and the American Medical Association: An Educational Journey

This is the story of the American Medical Association (AMA) and its role in continuing medical education (CME) and continuing physician professional development (CPPD) during its 163 years of existence. The AMA has been a major force in American medical education while serving its historic mission of representing US physicians. These historical struggles of the AMA around basic medical education allow us to better understand the AMA role in CME today.

The Beginnings

The AMA was founded at an evening meeting on May 7, 1847, in the hall of the Museum of Natural Sciences in Philadelphia, Pennsylvania. Approximately 200 delegates from 28 state medical societies gathered to establish a national association that would have more authority than any state society had singly and would represent all physicians to a growing national government. Nathaniel Chapman, MD, was elected the first AMA president, though most historians cite Nathan S. Davis, MD, as founder of the AMA. A 30-year-old New York physician, Davis had introduced successfully a resolution at the 1845 annual meeting of the New York Medical Association that led to the Philadelphia gathering. The resolution began: "It is believed that a national convention would be conducive to the elevation of the standard of medical education in the United States."[1]

That May 1847 meeting also saw the adoption of the original AMA constitution, which charged the AMA:

to give frequent, united and emphatic expression to the views of the medical profession in this country, must at all times have a beneficial influence, and supply more efficient means than have hitherto been available here for cultivating and advancing medical knowledge; for elevating the standard of medical education; for promoting the usefulness, honor and interests of the medical profession, for enlightening and directing public opinion in regard to the duties, responsibilities, and requirements of medical men; for exciting and encouraging emulation and concert of action in the profession, and fostering friendly intercourse between those who are engaged in it.[2]

By agreement, only two committees were formed at the first meeting: one on ethics and one on medical education. Prior to the AMA founding, state medical societies were proactive on behalf of the postgraduate education of the profession for many years. And so it was that the first focus of the Committee on Medical Education was on the basic education of doctors. Many of the decisions made by the committee over the next 50 years proved controversial. Numerous resolutions were introduced at the annual meetings—with none passed—that challenged the direction of the Committee on Medical Education. Some examples of these resolutions include the following:

1. The Association had not the power to control medical education.
2. The great objects of the Association were the advancement of medical science and the promotion of harmony in the profession.
3. The attempt on the part of the Association to regulate medical education had significantly failed in its object and had introduced elements of discord, and . . . any further interference on the subject would be useless and calculated to disturb the deliberations of the Association.[3]

Thus preoccupied by such challenges, the committee for the next 57 years focused on the issues of basic medical education and on the quality of the existing US medical schools. Early recommendations included a graded curriculum, some high school preparation for students before their admission to medical school, careful selection of medical students, and separation of education from licensure.

Because the quality of medical schools and their graduates varied greatly, the AMA defended the right of states to require examinations for licensure of medical school graduates and to not rely on the medical school. The committee persuaded the *Journal of the American Medical Association* (*JAMA*) to publish statistics on licensure examination failures of graduates by school. Such an act by the AMA led to its key role in the 1912 founding of the Federation of State Medical Boards of the United States, a voluntary organization of legally constituted licensing bodies.[4]

Until 1900, the AMA did not focus on continuation or postgraduate medical education though the committee recognized that many practicing physicians were graduates of inadequate medical schools. But several important events occurred around this time that began to change the medical education scene. In 1901, AMA reorganized to include the House of Delegates and a board of trustees with executive officers. In 1902, the AMA president appointed a new committee on education, which the House of Delegates in turn made into a permanent council on medical education (later known as the Council on Medical Education and Hospitals). The council branched out slowly, hindered by the resources available; the board of trustees could not find $5,000 to appropriate for the work of the first year.

Council efforts to stimulate interest in regular postgraduate education were ultimately unsuccessful; therefore, the new council continued to focus on the problems in medical schools and, in 1906, began inspections of medical schools. The first inspection of the 160 existing medical schools produced the following ratings: 82 were in Class A (above 70% or acceptable), 46 in Class B (50%–70% or doubtful), and 32 in Class C (below 50% or unacceptable).[5] Because of its findings, the council was attacked relentlessly by the medical schools who were not rated in Class A and sought help from outside the AMA. In a December 1908 New York City meeting, the council organized a meeting with the Carnegie Foundation for the Advancement of Teaching to design a national study of existing medical schools. Historically known as the Flexner Report, the study began in January 1909; it is named after one of the surveyors, Abraham Flexner of the Carnegie Foundation. Little remembered is the fact that N. P. Colwell, MD, secretary of the Council on Medical Education, served as co-surveyor.

In the report, Flexner wrote harshly about postgraduate education:

The postgraduate school as developed in the United States is an effort to mend a machine that was predestined to break down. It was originally an undergraduate repair shop. Its instruction was unnecessarily at once elementary and practical. There was no time to go back to fundamentals. . . . The training offered is calculated to "teach the trick" or to exhibit an instructor in the act of doing it. The part of the students is mainly passive; they look on at expert diagnosticians or operators. . . . The teaching has the air of handicraft rather than science.[6]

In retrospect, this harsh statement may have been responsible for coloring the nascent concepts of continuation medical education.

Postgraduate Medical Education Becomes an Interest

In 1906, prior to the Flexner Report, the Council on Medical Education and Hospitals asked J. N. McCormack, MD, to visit several states to stimulate interest in postgraduate education. Under this stimulus, several states began to organize educational courses. John Blackburn, MD, director of the Bowling Green Society in Kentucky, submitted a national plan in response to a request from the AMA and designed weekly programs on basic sciences and therapy for use by county medical societies.[7] By 1909, approximately 350 county societies sponsored these programs though they would not last: "the concept of continuation medical education as a third stage of medical education did not clearly emerge."[8]

But the seeds had been planted. Philadelphia physician J. M. Anders, MD, wrote a letter to the editor of *JAMA* in 1915 describing the evolution of a system of postgraduate medical education in Prussia (Germany) beginning in 1899. Said Anders:

If the practicing physician would either move forward, or prevent his falling behind the times, he must avail himself at intervals of postgraduate courses. The necessity for providing these has long been recognized, both at home and abroad, notably in the German Empire, but the task of properly organizing the work of postgraduate instruction is still unfinished.[9]

After describing what occurred in Germany, he concluded:

If there was a single reason for the creation of so complete an organization of graduate medical education as has been developed in Germany during the last decade and a half, then there are a dozen equally cogent reasons why the question of the reorganization of postgraduate education in America should be taken up with a view to bringing about a uniform and much extended system. I would suggest that the work already begun in this country under the auspices of the American Medical Association be promptly enlarged and promoted.[10]

Anders seems to wander between what is known today as *graduate medical education* and *postgraduate medical education*. But clearly postgraduate or continuing medical education was not a major concern of anyone. In the "History of the Council on Medical Education and Hospitals (1904–1959)," only one page is devoted to CME. Cited is the occasional report to the AMA House of Delegates and, beginning in 1938, the lists of postgraduate opportunities published quarterly in *JAMA*, which were reduced to an annual listing in 1955. Nevertheless, the council in 1952 appointed an additional member to its professional staff—Douglas D. Vollan, MD—to concentrate on a new study of continuation medical education and, two years later, established a committee on postgraduate medical education.

The Vollan Report

In 1955, the study titled "Postgraduate Medical Education in the United States" was published in *JAMA* and in booklet form.[11] Based on a national survey of approximately 5,000 practicing physicians, the report formed the basis for many AMA actions in future years. The report said:

The rapid rate at which the science and art of medicine are developing makes it apparent the undergraduate medical education can only lay the foundation upon which a lifetime of learning is to be erected. The continuing education of a physician throughout his professional life is absolutely essential if he is to use judiciously and effectively the new developments in the diagnosis, treatment, and prevention of disease that are necessary for adequate medical care.[12]

The council was shocked to find that almost a third of the physicians studied in the survey reported having received no formal postgraduate education for at least five years. However, of those who did, they reported an annual average of 667 hours (83.3 eight-hour days) devoted to all five of the areas of activity of learning they preferred. Vollan wrote that in the "motivated" group this represented about 22 percent of the average American physician's total professional activity—quite a remarkable statement.[13]

The five general types of learning activities reported were (1) reading of medical books, monographs, periodicals, and the abundant literature that every physician receives from pharmaceutical firms; (2) individual professional contacts between the physician and his colleagues, consultants, pharmacist, and the representatives of pharmaceutical firms; (3) attendance at hospital meetings such as staff meetings, clinicopathological and radiological conferences, and journal club meetings; (4) attendance at national, state, and local general or special medical society meetings; and (5) attendance at formal postgraduate courses. Vollan also noted reporting of other potentially educational activities such as research, individual study of patients, teaching, preparation of medical articles, etc., but did not include these because of the difficulty of obtaining significant data on these factors for a large group.

The report concluded:

At present, postgraduate medical education is suffering from a lack of clearly defined objectives . . . although there are many fine individual programs in the United States, the quality of postgraduate instruction varies considerably and all too frequently is poor. This is an important deterrent to physicians who wish to continue their education. It is largely due to undue emphasis on enrollment figures, haphazard preparation of course, and the practical limitations that often obstruct educational ideals. This malady of postgraduate education can only be corrected by an emphasis on quality. To improve the quality of postgraduate medical education, it must be recognized that the physician is a special type of student requiring special educational approaches. He is not motivated by a degree or certification as a reward. He is a mature individual with considerable prior knowledge of his subject. Although physicians expressed a marked preference for educational methods in which they actively participate—especially the seminar—didactic teaching in the forms of lectures and demonstrations is more useful in postgraduate education than in other phases of medical education because practicing physicians can readily relate information gained to experience in practice. Since those most in need are least likely to raise questions following didactic sessions, little is really lost by large attendance at such sessions. The faculty time conserved in this way could be effectively used in small group discussions or individual clinical case work with physicians. No one method can be expected to meet all the needs. At this stage flexibility is more desirable than standardization.[14]

In concluding the report, the council called for "a permanent national advisory council to be established to give guidance to the field."[15] The council stated that such a group should have representation from the AMA, the Association of American Medical Colleges, the Federation of State Licensing Boards, the American College of Physicians (ACP), the American College of Surgeons, the American Academy of General Practice, and any other groups vitally concerned with postgraduate education.

Pending the formation of such a group, the AMA formed an AMA advisory committee on postgraduate medical education. This committee worked diligently to implement some of the recommendations in the Vollan report. Thus, in June 1957, a guide regarding objectives and basic principles of postgraduate medical education was issued. Guidelines and principles for formal postgraduate medical education were announced, and it was urged that suitable appraisal mechanisms for evaluating such programs be developed. The advisory committee and the council decided that the names of sponsors meeting these standards, and their designated postgraduate educational programs, would be published regularly in *JAMA* as a service to physicians nationwide. This move was greeted with enthusiasm, and the first accreditation surveys of sponsors were completed in 1962.

In 1959, because of growing interest, the AMA House of Delegates recommended the adoption of the new term *continuing education* to replace the term *postgraduate medical education*. The new words were chosen to clearly separate the area of education of practicing doctors from the area of graduate medical education, which was rising in importance and had come to signify formal residency and fellowship training.

The AMA National Plan for Continuing Education

A little known story in the AMA involvement with CME has become known as the *Utah experiment*. It has been recorded by its organizers Patrick B. Storey, MD, John W. Williamson, MD, and C. Hilmon Castle, MD, in the monograph *Continuing Medical Education: A New Emphasis*. Storey, Williamson, and Castle had been asked by the AMA to oversee the development of a new project called the National Plan for Continuing Education. The demonstration project began in 1963 and lasted until 1966. Although it had a premature (and bitter) ending, the authors wrote, "Hopefully this experience may be of interest and value to others who are presently contending with the vexing problems of continuing medical education."[16]

The concept of a national plan was derived from the concept of a national academy for CME as proposed by Ward Darley and Arthur Cain in 1961 and amplified by Bernard Dryer in 1962.[17] The consensus of everyone was that only a national approach, using national resources, would be adequate to the solution of a national problem. A joint study group was convened and included the AMA, AAMC, ACP, American Academy of Pediatrics, American Psychiatric Association, American College of Gynecology and Obstetrics, and American Hospital Association (AHA). The

group recommended that a national academy be founded, but no financial means existed. However, the idea of a national plan was kept alive at the AMA within the Department of Postgraduate Programs headed by Storey, and major funding was approved by the AMA Board of Trustees to embark on a demonstration project.

Storey acknowledged the problems involved in the development of the idea, "not the least of which were those of a philosophical and methodological nature. These appeared to be fundamental to all the rest."[18] A grand concept was that the AMA effort could be devoted to developing the basic principles of the program "with the confidence that, as technological and instructional needs became evident, they would be met by the teaching resources of the country and the nation's communication industry."[19]

The plan proceeded with three steps: (1) organization of national faculties, (2) development of the criteria (or curriculum), and (3) development of practical means for applying the criteria in a physician's practice. In today's environment, it is worth recalling that everyone was committed to a key CME principle: to provide for constant improvement in medical care.

The AMA committed more than $1 million to fund the effort, a large amount of money for the 1960s. The faculty developed criteria for management of diseases or conditions in three predetermined areas of need in primary care: gastroenterology (GI), dermatology, and cardiovascular disease. Within these areas, teams were created, and only the GI disease team fulfilled the mission.

The initial subject matter for resource development was drawn from a study done in Washington State and published in monograph form, as well as hospitalization data from the Commission on Professional and Hospital Activities then located in Ann Arbor, Michigan. The GI faculty selected 10 subject areas to be developed: hiatus hernia, gastric and duodenal ulcer, hepatitis, cholelithiasis, regional enteritis, diverticulosis, pancreatitis (acute and chronic), and three others.

The goal was formidable: the development of *criteria* (a word chosen over the nearly synonymous *standards*) for optimal management of certain diseases that included reference to facts of place and circumstance where physicians and patients come together. Said Williamson and Storey:

The question is this: given a clinical situation involving management of a particular patient-type, what are the end results that should be obtained from proper management, and what are the actual characteristics of the flow of information between patient and physician at various points in time and place that are most likely to influence favorably the outcome of that relationship? . . . Expressed in the language of the cybernetic era in which we live, how does one move from relatively "soft" to relatively "hard" data concerning the clinical process? What, in fact, are the criteria of optimal physician performance?[20]

To apply this new emphasis on CME required a model of American medical practice to serve as a small scale demonstration project and template before rolling the program out on a national scale. The new emphasis stressed the implementation of a dynamic relationship between the program and practicing physicians. Such a relationship was established with Utah physicians. Utah provided an ideal environment: a single medical school—and its well-developed CME department—that had good relations with community hospitals and pioneered tools such as two-way FM radio and open circuit educational television; and motivated doctors.

The response from Utah physicians was quite remarkable. Out of a possible 907 licensed physicians, 476 (a response rate of 46 percent) completed and returned inventories about their practices and volunteered to participate.[21] Storey explains that many of the nonrespondents were specialists who already had opportunities to continue their education.

The details of the process and many examples are found in the monograph that is available in the Society for Academic Continuing Medical Education (SACME) archives and at the AMA. Un-

fortunately, the AMA stopped the project, probably due to the expense, and final results were never compiled. A 1969 report of the AMA Board of Trustees to the House of Delegates on the subject of audit and postgraduate study reads:

of even greater interest is the motivation of the physicians who participated and the implications that motivation has for the quality of care. Essentially, the physicians of Utah were given a mechanism whereby they could evaluate their skills and self-analyze their educational deficiencies. On the basis of their analyses, they were given an opportunity to update their skills in a priority sequence.[22]

It must have been an interesting time for the AMA Board. The association was dealing with strident calls for external regulation and outside audit of physicians. A 1969 report from the AMA Board described:

[an] external-audit-by-officialdom approach that was largely punitive and regulatory in nature. Under these circumstances, the best that can be expected of physicians is minimum compliance, and thus, in a very real sense of the word, the external audit is self-defeating. It is therefore in the interest of physicians and patients alike that efforts to perfect and widen the application of voluntary self-audit and postgraduate study be accelerated and that, to the extent possible, government health officials be convinced that the objectives they hope to attain by instituting their own audits are better achieved by voluntary means.[23]

As a result, the AMA House of Delegates adopted the following recommendations:

The AMA will

1. Endorse the principle of voluntary, life-long postgraduate study for all physicians and continue and accelerate the development of programs and incentives for such study.
2. Through the state medical societies, investigate the current status of in-hospital audit methods and make a similar investigation of the state of development of the evaluation of office services.
3. Encourage and assist the state medical societies and state departments of health and welfare to

develop uniform and effective methods of audit for office and in-hospital services, based on electronic data processing, to the maximum possible extent.

4. Request the Law Division to clarify the extent to which a physician's responsibility for the privacy of his patient's records will permit him to cooperate in an audit of his office practice.[24]

Yet, the pioneering Utah experiment had been canceled abruptly; no official reason was provided, though the AMA Board and House of Delegates had applauded the effort at an earlier time. Storey, Williamson, and Castle were left with a glorious concept—indeed a vision for the future—but not the expected outcome. But other developments soon occurred.

Certification of CME Activities and the Physician's Recognition Award

By 1967, a formal US system of approval of CME sponsors was in place and operated by the AMA. The AMA system has focused always on the accreditation of organizations and institutions that sponsor CME programs and never dealt with accreditation or certification of individual CME activities or courses; thus the AMA system differs from the system of family practice credit begun by the American Academy of General Practice in 1947.

In December 1968, the House of Delegates approved the establishment of a national award for physicians who participate in CME: the Physician's Recognition Award (PRA). The report establishing the award set out the following rationale and goals: to provide recognition for the many thousands of physicians who regularly participate in CME; to encourage all physicians to keep up to date and to improve their knowledge and judgment by CME; to reassure the public that US physicians are maintaining their competence by regular participation in CME; to emphasize the AMA position as a leader in CME; to emphasize the importance of developing more meaningful CME opportunities; and to strengthen the physi-

cian's position as the leader of the health service team by focusing attention on his or her interest in maintaining professional competence.

By establishing an award that could be achieved by all physicians, regardless of specialty, the AMA brought to a clearer focus its many efforts in advocating for increased visibility and a greater role for CME as the traditional third phase of the medical education continuum. After implementation of the PRA a universal US CME credit system was created, the PRA and AMA PRA credit were incorporated gradually into regulations and law as CME became mandatory, and CME continued to become a major force in the continuum of medical education.

In 1970, the House of Delegates adopted a set of revised "Essentials for the Accreditation of Institutions and Organizations Offering Continuing Medical Education" and formed an AMA Committee on Accreditation to conduct such surveys. Sensitive to the issues of making quality CME available in rural and isolated areas, the committee worked closely with state medical societies to develop equivalent standards of quality for smaller organizations (e.g., local hospitals) so that they could become accredited as well. These decisions helped the AMA PRA credit systems to evolve as a universal national credit system. From the beginning, AMA PRA credit could be designated by accredited providers with no difference between nationally accredited providers and state medical society accredited providers.

A brief look at how physicians earned the AMA PRA certificate in 1969 is interesting. At the start, the PRA recognized that this was really a process of *continuous* medical education and recognized the variety of learning experiences used by physicians. The requirements for attaining the AMA PRA were specified as learning in two categories: *required* (six learning formats) and *elective* (four learning formats).

In *required education* (a minimum of 60 hours was specified) the physician could report (a) hours from courses offered by AMA-accredited institutions, (b) hours from active participation as a teacher in any AMA-accredited medical education program (medical school, intern-resident programs, or continuing education), and (c) presentations at recognized professional bodies or publication of regional scientific papers in recognized scientific journals. Rules limited the amount to be obtained in each of these categories and each had to be listed and reported separately. The category of *elective education* was limited to 90 hours when applying for the PRA. Elective activities included attendance at scientific meetings of hospital staffs (50 hours maximum), preparation and personal presentation of scientific exhibits (30 hours maximum), and attendance at AMA scientific assemblies or the scientific meetings of major professional activities (50 hours maximum). The term *credit* was not used in 1969.

The earliest PRA rules also recognized the needs of younger physicians who would soon enter a practice. Physicians who had completed three years of graduate training in AMA-approved programs (there was no Accreditation Council on Graduate Medical Education at the time) or had the equivalent involvement and experience in research activity or in educational programs leading to further advanced degrees in medical science were immediately eligible for the award. These advanced degrees had to be applied for individually with appropriate documentation.

Establishing the System

As the number of accredited providers increased, and with increasing interest in CME, the hours of participation became formalized as AMA PRA credits. But the need for physicians to document their credits in CME within six categories was still required. In 1971, the AMA took action to require CME for physicians. The AMA Board of Trustees recommended that specialty boards and specialty societies require periodic recertification for their diplomates and members. The AMA proposed that doctors failing to engage in acceptable continuing education on an ongoing basis lose board certification or society membership. The AMA

Board also recommended that state medical societies require formal CME of physicians as a condition of membership. Several state medical societies immediately imposed such and licensing boards followed. The 1972 AMA annual meeting marked the first time that postgraduate courses for credit were offered at an annual convention program.

Emergence of a Coordinating Council on Medical Education

In 1972, the American Board of Medical Specialties, AHA, AMA, AAMC, and the Council of Medical Specialty Societies agreed to serve as parent bodies for a new Coordinating Council on Medical Education (CCME). This was a lifelong dream for C. H. William Ruhe, MD, director of the AMA Division of Medical Education. The grand design included an overriding council that had power to ensure continuity in medical education, utilizing three subcommittees for each of the three areas of medical education. These committees in turn would report to the CCME. Undergraduate medical education remained the purview of the Liaison Committee for Medical Education as formed in 1942, and two new committees were to be formed: the Liaison Committee for Graduate Medical Education and the Liaison Committee for Continuing Medical Education (LCCME).

The LCCME was formally constituted in 1977 by the CCME. The original intent of the AMA was to share its aims and interests in the further development of CME for the betterment of all physicians and patients. From the AMA point of view, the direction of the LCCME was of immediate concern. The AMA concept of the LCCME as a partnership with several new organizations was not realized because of several complex problems related to the organization of the LCCME. Many LCCME functions were contested by the AMA. The state medical societies who accredited local CME providers were particularly unhappy with the Chicago-based LCCME. At that time, the state medical societies were the dominant voting block in the AMA, and problems soon escalated.

In July 1979, the House of Delegates sent shockwaves through the CME community by withdrawing as a participating member of the LCCME and authorizing the AMA Council on Medical Education to resume its responsibility for the voluntary accreditation of CME providers. The council moved immediately to re-establish the AMA Committee on Accreditation of Continuing Medical Education (CACME). CACME was now the only AMA-authorized entity to function as an accreditor for providers wishing to designate AMA PRA credit. CACME had 22 members covering the interests of state medical associations, medical schools, specialty societies, hospital administration, hospital medical education, and the public. The list of members was impressive and included many of the thought leaders in CME at the time.

Meanwhile, the LCCME continued to operate with staffing services for the LCCME provided by the Council of Medical Specialty Societies. It was truly a time of turmoil. For CME providers in the field, a choice had to be made. If one did not seek accreditation from the AMA CACME, one could not award AMA PRA credit. Likewise, one did not want to jeopardize one's accreditation awarded by the newly formed LCCME. Most providers of CME viewed the situation as a true no-win dilemma.

Richard L. Egan, MD, secretary of the AMA Council on Medical Education, made an extemporaneous speech at the AMA Annual Congress on Medical Education on October 19, 1979, to explain the position of the House of Delegates: "The Council, in supporting the LCCME as an expression of AMA policy . . . was distressed that several states did not submit reviews to the LCCME, presenting a problem, both in the concept of the AMA as a Federation and in the compilation of course listings and the list of accredited sponsors for the AMA's PRA." Per Egan, members of the Council on Medical Education heard from many designated representatives of state medical socie-

ties that chose not to continue working with the LCCME. A conclusion needed to be reached.

Egan recalled that at the December 1978 meeting of the AMA House of Delegates the delegates adopted Substitute Resolution 27, which clearly defined AMA policy to declare that state medical societies should accredit intrastate organizations providing CME.

And I emphasize the precision of the words "State Medical Societies." This is one of the problems that has been of great concern to the Council on Medical Education. . . . In July 1979, resolutions from the medical societies of Arizona, Massachusetts and Connecticut expressed dissatisfaction with the lack of success on the part of the AMA in obtaining clear-cut recognition of state medical societies to accredit intrastate providers of CME. The resolution from Massachusetts, Resolution 66, also specifically asked that the AMA withdraw from LCCME. These resolutions were published in AMA NEWS and Dr. James Sammons, the AMA's Executive Vice President, notified the CEOs of the other sponsoring organizations of them.[25]

Egan outlined three major related problems as seen by the House of Delegates:

The first problem was the pervasive philosophy of CME exhibited by some of the other sponsors . . . you will find a significant and practical distinction between the accreditation of organizations and institutions to provide CME that meets course objectives and CME that meets learning objectives. . . .

Secondly, the role of state medical societies, a policy position of the AMA . . . differs significantly from the language used by the LCCME which speaks of "state or regional entities," constituted in accordance with criteria to be developed . . . the LCCME says it will permit states to grant accreditation to institutions and organizations within their jurisdiction, it does not say "state medical societies," it says "states" . . . LCCME will develop criteria and procedures for review of medical societies and/or other bodies granting accreditation . . . one of the significant policy issues as viewed by the Council on Medical Education.

The third problem was the failure of the LCCME to refer policy issues to its parent bodies, thus violating the very fundamental concept of a liaison committee. . . .[26]

Egan cites an example where the AMA asked that an LCCME decision be considered a policy question, and the LCCME—by majority vote—decided it was not a matter of policy: "What this does is to make the LCCME not a liaison committee, but a policy-making body which supersedes the policy-making power of each sponsor. . . ."[27]

And he concludes with a comment about financing:

It is as difficult to conduct a quality program of accreditation with financial support limited to fee income as it is difficult to maintain the quality of higher education if tuition income is to be the sole source of funding. Other sponsors of the LCCME had declared as a matter of policy that in the future they would not commit money to the support of accreditation activities. The AMA supported all of the cost of accreditation until the current year. During fiscal 1979, after the costs of survey visits were increased by the LCCME, the AMA contributed only about 60 percent of the cost . . . the AMA representatives to the LCCME were confronted with a proposal to tax participant hours of CME to accrue a considerable sum of money, in excess of those needed in the accreditation process, in order to fund research on CME. This, too, troubled the Council.[28]

Coming Together: Reconciliation

In 1981, representatives of the AMA, after informal and later formal discussions with representatives of remaining parent organizations of the former LCCME, agreed to participate as members of a newly constituted organization: the Accreditation Council for Continuing Medical Education (ACCME). The basic conflicts that had caused the AMA withdrawal from the LCCME in 1979 were resolved as a condition for the new council. It was also agreed that AMA PRA credit could be offered in the United States by institutions and organizations accredited by the ACCME. At the present, the AMA continues to grant organizations accredited by the ACCME or by state/territorial medical societies the privilege to certify activities for AMA PRA Category 1 Credit while reserving the right to withdraw that privilege if the organization violates the AMA PRA rules.

In 1981, the AMA also discontinued its Council on Continuing Physician Education, a council that had been established separately from CACME to plan regional CME seminars for the nation. The board believed this action would be more consistent with the new AMA role in CME but it also recognized the roles of the medical specialty societies in CME programming.

Reflecting on all that had happened, Ruhe, the AMA senior official in medical education, offered the following comments at the 1987 SACME spring meeting:

Continuing medical education is a young child in the field of education. It is a vigorous growing child, but it has many of the growing pains and delinquency problems of the adolescent. Its exact age cannot be determined, for it was born out of wedlock (and is still regarded as illegitimate in many polite circles), its parents were reparative education and specialty training and before 1930 the three were hopelessly intertwined. . . .[29]

The Evolution of the AMA PRA Credit System

The PRA has been continuously evolving since its inception and has changed enormously over the years. The 11 different categories of education and learning, grouped as formal and informal, for reporting CME participation in 1969 were gradually reduced to six categories. Even so, many physicians applying for the PRA complained about the overly burdensome requirement to document credits or hours in six different categories. In 1985, the Council on Medical Education recommended the collapse of the six categories into two—Category 1 (formal CME) and Category 2 (elective, informal CME)—and the removal of the requirement to balance one's education in various categories. As such, a physician could report all of his or her CME in Category 1 and from a single type of format (e.g., lectures) to achieve the AMA PRA.

Because Category 1 credit was documented PRA credit and Category 2 was not, doctors began to view Category 2 credit as less important and desirable second-level CME. The various states with CME licensure requirements reinforced this view, seeing documentation of Category 1 credit as verifiable. The pendulum had swung in an unanticipated way.

These changes were not lost on the council. It asked its CME Advisory Committee to study the issues and in 1992 the House of Delegates reaffirmed that the areas of learning and CME captured in Category 2 were as important as those in Category 1. For a while, the AMA PRA program even required a minimum number of hours in Category 2. At the same time, a new requirement was instituted: physicians applying for the AMA PRA had to affirm their reading of the medical literature for at least two hours a week (reading that was not reportable as credit). And, finally in 1993, extra recognition was given to physicians who documented their self-directed learning by awarding them an AMA PRA "With Special Commendation for Self Directed Learning." Concomitantly the AMA PRA referenced two ethical opinions from the Council on Ethical and Judicial Affairs that were adopted by the House of Delegates. Now, adherence to the AMA Ethical Opinions 8.061 (Gifts to Physicians from Industry) and 9.011 (Continuing Medical Education) was made mandatory whenever activities were certified for AMA PRA credit.

Several other changes happened in 1992. The AMA PRA was made available upon request to physicians who had obtained specialty board recertification. Teaching was reinstated as worthy of credit but was limited to teaching in certified CME activities, and recognition was given for physician attendance at certain international CME conferences.

The AMA PRA program also responded to practice changes. In the mid-1990s, a small crisis arose as the laparoscopic surgery techniques exploded around the country. Hospital credentialing committees were suddenly confronted with requests from a surgeon for expanded clinical privileges, e.g., to perform laparoscopic surgery, but the only evidence of competence provided by the surgeon was the standard certificate of AMA PRA CME credit. Working in cooperation with the AHA, the AMA responded by establishing a new system of designating credit for training and education in new skills and procedures that would be used to gain new clinical privileges. All providers of such courses who designated AMA credit were informed they had to use the system. It was a major change of direction for the credit system, as participant outcomes were actually to be measured. Under the program, CME activities are graded into four levels of outcome; these identify the depth and complexity of the course and document the level of skill acquired by the physician learner. It was a major step forward for CME because the end result was teacher-learner accountability.

The evolution continued, championed by the Council on Medical Education. Most of the new changes to the AMA credit system were directed at making CME more relevant and integrated with a physician's daily work and an increasingly hectic life. Thus AMA PRA Category 1 credit was made available for journal-based CME (reading), for authors who published in a peer-reviewed journal that was indexed in MEDLINE, for obtaining a medically related advanced degree, for participation in actual manuscript review for peer-reviewed journals, for test item writing for significant major national board examinations, for participation in performance improvement activities, for point-of-care learning using the Internet, and for participation in independent learning plans and committee work of an educational nature. A major breakthrough was to remove the long-standing formula of one credit for each hour of CME, in which the AMA was joined by the American Academy of Family Physicians (AAFP).[30] The concept of credits, instead of hours, remains linked to a time metric in live activities and enduring materials. But the change allowed both credit systems to allocate credit more appropriately to other CME formats, in particular performance improvement CME (PI CME) and Internet point-of-care CME (PoC CME).

These two new formats for learning were approved by the council after pilot programs beginning in 2001 demonstrated their validity. PI CME brought together educational principles with process improvement, recognizing that physicians work in a health-care environment that impacts their ability, positively or negatively, to provide the best possible health care to patients.

Internet PoC CME was approved in March 2005 by the council and took advantage of current technologies that brought useful information to the physician at the time of interaction with the patient and offered recognition for the learning that takes place. In both cases, the AAFP actively participated in the promulgation of the rules regarding both formats. The development of these two new learning formats earned the AMA a 2006 Alliance for CME award in recognition of Significant Contribution to the Field of CME and to the Future of the Profession.

In retrospect, it seems that the whole process of evolution of the AMA PRA credit system and many, if not most, of the changes made in recent years have in fact restated the original concepts of individual learning recognized by the original 1968 AMA PRA. Perhaps the attempt to simplify the PRA system in 1985 simply did not work.

An important contribution by the AMA to the evolution of CME came from the Council on Ethical and Judicial Affairs (CEJA) of the AMA. CEJA recognized the importance of addressing the potential for commercial influence on practicing physicians and on CME activities. Two CEJA documents—CEJA Ethical Opinions 8.061 and 9.011—relate to both of these topics. Opinion 8.061 reflects concerns about gifts from industry to physicians that may not be consistent with the Principles of Medical Ethics.[31] It sets guidelines to avoid the acceptance of inappropriate gifts. Opinion 9.011 sets guidelines for physicians (be they learners, faculty, or CME developers) related to a physician's ethical obligation to maintain his or her medical expertise through CME and to also ensure that the content CME is appropriate. The Council on Medical Education made explicit that there is a logical and inescapable link between the AMA PRA Credit system and the CEJA opinions: CME activities for Category 1 Credit must always be in compliance not only with the PRA rules but also with the pertinent CEJA opinions. The AMA has also contributed to the development of contemporary research in CME and CPPD by sponsoring and publishing two important books: *The Physician as Learner, Linking Research to Practice* and *The Continuing Professional Development of Physicians, from Research to Practice*.[32]

AMA International Efforts

The AMA is active in the international development of CME and CPD. The Division of Continuing Physician Professional Development and the board of trustees have actively cooperated with foreign organizations that are in the process of developing a formal CME system, including efforts through the World Medical Association. Because the United States has a mature CME system, other countries often study the history of US CME to determine what did and did not work. For many years the AMA has authorized the accredited medical schools in Canada to certify activities for AMA PRA Category 1 Credit. More recently a formal agreement permitting exchange of CME credits with the Union of European Medical Specialists European Accrediting Council for CME was reached in 2002 and reconfirmed in 2007.

Recent Initiatives from the AMA

The AMA continues to explore ways to improve the education of physicians. The goal of AMA's new Initiative to Transform Medical Education is to "promote excellence in patient care by implementing reform in the medical education and training system across the continuum, from premedical preparation and medical school admission through continuing physician professional development." A June 2007 council report made 10 recommendations to improve medical education, many of them dealing with education after residency/fellowship training.[33] Subsequent reports have addressed topics such as lifelong learning and physician re-entry and retraining, and the initiative is ongoing.

Interesting but Abandoned AMA CME Projects

AMA has had its share of success over the years. But not all experiments and innovations can be so lucky. Some CME and CPPD efforts have proven unsuccessful or unsustainable. Perhaps some were even ahead of their time. Four endeavors that fall into the category of abandoned projects include a physician CME tracking system, AMA/NET, American Medical Television, and the National Institute for Continuing Physician Education.

Proposals for a CME credit tracking system were delivered in 1971 and 1994. The first proposal called for a credit card–like membership card linked to a central AMA database. The second proposal also relied on electronic recording and allowed for a central database and information sharing with state licensing boards. Neither proposal obtained the approval of AMA management.[34]

In 1980, the AMA launched AMA/NET, one of the earliest computer-assisted programs directed at practicing doctors. While CME was only a small part of AMA/NET, it did allow for patient simulations, tutorials, electronic conferences, clinical decision assistance applications (e.g., Dx-Plain), examinations on written or video material, and e-mail for administrative communication on such topics as registration for CME courses, communication among CME providers, and announcement of CME opportunities.[35] Physicians subscribed to AMA/NET for a modest fee and accessed the system through a telephone connection via a modem to a central computer located in Denver. By 1989, AMA/NET had approximately 40,000 physician subscribers. But due to escalating operating costs, AMA management ended the service in 1990, stating:

> After ten years of operation, the AMA is discontinuing AMA NET. This decision is the result of the substantial costs of operating a national on-line information system versus the fiscal and business needs of the organization. We have searched for many months to find a long-term investment partner with complementary strategic business objectives, in order to continue operation of the network. Regrettably, we have been unsuccessful in our search.[36]

In the 1980s, the AMA released a series of VHS videotapes called "AMA Video Clinics" about selected disease entities and diagnostic tips for primary care doctors. The Video Clinics proved useful to not only practicing physicians but also US licensed physicians stationed outside of the United States as a means of obtaining needed AMA PRA credit. Physician interest in the Video Clinics led to AMA's entry into live television in 1984. In partnership with Lifetime Television, the AMA provided the content for a series of CME programs aimed at practicing physicians. By 1989, the AMA worked out a new arrangement with the Discovery Channel that included medical programming for CME credit and a 30-minute segment directed at consumers. Although successful, the programs failed to attract

The Division of CPPD actively participates in international forums, such as the Rome Group and others.

financial support. In 1992, AMA entered an arrangement with the cable network NBC Television (today known as CNBC) to provide five hours of weekly programming. Three hours were dedicated to CME activities and two hours provided consumer health education. Initially well received by the profession and the public, the project ultimately failed to generate the needed revenue and came to an end in 1994.[37]

Recognizing that coordination would be needed as CME expanded exponentially, the AMA chartered a National Institute for Continuing Physician Education in 1992. The Institute was registered as an Illinois corporation in 1992; it then became a 501(c)(3) (not-for-profit) organization. The purposes of the Institute as found in the initial bylaws were (1) to provide coordination and advocacy for the discipline of continuing physician education in the USA (*the name CPE was chosen deliberately to change the paradigm from CME*), (2) to foster research in CME/CPE, and (3) to create a continuum of medical education that dealt with the lifelong educational needs of US physicians.

The concepts of the Institute were presented to a variety of CME stakeholders over the next two years. In 1993, Dennis Wentz spoke to the fall meeting of the Society of Medical Directors of CME in Washington, DC, and outlined the following possible goals and potentials for the Institute:

- Initiate a comprehensive study of CME, perhaps in context with the SMCDCME, the AAMC and others, a Flexner-type report on CME.
- Develop a pool of funds to stimulate CME research.
- Provide advocacy for a better public image of CME.
- Develop enabling tools for a national CME needs assessment process.
- Develop a national curriculum as a point of reference for physicians, in conjunction with national specialty societies.

- Work with the communications technology industry to position delivery and availability of CME.
- Link CPE to performance and competence by fostering the use of clinical guidelines, evidence-based practice, and actual performance in practice, with development of systems to measure practice outcomes.

A summary document about the Institute was widely circulated to organizations active in CME. While some early expressions of support emerged, they were few. Individuals and several organizations feared that the AMA was trying to engineer a "take-over" of the field of CME. But funding was the major problem: major foundations were not interested in the concept, nor did industry embrace the Institute, perhaps because most of funding and support for CME related to specific disease groups.

Conclusion

The recognition of the critical role of CME and CPD in a physician's professional development has long been codified in the AMA Principles of Medical Ethics:

> A physician shall continue to study, apply, and advance scientific knowledge, maintain a commitment to medical education, make relevant information available to patients, colleagues, and the public, obtain consultation, and use the talents of other health professionals when indicated.[38]

The inclusion of these concepts in the AMA Principles of Medical Ethics elevates the lifelong educational commitment of a doctor to the level of an ethical imperative and makes it one of the standards of conduct that defines the physician as a professional.

The AMA definition of CME adopted many years ago remains appropriate today. The scope of CME, and CPPD, is broadly defined as all of the areas of learning that assist a physician in fulfilling his or her professional responsibilities, clinical and nonclinical:

> CME consists of educational activities which serve to maintain, develop, or increase the knowledge, skills, and professional performance and relationships that a physician uses to provide services for patients, the public or the profession. The content of CME is the body of knowledge and skills generally recognized and accepted by the profession as within the basic medical sciences, the discipline of clinical medicine, and the provision of health care to the public.[39]

To fulfill organized medicine's professional responsibilities to physicians, the three major CME credit systems in use in the United States must continue to evolve. Regardless of what other regulatory, accrediting, or licensing bodies may do or of what the government or insurance companies might require for payments for services, the collective profession of medicine owns the responsibility for what makes physicians worthy to be called professionals. We owe it to society, to our patients, and to ourselves to lead the process by which we define and award recognition for continuous learning and improvement, recognition that is credible to all stakeholders who now or in the future will ask for such documentation.

Notes

1. American Medical Association Archives, http://www.ama-assn.org/ama/pub/article/1916-4493.html (accessed March 23, 2010).

2. Ibid.

3. American Medical Association House of Delegates Minutes (1880–1900).

4. American Medical Association, *A History of the Council on Medical Education and Hospitals of the American Medical Association* (Chicago: AMA, 1959), 24–25.

5. American Medical Association, *A History of the Council,* 26–27.

6. A. Flexner, *Medical Education in the United States and Canada. A Report to the Carnegie Foundation* (Boston: Merrymount Press, 1910), 174.

7. P. R. Manning and L. DeBakey, *Medicine: Preserving the Passion* (New York: Springer-Verlag, 1987), xxvi; J. D. Bruce, "Postgraduate Education in Medicine," *Journal of the Michigan State Medical Society* 36, no. 6 (1937): 369–377.

8. American Medical Association Council on Medical Education and Hospitals, *Continuation Study for Practicing Physicians* (Chicago: AMA, 1940), 216; G. R. Shepherd, "History of Continuation Medical Education in the United States since 1930," *Journal of Medical Education* 35 (1960): 740–758.

9. J. M. Anders, "Postgraduate Education," *Journal of the American Medical Association* 63, no. 22 (1915): 1969–1970.

10. Ibid.

11. D. D. Vollan, "Scope and Extent of Postgraduate Medical Education in the United States," *Journal of the American Medical Association* 157 (1955): 701–707.

12. Ibid.

13. Ibid.

14. Ibid.

15. D. D. Vollan, "Scope and Extent of Postgraduate Medical Education in the United States," *Journal of the American Medical Association* 158 (1955): 395–396.

16. P. B. Storey and others, *Continuing Medical Education: A New Emphasis* (Chicago: American Medical Association, 1968).

17. W. Darley and A. S. Cain, "A Proposal for a National Academy of Continuing Medical Education," *Journal of Medical Education* 36 (1961): 33–37; B. V. Dryer, "Lifetime Learning for Physicians: Principles, Practices, Proposals," *Journal of Medical Education* 37, no. 6 (1962): 1–134.

18. Storey and others, *Continuing Medical Education.*

19. Ibid.

20. Ibid.

21. Ibid.

22. American Medical Association House of Delegates Proceedings (Clinical Convention, 1969).

23. Ibid.

24. American Medical Association House of Delegates Proceedings, June 1969.

25. R. L. Egan, "Extemporaneous Remarks on AMA Withdrawal from LCCME," *AMA Continuing Medical Education Newsletter* 8, no. 12 (1979): 8–12.

26. Ibid.

27. Ibid.

28. Ibid.

29. C. H. William Ruhe, "Continuing Medical Education in the United States: The Present Picture" (address given to the Society of Medical College Directors of CME, spring meeting, 1987).

30. D. K. Wentz, *Forty Years for the AMA PRA: Still Relevant in 2008. The AMA CPPD Report* (no. 26, summer 2008).

31. AMA Code of Medical Ethics (adopted by the AMA House of Delegates, June 17, 2001).

32. D. A. Davis and R. D. Fox, *The Physician as Learner: Linking Research to Practice* (Chicago: American Medical Association Press, 1994); D. Davis and others, *The Continuing Development of Physicians: From Research to Practice* (Chicago: American Medical Association Press, 2003).

33. American Medical Association, "Initiative to Transform Medical Education," AMA Web site, http://www.ama -assn.org/ama1/pub/upload/mm/16/itme _final_rpt .pdf (accessed May 19, 2009).

34. C. W. Mangun, Jr., memorandum dated of Sep-tember 2, 1971, to C. H. William Ruhe; G. Paulos, business plan for an AMA CME-Tracker, presented to the AMA Board of Trustees (1994).

35. W. A. Yasnoff, presentation to the AMA CME Advisory Committee, July 26, 1988.

36. J. F. Rappel, memorandum to AMA Executive Staff, July 13, 1990.

37. R. M. Evans, telephone conversation, January19, 2010.

38. AMA Code of Medical Ethics.

39. American Medical Association, "Council on Medical Education Report A, House of Delegates Policy 300.988" (1982).

Delores J. Rodgers, Diane Burkhart, and W. Douglas Ward

CHAPTER 6

The American Osteopathic Association Continuing Medical Education Program

The American Osteopathic Association (AOA), originally called the American Association for the Advancement of Osteopathy, was founded in 1887. The name was officially changed to the AOA in 1901. The AOA is a member association representing more than 70,000 osteopathic physicians, or doctors of osteopathic medicine (DOs), as of July 2010. The AOA serves as the primary certifying body for osteopathic physicians and is the accrediting agency for all osteopathic medical colleges and residency training programs. The AOA mission is to advance the philosophy and practice of osteopathic medicine by promoting excellence in education, research, and the delivery of quality, cost-effective health care within a distinct, unified profession.[1] The objectives of the AOA are to promote public health, to encourage scientific research, and to maintain and improve high standards of osteopathic medical education.[2]

Governance

There are four governing bodies that provide oversight to the AOA program of continuing medical education (CME). The AOA House of Delegates is the policymaking body of the AOA that is responsible for establishing the overall direction for the AOA and its programs. The board of trustees is an executive body of the House of Delegates responsible for the day-to-day opera-

tions of AOA programs and policy. The Bureau of Osteopathic Education (BOE) serves as a reviewing body of existing policy documents or of proposed policy changes originating within the Council on Continuing Medical Education (CCME).

In this capacity, the bureau makes recommendations to the AOA board for its final action. The CCME is responsible for recommending administrative changes in the CME program, determining category credit for CME courses, reviewing document surveys for accreditation decisions, and determining decisions on individual member requests for CME waivers and exemptions.

The CCME also responds to requests by CME sponsors for clarification of CME policies. CME policy, changes to policy, clarifications on CME, and frequently asked questions are published through a variety of recognized methods of communications and osteopathic publications such as *The DO*, a monthly magazine containing news of the osteopathic profession and its members; the *Journal of the American Osteopathic Association (JAOA)*; and periodic newsletters from the CCME chair to sponsors and other stakeholders.

In July 1979, the AOA board of trustees was designated to be the only body entitled to establish accreditation policy for osteopathic CME sponsors. All policy recommendations originate from the CCME and move forward to the BOE.

The BOE reports its deliberations and actions directly to the AOA board of trustees, which serves as the final decision body for policy change.

The primary and continuing function of the staff of the AOA department of CME is to implement the regulations, guidelines, and procedures of the CME program, as approved, guided, and directed by the council and its chairman.

It is the responsibility of staff to handle all data recording as quickly as possible, reply to all correspondence as soon as it is received, and allow as little time as possible to lapse between the time correspondence is received and data are permanently recorded. All correspondence is coded and permanently filed through microfilming.

Establishment of Osteopathic CME

Before the AOA adopted requirements for CME, the osteopathic profession had a long history of instituting CME requirements for state licensure for osteopathic physicians practicing in the state. It appears that Michigan was the first state to require CME as early as 1949. DOs practicing in Arizona, Florida, Maine, Michigan, Nevada, New Mexico, Oklahoma, Tennessee, Vermont, and West Virginia were required by state legislation to complete CME to assure the public that DOs were up-to-date in medical knowledge and skills.[3] In 1950, the American College of General Practitioners in Osteopathic Medicine required an annual postgraduate requirement for CME. The osteopathic profession relied on the state licensure system to require CME for its physicians until a resolution came for discussion and approval to the House of Delegates in 1972. At that time, it was agreed that CME needed to be expanded for osteopathic physicians in order to meet the rapid advancement of modern medical practice.

During the 1950s and 1960s, public and professional interest grew in regard to establishing professional standards throughout the United States. This was especially true in the field of medicine. In the 1960s, the AOA Bureau of Professional Education (BPE) became recognized as the accrediting body for the DO degree, and federal recognition provided funding for osteopathic postdoctoral training programs approved through the BPE and the Council on Postdoctoral Training (COPT). Ultimately, the CME program was under the authority of the BPE. These early CME programs were conducted in osteopathic hospitals and taught by osteopathic program directors and faculty physicians. During the 1970s, it became clear that the credentials of all osteopathic physicians needed to be validated before public opinion. The American Medical Association (AMA) and the Accreditation Council for Continuing Medical Education (ACCME) had already established a voluntary CME program for doctors of medicine (MDs). In 1973, the AOA House of Delegates went a step further and mandated a universal CME requirement for all DOs.

Most DOs were practicing in osteopathic hospitals at this time. Few medical education programs were available to DOs other than osteopathic CME programs. For the most part, allopathic CME was not made available to DOs in the early years of formal CME. When the AOA CME plan was first adopted, all DOs were included, regardless of whether they were members of the AOA. All DOs were eligible to enter the AOA CME program, and most took advantage of the opportunity at that time.

As colleges of osteopathic medicine expanded during the 1970s and 1980s, they became osteopathic CME providers and teaching sites. Over time, the osteopathic hospital systems throughout the United States phased out and AOA CME evolved into the current system.

Establishment of the AOA CME Program and Infrastructure

The guiding principles and format of the AOA CME program were first adopted by the AOA House of Delegates in July 1972 and placed for evaluation and implementation on an annual calendar year basis. The first CME cycle of the program officially began in June 1973 and ended in

December 1974. The cycle was expanded to become a three-year annual cycle requiring 150 credit hours by its members ending December 1976. The board of trustees organized a special committee to create the operations for the AOA CME program in October 1972.

Original members on the CCME included representatives from the following osteopathic groups: state executive directors, practice affiliates, the American Association of Colleges of Osteopathic Medicine (AACOM), members from the AOA House of Representatives, and a member-at-large chair to be appointed by the AOA president.

The CCME was granted broad discretionary powers for reviewing individual cases where mitigating circumstances prevailed. It also establishes criteria for CME program attendance and a list of acceptable courses and programs that are published at the start of each three-year CME cycle.

Orthopedic surgeon Donald Siehl, DO, was the first chair of the AOA CCME. In addition to Siehl, the original AOA CME committee members included: R. William Bradway, DO; Edward H. Borman, DO; John P. Goodrige, DO; Joseph J. Namey, DO; Mahlon L. Ponitz, DO; and Margaret D. Willard, EdD. Member selection was based on organizational affiliation, educational background, and areas of expertise in an effort to represent all segments of the profession.

The first meeting of the CCME was held at the AOA central office in Chicago on January 12, 1973, with many consultants in addition to members. The initial aim of the CME program was to stimulate attendance in CME. It was determined that the AOA CME program should focus on each member's clinical practice and related specialty area.

The CCME defined the purpose of the AOA CME program as the growth of knowledge, the refinement of clinical skills, and the deepening of understanding for the osteopathic profession.[4] The CCME recognized the ultimate goals of CME as providing excellent patient care and improving the health and well-being of the individual patient and the public.

The design of the AOA mandatory CME program encouraged and assisted osteopathic physicians to achieve the AOA mission and specified CME objectives and goals. The AOA CME system was implemented by granting credits to osteopathic physicians for their participation in approved CME activities sponsored by recognized organizations, institutions, and agencies. The clinical credit hour for the CME program was defined as a *clinical session hour*.

Approved educational activities were sorted as formal or informal and full-time or part-time. These included, but were not limited to, scientific seminars; workshops; refresher and postgraduate courses; lectures; home study; and local, state, regional, and national medical meetings. Specifically excluded from CME credit, then and now, are educational programs leading to any formal advanced standing within the profession. Programs, clinical rotations, or coursework leading to a degree (doctor in osteopathic medicine) or required in a postdoctoral training program (internship, residency, and fellowship) are not eligible for CME credit.

In 2010, the AOA continued to award CME credit to osteopathic physicians for their participation in educational activities meeting specific criteria. The criteria have continued to develop and be redefined over the past 40 years. These criteria, depending on the type of activity, are described in a document titled "AOA CME Guide for Osteopathic Physicians." The guide is updated each cycle with newly approved criteria and specifications.

CME and Licensure

Since its inception, the AOA CCME has encouraged that CME continue to be a requirement of state licensing laws and a condition of periodic relicensure. In July 1997, the AOA went on public record to support the standards developed and established by the AOA CCME as early as 1972.

The CCME encourages divisional societies recognized by the AOA to work with their state licensing boards to include appropriate amendments in consultation with the Bureau of State Government Affairs. Together they recommend appropriate strategies and legislative language to support the passage of CME requirement language into state laws.

CME Activity Reports

In 1973, the CCME requested a statistical analysis to evaluate what would be required to provide each member a CME activity report. Producing this report would provide information acceptable by state licensing boards as evidence of CME compliance. Many hospitals require documented CME before allowing physicians to have privileges at the hospital. After analysis, the CCME determined that a status report would be provided via a computer printout to each individual DO participating in the program. Physicians could monitor their individual CME activity and access a printed report as documentation for licensing boards and hospitals.

It was determined in January 1975 that AOA staff would compile and mail individual status reports of recorded CME credit to all AOA-member DOs who had reported CME activities since June 1973. The first CME activity report was mailed the third week of January 1975. The AOA board of trustees approved a resolution to mail activity reports annually in July and December. In 2004, twice-yearly mailings ended because AOA members were given daily, 24-hour access to their activity reports through the members-only portal of the AOA Web site (www.do-online.org).

Once a report is available to the member, it is the physician's responsibility to forward copies of his or her status report to agencies and institutions. In April 1974, the CCME agreed that the CME activity report would not be mailed automatically to AOA nonmembers. Until July 1998, nonmembers could obtain a copy of their CME activity report for a $225 fee to reimburse the

AOA for computer and administrative costs. By July 1998, nonmembers were no longer eligible to receive CME activity reports. The AOA CCME determined that this popular service be reserved strictly as a benefit of AOA membership.

Developing the CME Cycle Based on Lessons Learned

In April 1976, the CCME developed strategies based on the evaluation of phase I and implementation of the CME program since its 1973 inception. The goal of the April meeting was to prepare resolutions that would go before the BPE, board of trustees, and House of Delegates for final action in July 1976. Phase II included consideration of guidelines for individual waivers and reductions for health and other reasons, a plan on how to handle the end of the first complete CME cycle, deadlines for submissions, an accounting of those physicians who did not fulfill CME membership requirements and recommended actions for those physicians, and the development of recommended changes for the second cycle that should be published in advance to all members.

The first assignment for W. Douglas Ward, PhD, AOA director of education, from 1977 through 1996, was to rewrite the AOA CME manual with the assistance of CCME chair Siehl. Later, Ward recommended the categories be reduced from 13 to four: 1-A, 1-B, 2-A, and 2B. These four categories remain in effect today. This major administrative accomplishment simplified the annual reports, greatly reduced the administrative workload, and made the process much more understandable to DOs and licensing boards.

Waiver Criteria

It was determined in 1976 that CME requirements would be waived for AOA members in meeting one or more of the following criteria: life members, retired members who do not hold an active license to practice medicine, physicians not engaged in active clinical practice, physicians on active duty in the uniformed service or Veterans Administration, osteopathic physicians located outside of the continental limits of the United States, and physicians in missionary service. These categories remain in effect for physicians who are in active clinical practice today. It was clarified that *active clinical practice* would include any DO who is treating patients on a full-time or part-time basis. The council on CME was given "broad discretionary powers" by the AOA board of trustees to review individual requests for exemption based on hardship of any DO member. The council may grant or deny CME credits based on its evaluation of the content, faculty, and educational quality of programs submitted for CME credit.

AOA Credit Hour CME Requirements

In July 1998, the requirement for Category 1-A CME was reduced from 60 credit hours to 30 credit hours. Category 1-A continues to be defined as "formal live didactic educational programs that are sponsored by an AOA Category 1 CME Sponsor and meet requirements in the AOA CME Guidelines for Category 1-A."

Starting with the 2004–2006 CME cycle, the AOA board of trustees approved a resolution for a change of the total required credit hours for membership from 150 to 120 credit hours, of which 30 hours must continue to be Category 1-A. As of 2010, this is the credit hour requirement for all osteopathic physicians.

The AOA Council on CME did not make lightly the decision to lower the total number of credit hour requirements. The decision was made in light of the competing requirements physicians have to make in the economy today, changes in how physicians obtain CME credit, and other demands. At the end of the 1998–2000 CME cycle, it was apparent that the changing environment of osteopathic medicine was making it increasingly difficult for members to meet the AOA CME requirement for membership. Specialties within the AOA have voluntarily

TABLE 6-1 *2010 AOA CME Categories of Credit*

Category	A: Formal or live	B: Less formal
Osteopathic	1-A	1-B
Nonosteopathic (i.e., AMA or AAFP)	2-A	2-B

continued with a 150 credit hour requirement, which is allowable. Concerned that it may be perceived that the AOA diminished the value of CME by reducing the credit requirement to 120, the Council on CME reviewed the entire CME program and affirmed that the goals of the CME program remained valid, that the three-year cycles should continue, and that the CME categories of credit should remain intact.

In 2003, the AOA board of trustees and House of Delegates approved the 120 CME credit hour requirement for membership, of which 30 hours must be in Category 1-A. The remaining hours can be met in any category (see Table 6-1). State licensing boards may require specific categories in any of the four categories, but the AOA does not regulate CME state licensure credit.

Category 1-A formal educational programs are designed to enhance clinical competence and improve patient care, and they must be sponsored by an approved AOA-accredited Category 1 CME sponsor. Category 1-B programs are less formal osteopathic-related educational activities that include credits for obtaining recertification or a Certificate of Added Qualification (CAQ), precepting osteopathic medical students, writing for peer-reviewed publications, developing examination questions, serving on educational committees, and reading osteopathic medical journals. Category 1-B is awarded to osteopathic physicians who participate in the AOA Clinical Assessment Program (CAP), which is an option for Component 4 that will be in the Osteopathic Continuing Certification (OCC) program and will be required for all AOA board specialties by 2013. Component 4 is similar to the Maintenance of Certification program required by all specialties recognized by the American Board of Medical Specialties (ABMS). Like 1-A, Category 2-A is formal education, but the AOA accepts AMA and American Academy of Family Physicians (AAFP) credit in the total requirement of 120 CME credit hours. Category 2-B is less formal educational activities similar to those in 1-B but unrelated to the osteopathic profession.

AOA leadership considers its CME system as two equally important tiers. In the first tier, programs are designed to ensure osteopathic physicians maintain a strong connection to the osteopathic profession, its philosophy, and the member community through the AOA. In the second tier, osteopathic physicians maintain a commitment to lifelong learning and quality patient care through CME.

The first tier remains a requirement in the current system of osteopathic CME. Leaders in the osteopathic community insisted from the early years of CME that osteopathic principles and practice be integrated throughout the CME program for Category 1.

The basic requirement for osteopathic CME is that it remain unique to the osteopathic medical profession. The philosophy of osteopathic medicine has always meant more than manipulative medicine, but osteopathic manipulative treatment (OMT) is certainly a component. OMT is incorporated into the training and practice of osteopathic physicians. With OMT, osteopathic physicians use their hands to diagnose illness and injury and to encourage the body's natural tendency toward good health. By combining all other available medical options with OMT, DOs attempt to offer patients the most comprehensive care possible.

The CCME believes that members should be required to earn 30 hours of Category 1-A credit to meet the intentions of the first tier. The Category 1-A requirement has several purposes that are fundamental to the goals of the CME program. Category 1-A CME programs are formal didactic educational programs that promote a deeper understanding of the profession. This purpose was built into the initial construction of the CME system and remains as valid today as it did more than 30 years ago. Other significant purposes of maintaining Category 1-A CME is to encourage osteopathic physicians to maintain osteopathic manipulative medicine skills, develop research skills, and educate other osteopathic physicians.

CME Certificates

In February 1975, AOA leaders considered providing osteopathic physicians a certificate for completion of their AOA CME requirement. Five months later, the AOA board of trustees adopted a resolution that CME certificates be made available at a minimal cost to those members who request one. Although this service remains an option, the ability to print one's own CME activity report has gained wider acceptance.

After the decision in 2003 to reduce the credit hour requirement from 150 to 120, the AOA agreed that members who continued to obtain 150 CME credits would be recognized with a CME Certificate of Excellence at the end of the three-year cycle. Any eligible member who obtains 150 hours or more of AOA-approved CME credit in a three-year CME cycle may print a Certificate of Excellence directly from the members-only side of the AOA Web site www.DO-online.org. The physician must have met his or her AOA CME requirement by December 31 at the end of the CME cycle.

CME Requirements for AOA Board Certification

In addition to CME requirements for AOA membership, the AOA board of trustees adopted a resolution in February 1996 that all certified members of the AOA were to obtain a minimum number of CME specialty credit hours during the three-year cycle. Since then, 50 credits must be earned in the physician's primary specialty (Category 1 or 2). The regulatory body for certification, the Bureau of Osteopathic Specialists, oversees adherence to this requirement, which is documented on the AOA CME activity report as a service to certified members.

AOA System for Recognition of Category 1 Sponsors and CME Policy

The AOA began recognizing Category 1 sponsors in 1992. The CCME was delegated authority by the AOA board of trustees to award Category 1 accreditation status to osteopathic CME sponsors, develop policy, ensure sponsors adhere to osteopathic CME requirements, and conduct accreditation document surveys and on-site surveys of CME sponsors as part of that process. To qualify to be a sponsor, applicants are required to be an AOA-recognized affiliate. In 1992, the AOA recognized more than 200 sponsors. Over time, many sponsors consolidated into consortiums, and in the mid 1990s, many osteopathic hospitals closed or partnered with larger hospital corporations for economic reasons. There were approximately 160 Category 1 AOA sponsors in 2010.

The AOA board of trustees adopted a policy that the AOA would develop and implement a system for monitoring CME sponsors and their compliance with uniform guidelines. The AOA board of trustees adopted the "Uniform Guidelines to Be Followed by Accredited Sponsors of Continuing Medical Education" in principle, pending approval of the final version.[5]

The uniform guidelines were updated in 1993 after the AOA participated with the Task Force on CME Provider/Industry Collaboration, which included 31 major national CME organizations and the US Food and Drug Administration (FDA). In March 1993, the AOA published draft accreditation requirements that encompassed the uniform guidelines and the FDA policy statement. These guidelines are updated continually to provide a consistent policy for CME accrediting agencies, industry, and the FDA to assess the compliance of accredited CME sponsors with basic principles of good practice in the delivery of CME programs. In 1993, a companion manual titled "Accreditation Requirements for AOA Category 1 CME Sponsors" was created and includes the fee structure to implement and operate certified CME programs by Category 1 CME sponsors.[6]

The CCME and AOA staffs monitor AOA CME Category 1 sponsors for adherence to these policies and procedures, audit CME programs for compliance with AOA policies, and investigate all written complaints of deviation from AOA policy using a standard complaint review procedure. The AOA solicits regular feedback on related policies and procedures.

In February 1993, the AOA conducted its first AOA National Conference of Osteopathic CME Sponsors at the O'Hare Hilton Hotel, Chicago. This conference was developed to inform CME providers of changes in CME policy and informed recognized osteopathic organizations how to become an AOA-accredited CME sponsor under the new policy. Today, this annual conference includes topics on CME from a global and AOA perspective and assists sponsors in providing quality programs. Sponsors must attend the national conference at least once during a three-year cycle, but many attend annually.

In 1994, the AOA CCME considered policy for surveying CME programs and using on-site reviews to monitor program quality. By February 1995, a document survey protocol was approved by the AOA board of trustees as a means of conducting reviews of CME sponsors. The CCME determined that on-site inspections would be conducted only if authorized by the CCME when there was evidence of noncompliance. Document surveys continue to be used as the primary evaluation tool of sponsors to ensure a continuous review of policy adherence. The CCME reviews document surveys of CME sponsors at its regularly scheduled council meetings.

Activity in the National CME Community

In 1990, Ward was invited to become a member of a coalition of CME groups composed primarily of allopathic CME agencies. He was the only osteopathic representative in a group of approximately 25 agencies. The coalition met in Chicago twice yearly to discuss cross-agency and nationwide matters of CME interest. As a matter of course, the meetings would not end until the AOA's policy positions on the national CME issues under discussion had been heard. In 2010, the AOA director of education filled a membership position on the National Task Force on CME Provider/Industry Collaboration and is treated with the same respect and consideration. Representatives from the AOA board of trustees serve on the CMSS Conjoint Committee on CME and the AAFP Clinical Content Committee. Although the AOA CME credit system is separate and distinct, CME leaders in the osteopathic profession monitor and evaluate policy and changes made by the ACCME, AMA, and AAFP.

Summary

The AOA CME program has existed since June 1973 and continues to thrive. There have been major changes within the CME program since its inception, and changes will continue in an effort to meet the needs of osteopathic physicians and AOA Category 1 CME sponsors. Currently, changes are underway to the online calendar that will give Category 1 CME sponsors direct access to enter their own Category 1-A events through a secure online interface.

CME leadership in the osteopathic profession believes that the AOA must ensure that physicians continue to receive cutting-edge, certified CME programs and services that address validated educational needs and that the benefits of CME to society are transparent. All CME providers—osteopathic and allopathic—have an obligation to the medical profession and society-at-large to maintain standards for CME, establish clear and concise roles and responsibilities, and identify quality indicators of CME programs that are developed, implemented, and evaluated. CME must ultimately benefit patients, and providers must seek methods to evaluate improved patient and community health outcomes.

Notes

1. "About the AOA," American Osteopathic Association Web site, http://www.do-online.org/index (accessed July 13, 2010).

2. "American Osteopathic Association Basic Documents, Constitution and Bylaws (2007)," American Osteopathic Association Web site, http://www.do-online.org/pdf/aoa_conbylaw.pdf (accessed July 13, 2010).

3. "Continuing Medical Education, Phase I Editorial," *Journal of the American Osteopathic Association* 72 (1973): 666.

4. "American Osteopathic Association CME Guide for Osteopathic Physicians, 2010–2012," American Osteopathic Association Web site, http://www.do-online.org/index.cfm?PageID=edu_main&au =D&SubPageID =cme_main&SubSubPageID =cme_guidemain (accessed July 13, 2010).

5. D. K. Wentz and others, "CME, Unabated Debate," *Journal of the American Medical Association* 268 (1992): 1118–1120.

6. "American Osteopathic Association Accreditation Requirements for AOA Category 1 Sponsors (2008)," American Osteopathic Association Web site, http://www.do-online.org/pdf/cme_accredreqs.pdf (accessed July 20, 2010).

CHAPTER 7

Continuing Medical Education at the Association of American Medical Colleges

A membership association reflects the values, experiences, and needs of its members. The Association of American Medical Colleges (AAMC)—with 125 years of history—is no exception to that rule. The story of continuing medical education (CME)—the last, longest, and arguably the most complex of the three phases of medical education—exemplifies this notion, as it played out in the setting of the medical school or academic medical center.

Silence on CME

Recognizing the need for an association to represent at least a portion of the nation's medical school enterprise, a group of 22 schools founded the association that would eventually become the AAMC in Philadelphia in 1876. Despite changes in the group's mandate and membership over several years, the association continued to grow, expanding its membership and, in 1890, reconstituting itself with new governance and organizational structures.

We note no mention of CME during these early years. This absence was not through any oversight on the part of the AAMC; other organizations were similarly silent on continuing education or the need for learning post graduation. This silence represents a relatively stable body of knowledge needed to practice medicine, thus

.directing medical schools to concentrate solely on the preparation of the physician and not his (rarely her in that period) ongoing education. Several events and concepts changed how medical education was viewed, some of which would have later implications for CME and lifelong learning.

First, Sir William Osler, exhibiting a portion of his profound impact on medical education at Johns Hopkins (and elsewhere in North America and Great Britain) delivered a speech in early 1900, offering the first modern articulation of the principles of lifelong learning for physicians. In his speech, he indicated that "the hardest conviction to get into the mind of a beginner is that the education upon which he is engaged is not a college course, not a medical course, but a life course, for which the work of a few years under teachers is but a preparation."[1]

Second, the Flexner Report, issued in 1910, dramatically altered the nation's model of medical education. While not specifically mentioning CME, it established a sounder basis of undergraduate medical education, moving it from a relatively unscientific and proprietary enterprise to one which espoused best scientific principles, was based in universities, and was nonproprietary. It would be difficult to refute the notion that this report and its consequent reforms have provided a platform for a solid, reproducible, and more standardized basis for medical training. By the 1920s, as a result of the Flexner Report, "medical schools had become an integral part of the university community" thereby exhibiting a firm investment in medical education and the academic community.[2]

Third, World War I, with its emphasis on battlefront surgery and its profoundly dislocating influence on society, challenged the notion that undergraduate medical education could provide an unchanging knowledge base for practice. This period witnessed the rise of the medical specialties and their influence on and recognition of CME as their raison d'être.

Fourth, in 1932, the AAMC issued its report on medical education. It is interesting to note that while still silent on the question of CME, the report stressed the need to prepare the student for a lifetime of learning with the appropriate skill set and attitudes to accomplish that task. The report echoed Osler and added:

> There is a distinct shift in many medical schools now toward placing greater responsibility on the student for his own training in an effort to emphasize learning by the student in contrast to teaching by the faculty. . . . The aim is to develop minds capable of appraising evidence and drawing conclusions based on logical reasoning and to help provide a permanent intellectual equipment, resourcefulness, judgment, and proper habits as well as methods of study, which will prepare the student to continue his own self-education throughout his professional life.[3]

While undergraduate education was characterized as the developer of an individual skilled in lifelong learning and the AAMC as virtually its sole spokesman, the question of graduate education and its ownership was less clear. This situation generated rigorous debate between the American Medical Association (AMA) Council on Medical Education and the AAMC. This dialogue culminated in the AMA and the new specialist boards laying claim to hospital internship and graduate training. Kenneth Ludmerer has suggested that this was a missed opportunity: one

can imagine that more attention might be paid to education and subsequently to lifelong learning and continuing professional development had the medical schools and the AAMC been able to establish ownership.[4] Instead, the focus, however appropriate and utilitarian, was on training towards a finite certification endpoint, with the creation of training and regulatory rules surrounding the residency experience, and possibly in continuing professional development. This ambivalence about CME in the AAMC in some ways parallels its mixed commitment to its cousin graduate medical education (GME).

The Flexner Aftermath

The period following the release of the Flexner Report produced an increased focus on undergraduate medical education (UGME) (and some early interest in GME and on CME) on the part of the AAMC.

First, along with the growing recognition of the importance of UGME, the advent of World War II brought with it the need to train more physicians more rapidly. This accelerated and abbreviated training gave rise to concerns about the quality of medical education, ultimately culminating in an accreditation process. The question was, who would undertake such an effort?

Given the inherent difficulties in being both a membership and constituent body, the AAMC by itself seemed an unlikely yet important candidate. On the other hand, the AMA—also a potential candidate—lacked the educational expertise and ownership of UGME. Hence, with increased wartime collaboration between the AAMC and AMA, the Liaison Committee on Medical Education was formed. Its creation marked the beginning of an accreditation process and organization, instructive to the creation of similar processes in GME and CME.

Second, post-World War II, concerns were raised about the rise of specialization, the deemphasis of the patient in medical education, and the quality of teaching. These concerns led to the development of two entities within the AAMC framework. In 1950, the AAMC created its first committee on CME and a subcommittee on research and evaluation that led to an early faculty development project termed the *Teaching Institute* in 1951. As such, innovation in medical education was highlighted, allowing, perhaps for the first time, the UGME curriculum to reflect the problem-solving needs of the practicing physician—the ultimate product of a UGME curriculum.

Ambivalence about CME

The period from the 1960s to the 1970s witnessed some interest in CME, perhaps best described as approach-avoidance. In this era, the AAMC took several steps in the direction of ownership of CME as a legitimate medical school enterprise, then—recognizing its complexity, political nature, and the important demands of other segments of academic medicine—backed away from it.

Archived minutes of a 1960 AAMC medical education committee meeting identified only 18 medical schools with a CME program. In contrast, the notes indicate that many specialty societies had grown to meet the ongoing educational needs of their members.[5]

Among many changes developed in the 1960s, perhaps none was more important to the life of the AAMC and to medical education than the April 1965 Coggeshall report titled "Planning for Medical Progress through Education." The report was framed "in the context of the changes proposed by President Johnson in 1965 creating Medicare and Medicaid," and its publication had a profound influence.[6] Coggeshall called for a thorough review of AAMC governance and a move from Chicago to Washington, DC. Beyond the organizational and geographic changes outlined by Coggeshall, major recommendations were made with regard to medical education that, for the first time, clearly articulated its cross-

continuum nature. Many of these presaged current developments in continuing education and urged that medical schools, rather than specialty societies, undertake more responsibility for CME. It also suggested that physicians' needs, and thus learning, be more linked to the health-care demands of society.[7]

In 1969, following the major transformation of the AAMC generated by Coggeshall, the AAMC formed a committee on CME that recommended that it place CME among its primary concerns, that its member schools recognize CME among their major responsibilities, and that it establish an administrative unit to support CME activities arising within its component medical schools. Exemplifying the ambivalence with which CME was regarded in that decade, these recommendations went unaccepted and, in the early 1970s, the AAMC discharged its CME committee.

Founded in 1969, the Group on Medical Education, subsequently called the Group on Educational Affairs (GEA), offered a potentially vibrant vehicle for faculty development and ultimately for continuing education. The GEA served then, as it does today, a heterogeneous constituency. In 1974, despite rejection of the notion that academic medical centers accept responsibility for CME, the steering committee of the GEA responded to growing CME pressures and expanded its interests to include the continuum of medical education, thus including CME in its administrative and programmatic purview. Although its charter encompassed the continuum of medical education, the activities of the GEA focused on UGME and the Research in Medical Education conference.

In addition to the General Professional Education of the Physician Report, several other reports called for change in medical education during the 1980s. GEA activities during this decade included expanded programming during the national AAMC annual meeting and in the four regions of the GEA. Members developed an annotated bibliography on professionalism across the continuum and began a program to promote the scholarship of teaching that continues today.

In 1994, the GEA chair appointed a task force (comprising representatives of UGME, GME, CME, and research in medical education) to review the GEA and its membership and activities. The charge to the task force was to (a) review the GEA and AAMC mission statements and make recommendations for needed alterations and revisions; (b) identify the GEA functions and activities that serve the needs of its members; (c) identify GEA constituents and recommend mechanisms for continuous updating of constituent groups; and (d) describe two or three organizational frameworks that are suitable for serving the GEA mission and functions and the advantages and disadvantages of each proposed organizational framework. The review was necessary because it had become difficult to articulate the mission of the GEA and how it is integrated across levels of medical education. It was equally difficult to integrate the activities of its members, ranging from undergraduate through continuing education. In addition, some GEA members expected more from the GEA than they were experiencing, while potential members did not know the GEA existed.

The GEA constituency includes teaching faculty, curriculum managers, course or clerkship directors, continuing education directors, deans, researchers in medical education, and GME directors.

As a result of the GEA self-study process, the GEA was reorganized in 1996 around four sections that represent the continuum of medical education: UGME, GME, CME, and research in medical education. In addition, the regional organization of the GEA was retained and strengthened with section activities occurring within the regions and throughout the nation. Representation from the Organization of Student Representatives and the Organization of Resident Representatives was added to the GEA steering committee. The goal of the reorganization is to make the continuum of medical education real and more than an expression.

An active component of the GEA, the Research in Medical Education (RIME) conference has been part of the AAMC annual meeting since 1964. Recognizing the importance and relevance of CME research to UGME and GME, beginning in 1975, the six-member GEA Steering Committee always included a representative of the CME community and a section of the RIME program and proceedings for CME research. The RIME Invited Address, presented yearly at the association's annual meeting, included more than one perspective from CME. However, with the introduction of the Research in Continuing Medical Education conference of the Society for Academic CME and the rise of other competing demands and interests, the synergy between CME and the wider medical education research community has diminished. The potential for fuller collaboration across the continuum remains.

Currently, the GEA activities are prioritized by an evolving and proactive "Agenda for Action" in which CME activities are represented.

Investing in CME

Two major developments in the last half of the 1970s generated sizable support for academic CME. First, in 1975, a group at the annual meeting of the AAMC "generated much enthusiasm for forming an independent membership organization."[8] This group, then called the Society of Medical College Directors of CME (SMCDCME), became the single body representing academic CME in the United States and Canada. Today called the Society for Academic CME (SACME), it is one of two North American groups devoted to CME; its influence in supporting research in CME, its journal, and its other endeavors have been enormous. SACME has been supported by AAMC staff through a portion of this period, and is once again closely aligned with current activities in academic continuing education.

Second, 1977 saw the formation of the Liaison Committee on CME (LCCME), the accreditation body for continuing education. The AAMC was a formal founding member organization with the Council of Medical Specialty Societies, the Federation of State Medical Boards, the AMA, the American Hospital Association, the American Board of Medical Specialties, and the Association for Hospital Medical Education. Not unlike other similar organizations, the LCCME ultimately evolved into a different structure, becoming today's Accreditation Council for CME.

The late 1970s and early 1980s also exemplified growing scholarly and developmental interests of AAMC in CME as witnessed by several projects that analyzed continuing education from both theoretical and practical perspectives. These included the Continuing Education Systems Project, designed as a project to focus AAMC goals in the area of CME; the Adult Learning Working Group of the LCCME; the Illinois Field Test of assessment measures in CME; and, of importance to the formation of a skilled lifelong learner, the General Professional Education of the Physician Report.

The late 1970s witnessed the establishment of and report from an ad hoc committee on the continuing education of physicians. Formed in 1976, the report was accepted by AAMC governance in 1979. It had, if not an immediate, then a fairly profound influence on the AAMC role (and thus that of medical schools) in CME. It identified several major issues in CME: the growing need for continuing education expressed by licensing and specialist boards; the inadequate resources devoted to CME on the part of medical schools; the lack of application of an adult learning model to CME; and the need for a research agenda to identify the causal links between CME activity and physician performance.[9] Among its recommendations, it urged adoption of policies to support CME and its accreditation process by the AAMC;

assistance of medical schools with the provision of adult- and performance-based CME; and provision of a national forum for CME.

If CME is to be effective, the preparation of the physician undertaking ongoing learning, reflection, and application is important. In this area, the General Professional Education of the Physician report of 1983 presented five significant recommendations with ultimate reliance for the education of the practicing physician. These included, among others, the de-emphasis of memorization and an emphasis on the acquisition of skills; value and attitudes that would enable continued competence; broad liberal arts preclinical training; the acquisition of learning skills; and a focus on patients and patient families.

Integrated Continuing Education and Performance Improvement

Viewing the AAMC history regarding CME across more than a century of activity generates a somewhat mixed picture. On one hand, it reveals a natural, exclusive focus on UGME not unlike that of the profession itself. On the other hand, it reveals a process that progressively, if sporadically, considered the creation of the lifelong learner and CME as a focus of the efforts of academic medical centers. In this regard, the relatively slow uptake of CME as a core function of academic medical centers and the AAMC itself is both understandable and perhaps necessary.

Signs of a growing commitment to CME on the part of the AAMC became more notable by the late 1990s. Like the profession itself, the AAMC had more fully evolved a picture of the continuum of medical education and, like health-care systems, had begun to develop an understanding of quality improvement; apply better principles of continuing professional development; consider team training; and weigh the influence of commercial support on CME content—all major strands in the development of CME.[10]

An identifiable tipping point in its commitment to CME was the work of a group commissioned to write a report on the state of CME and its role in the academic medical center in 2000. The white paper, authored by N. L. Bennett and her colleagues, articulated in greater detail the role of medical schools in CME and outlined what was to become, by 2006, the guiding principles for continuing education and performance improvement—characterizing CME in a manner emphasizing outcomes beyond competence.[11]

The paper outlined several goals for continuing education. First, it articulated a new CME paradigm, one that (a) moved CME from its traditional conference-producing role to one that provided an effective communication vehicle to deliver best evidence at the point of care and (b) stressed clinical outcomes and thus a more meaningful integration into the missions of the academic medical center. Second, it argued that such a paradigm could not be created without a strong commitment to academic development, stressing scholarship and research in the field—thus urging a commitment to faculty and staff development. Third, it put forward the notion that CME should include a focus on the training of the learner, urging those in CME to be supportive of UGME and GME as the training ground for next-generation practitioners.

A further tipping point came in 2005 with the first meeting of a body known informally as the Joint Working Group—comprising the GEA CME section steering committee and the leadership of SACME. Together, these elements (i.e., the advice of the Joint Working group, the directions of the Bennett paper, and the results of a rapidly growing literature on the effect of CME) produced an initiative within the academic affairs committee that the AAMC termed *continuing education and performance improvement*. Broadly reflecting a new paradigm and aimed at integration, efforts of the AAMC academic affairs committee in this context focus on several of the following areas:

- *The research enterprise.* Efforts to increase the notion of research in medical education across the continuum are visible, though as yet—given somewhat different research paradigms and history—more sporadic than functional. Offering equal potential for development (and more potential for funding) is the amalgamation of outcomes-oriented CME research with the fields of implementation science or knowledge translation—an increasing area of interest on the part of the Agency for Health Research, the National Institutes of Health, and the Veterans Administration. These have been heavily emphasized in reports
- *The clinical enterprise.* A progression towards outcomes-oriented CME activities (now a requirement of the ACCME) shows sizable promise for increased collaborative activity between CME providers (and their colleagues in faculty development and continuing professional and staff development) and quality improvement managers, committees, and activities.
- *The continuum of medical education.* Efforts to increase the awareness of UGME and GME program planners about current needs of the practicing physician and the health-care system have resulted in calls for understanding the competencies of lifelong learning and their incorporation into pre-practice education and areas *of quality improvement and patient safety, among others.*[12]
- *Other issues.* Among many other logistical and functional issues, that of commercial conflicts of interest has risen to the surface. Lessons learned in CME have implications for the governance and funding of the academic medical center.

These activities aimed at moving from a paradigm of CME-as-conference to a more holistic provider of best evidence at the point of care have shown promise at the association level and within an increasing number of academic medical centers.

Summary

A product of the traditional medical school, the AAMC was formed in the late 1800s representing what then were its key elements: UGME and its relationship (or lack of such) with an affiliated university. As medical schools or the construct of the academic medical center grew so, too, did the AAMC. In the early 1900s, following the release of the Flexner Report and the demise of non-scientific proprietary schools, the AAMC demonstrated its commitment to a scientific basis, adding research to its agenda. Following both world wars in the early and mid 1900s and the need for specialty training, the AAMC developed its interest in residency education and—ultimately in the setting in which this would occur—the beginnings of the division of health care affairs.

Absent from the medical school until the early to mid-1900s, however, was an expressed and consistent need to consider CME as a part of the educational continuum. Most schools at that time would agree that CME was not in their domain. When considered at all, it was in the nature of an update, offering new advances (relatively few in the first half of the last century) or as a refresher program for those returning from the two world wars and whose preparation for basic medical training may have been rushed or insufficient.

As J. R. Buchanan states, however, the "past is prologue," in this way emphasizing the strong commitment to medical education, research, and health-care delivery on the part of the AAMC and the creation of a platform from which a meaningfully integrated and effective CME presence might be realized.[13] Awareness of the need for CME, discussions about its importance, and its role become more commonplace in the late 20th century and—with greater emphasis and attempts at integration—the early 21st century.

Notes

1. *Aequanimitas and Other Addresses* (Philadelphia: P. Blakiston's Son & Co., 1904), 400.

2. Mark Bowles and Virginia Dawson, *With One Voice, The Association of American Medical Colleges, 1876–2002* (Washington, DC: Association of American Medical Colleges, 2003).

3. A. Lawrence Lowell, *Final Report of the Commission on Medical Education* (New York: Office of the Director of Study, 1932).

4. Kenneth M. Ludmerer, *Time to Heal: American Medical Education from the Turn of the Century to the Era of Managed Care* (New York: Oxford University Press, 2004).

5. Archived minutes, Medical Education Committee of the Association of American Medical Colleges, Washington, DC (accessed April 2009).

6. Lowell T. Coggeshall, *Planning for Medical Progress through Education* (Association of American Medical Colleges, 1965).

7. W. G. Anlayan, "What Has Happened to the AAMC since the Coggeshall Report of 1965," *Journal of the American Medical Association* 210 (1969): 1897–1901.

8. Archived minutes, Society of Medical College Directors of CME of the Association of American Medical Colleges, Washington, DC (accessed June 28, 2009).

9. W. D. Myer and others, *Ad Hoc Committee on CME: CE of Physicians—Conclusions and Recommendations* (Association of American Medical Colleges, 1979).

10. Archived minutes, Group on Educational Affairs of the Association of American Medical Colleges, Washington, DC (accessed July 2009).

11. Nancy L. Bennett, "Continuing Medical Education: A New Vision of the Professional Development of Physicians," *Academic Medicine* 75, no. 12 (2000): 1167–1172.

12. Association of American Medical Colleges and American Association of Colleges of Nursing, *Lifelong Learning in Medicine and Nursing* (Josiah Macy, Jr. Foundation, 2010), http://www.aamc.org/meded/cme/lifelong/macyreport.pdf.

13. J. R. Buchanan, "The Past as Prologue," *Academic Medicine* 68 (1993): 173–177.

Pamela M. Mazmanian, Robert K. Richards,
Robert L. Tupper, and Dennis K. Wentz

CHAPTER 8

The Key Role of the State Medical Societies in Continuing Medical Education

Prior to 1900, a doctor usually apprenticed with a practicing physician and took medical school lectures to complement years of practice. Proprietary medical schools augmented a number of university associated medical schools. Medical education included lectures, with formal clinical or laboratory teaching virtually nonexistent and no requirement of internship. This approach to training, while woeful by current standards, provided general practice physicians for many communities. Since there was little scientific base for medicine, the physician's lack of a university education was not considered a significant deficiency, but as early as the 1700s physicians showed concern for developing the practice of medicine.

In "Documentary History of Philanthropy and Voluntarism in the United States, 1600-1900," editor Peter Dobkin Hall presents a letter written ostensibly by a doctor and circulated in 1765 throughout the Massachusetts medical community.[1] It clearly expressed the concerns of physicians of the time. They desired to establish an association to advance the field of medicine.

SIR: There has been [for] some time on foot a proposal [for] forming medical Societies or Associations of Doctors analogous to those of the Clergy for the more speedy Improvement of our young Physicians; as by communicating to each other any Discoveries in any of the Branches of Physick, especially Botony, for

which this Country is an ample Field. To get the Profession upon a more respectable footing in the Country by suppressing this Herd of Empiricks who have bro't such intolerable contempt on the Epithet *Country Practitioner*. And to increase Charity & good Will amongst the lawful Members of the Professional that they may avoid condemning & calumnating each other before the Plebians as it is too common for the last that's call'd in a difficult Case to do by those that preceded him which we apprehend to be highly detrimental to the Profession and the chief Root from whence these very Empiricks spring.[2]

The originator of the letter remains anonymous. It concludes with an invitation for select Boston area physicians to meet on the third Monday in March 1765, instructing the reader:

Presuming upon your Concurrence we desire you to promote the Design by circulating this Paper thro' the Hands of all the undermentioned Physicians, or others beyond their Limits, but we must be careful that it falls not into the Hand of any but orthodox Physicians, and to prevent it your [sic] should deliver it yourself or send it by a trusty Person carefully sealed and superscribed lest a teltale Wife or Child divulge that which must be as secret as Masonry till some Societies are established.[3]

Physicians of late eighteenth-century New England were forming associations and petitioning their legislatures unsuccessfully for charters of incorporation. Finally, in 1781, as described by Aghababian and Tulgan, a small group of physicians and surgeons from the Boston area successfully petitioned the Massachusetts legislature to incorporate the Massachusetts Medical Society (MMS), a year before Harvard Medical School was founded.[4] The authors report that the formation of the MMS was likely inspired by medical societies known to exist in European cities, such as Berlin, Edinburgh, Göttingen, London, Munich, and Paris.

Limitations and restrictions on membership in the MMS led to the development of other medical associations in Massachusetts, such as the Berkshire Medical Society and the Worcester Medical Society. The Berkshire Medical Society met for the first time in 1787 at Widow Bingham's Tavern in Stockbridge "to form an association for the purpose of observing and communicating those things which may be for the improvement of the art of the Physic, and of encouraging a spirit of union with those of the Faculty, and rendering the Faculty more respectable."[5] The Worcester Medical Society, formed in 1794, required its members to attend semi-annual meetings and orations. According to the 1837 publication "History of Worcester, Massachusetts":

The Mass. Medical Society, intended to produce that harmony and mutual effort necessary to elevate the profession to the standing and usefulness which the interests of the community required, failed of its object, by the limitation of its members to eighty in Massachusetts and Maine, and the restriction on their consultations with any, except those who obtained the qualifications they required. . . . At an early meeting [of the Worcester Medical Society] a petition was referred to the state legislature for incorporation, referred to a joint committee of physicians, and resulted in an arrangement to enlarge the number of the general society, and a proposal to create district associations. This system removing the evils which had been felt, and mutually satisfactory, was carried into effect, and on the 20th of Sept. 1804, the Worcester District Society was organized.[6]

State legislative approval of a reorganization of the MMS in 1804 permitted the district societies to become incorporated into the MMS.[7]

The formation of medical societies during the eighteenth century was concentrated in the eastern United States and extended beyond New England. New Jersey physicians formed a society in 1766 and unsuccessfully petitioned the legislature to seek incorporation. The society remained inactive until 1786 when it reorganized and was granted a charter for incorporation. In 1799, the Maryland Medical Society became incorporated to "prevent the citizens [of Maryland] from risking their lives in the hands of ignorant practitioners or pretenders to the healing art."[8]

AMA and State Medical Society Initiatives in Educating Physicians

The American Medical Association (AMA), founded in 1847, and the Association of American Medical Colleges (AAMC), founded in 1876, each tried to encourage and upgrade standards for physician education. Development of the AMA resulted from the efforts of state medical societies who were already functional and proactive on behalf of the profession. After the AMA appointed its new Council on Medical Education and Hospitals in 1904, the council's annual ratings of medical schools and their graduates' success in passing state licensing exams was an important step in the reform of medical education. However, the 1910 study of medical education commissioned by the Carnegie Foundation for the Advancement of Teaching and conducted by educator Abraham Flexner, MD, led to a science-based revolution, including accreditation of medical schools by the AMA Council, acceptance of medical education responsibility by universities, and the merger and/or closing of 65 medical schools by 1915.[9]

The AMA, through its component state and county societies, and along with a few pioneering university medical schools, became the first organizing structures for continuing medical education (CME). The early leaders of the CME movement were the scientific and educational leaders of medicine. As the physician-learners of this era were mostly general practitioners without internship training, the primary goal of CME was to correct their educational deficiencies in order to make them more competent. The 1907 report of J. C. McCormack, MD, chairman of the AMA committee on organization, stated:

The necessity of doing something in this direction [CME] and the magnitude of the problem, will be appreciated when it is known that a large majority of the licensed physicians who are treating sick people every day do not attend medical meetings, and that a large percent of this element do not read research periodicals or standard literature.[10]

Since many general practitioners were in solo practice, and modes of communication and transportation were limited, it was vital to bring CME to doctors via systematic CME programs. McCormack, commissioned by the AMA, visited several states to "perfect medical organization and stimulate interest in postgraduate education."[11] Following one of McCormack's promotional state visits, the Tarrant County Medical Society of Texas developed and offered 12 courses in the basic sciences, physical diagnosis, and surgery. The plan served as the basis for a county medical society CME program organized by John H. Blackburn, MD, in Bowling Green, Kentucky. It offered an extensive plan of study designed for general practitioners and distributed to all county societies. Publicized by the AMA in 1907 as a model, the Blackburn Plan led approximately 350 county societies in 29 states to emulate it by 1909.[12]

Another pioneering effort to provide CME systematically was the North Carolina Extension Plan started in 1916 by W. S. Rankin, MD, the state health officer. Following strategies first worked out by the Fourth District Medical Society, the process included two predominantly rural circuits in which clinician taught pediatrics each week for 12 successive weeks. Subsequently, the North Carolina Extension Plan was adopted with modification in Missouri, West Virginia, and Oklahoma.[13]

The AMA Council on Medical Education and Hospitals called attention to the increasing opportunities afforded to county, state, and district medical societies to organize and operate, once or twice each year, diagnostic clinics as well as extension courses of lectures and clinics. The June 1927 *American Medical Association Bulletin* featured an example of a successful program: the Brooklyn Idea. Originating in 1922, the Medical Society of the County of Kings adopted as one of its functions the supplying of postgraduate medical education and arranged with Long Island Hospital for a joint committee to offer courses for general practitioners. The chief types of courses developed by the joint committee were called extension courses, and it is reported that "they grew out of the weekly lectures in an effort to supply the indispensable element of bedside teaching."[14]

In part because of the Brooklyn Idea, in the 1920s the Medical Society of the State of New York embarked on the most extensive state-wide program for medical education of practicing doctors in the country through its Committee on Public Health and Medical Education. Very prominent were a number of extension courses offered to county societies. Some addressed obstetrics and pediatrics with support from a New York State Board of Health special appropriation. The aim of the state society program was not to train specialists but to raise the standards of local physicians in general practice. Courses were open to all physicians, regardless of membership in the society. The instructors were members of medical faculties and selected practitioners, and they were paid a $25 honorarium for each day of service. The average cost per course was $215.40, which translated into a cost of $1.38 per physician enrolled.[15] The society also invited the local units to "ask for anything they want" from single lectures to a course of any length, and usually the demand was met. Educational materials were also distributed, such as notes from the courses and special items, including 12,000 copies of the AMA

"Manual on Periodic Health Examinations" sent to all doctors in 1925.[16]

The Michigan Plan grew out of efforts begun in 1919 from "recognition of the fact that the public was demanding the services that scientific medicine held for them." The purposes of the plan, in the words of F. C. Warnshuis, MD, Secretary of the Michigan State Medical Society, were to reach the "large number of our members who were content to travel along in the old rut" and to "bring to these men the progress of scientific medicine." The efforts involved faculty from the University of Michigan and other physician leaders, taking education to the "door step of the physician." Several strategies were employed, including organized clinical tours to go to county society meetings; two- and three-day clinics in leading hospitals; and district one-day postgraduate conferences that reportedly attracted between 500 to 1,200 physicians each.[17]

Despite the success of these educational efforts, a 1933–1934 survey by the Michigan State Medical Society reported:

Only 29 percent [of physicians] had participated in postgraduate study for one month or more during the previous ten years. About 40 percent attended less than six medical meetings a year and, of this number, 15% attended none. The principal reasons given for this failure to engage in postgraduate study were inaccessibility of courses, cost, reluctance to leave practice for the length of time involved in the average course, lack of appeal of the programs, and not infrequently, indifference.[18]

By the 1930s, the emphasis in CME was changing from attempts to remedy the deficiencies of poorly educated practitioners to a new focus on keeping physicians up to date with an expanding body of medical knowledge. A key study and survey emerged from the Medical Society of Virginia (MSV).

In conjunction with a special committee on postgraduate study of the MSV, the extension division of the University of Virginia conducted a survey on postgraduate medical education in Virginia compiling the results and publishing a 1930 report.[19] A questionnaire was sent to all members of the society, of which 397 physicians completed. (The n is unknown, but the authors suggested it was a significant response.) In a May 10, 1928, cover letter included with the questionnaire, J. W. Preston, MD, president of the MSV and MSV special committee chair on postgraduate study, asked members whether they believed a plan should be devised that would "make some form of clinical work available throughout the State":

As you doubtless know, the University of Virginia and the Medical College of Virginia have already undertaken or are planning to undertake graduate courses. Supplementing this intramural work, the Council [of the MSV] recognizes that there are those who cannot leave their practices just when desired, even for short courses, and is at this time giving consideration to working out some plan which in addition to stimulating attendance upon these courses, may make some form of clinical work available throughout the State, or in such sections as appear more interested.[20]

The response was encouraging. According to report authors, George B. Zehmer, director, and George Eutsler, associate director of the extension division at the University of Virginia:

The impressive fact revealed is that a large majority of the physicians, almost ninety per cent, approved the plan to make clinical work available to them. Nearly all of this large majority indicated their belief in personal benefit from such study, their willingness to make an especial effort to attend clinics in their neighborhood and to cooperate in securing material for demonstration, and their entire approval of the undertaking on the part of the Medical Society of Virginia. The opposition expressed in these returns was negligible.[21]

In the introduction, the authors state that "post-graduate medical education is an ambiguous term." The report quotes a definition provided by a speaker during a January 1928 symposium at the New York Academy of Medicine: "Graduate Medical Education is the organized, planful [*sic*] opportunity and guidance of physicians in their mental and technical development after graduation. In this definition emphasis is placed on the word guidance."[22]

The authors were struck with the idea of postgraduate medical guidance and went on to elaborate:

[I]f it is exact enough to exclude extensive and rigorous specialization and is yet distinctive enough to dignify even the most elementary purposeful attempts on the part of the physician to keep abreast of the new developments and advances in the profession—in that case, post-graduate medical guidance is the sole concern of this paper. . . . Its task is that of helping the physician to keep alert to the progress of medical science. . . . A physician who has taken no graduate work for five years may still catch up, so to speak. After ten years only the exceptional man can find contact with the advancing front and after fifteen years he is hopelessly behind times.[23]

The final report addressed a discussion of various plans of continuing interest for the general practitioner; the needs and desires of Virginia physicians in relation to postgraduate education, as revealed in their answers to a questionnaire; and a proposal for a program of postgraduate medical education in Virginia. The rich details in the report and its appendices are beyond the scope of this chapter, but they represent one of the earliest high-quality studies.[24]

In 1936, the AMA House of Delegates approved a study proposed by the AMA Council on Medical Education and Hospitals on "opportunities for practicing physicians to engage in further training." Based on visits to 24 states, findings suggested medical societies had taken on leadership responsibilities in CME. The report noted that "the success of such programs [of CME] seemed dependent on the sustained interest and activity of component medical societies. With few exceptions it may be said that the most practical educational projects encountered thus far have been found in active, progressive and well organized medical societies" and that it "was especially true in rural communities." The study found that in 20 states the chairmen of the state society medical education committees directed some or all of the courses in their states.[25] In 12 of those 20 states, the committees maintained "fairly accurate records of attendance" showing approximately 25 percent of practicing physicians engaged annually in some form of CME.[26]

For the next 40 years, CME filled the role of reinforcing, updating, and expanding the practitioner's scientific knowledge base, with state and county medical society meetings and outreach efforts an important, if relatively declining, source of CME for practicing physicians. Frequently, medical societies worked with the medical schools supporting CME initiatives, as exemplified by the California Medical Association (CMA). From the 1950s through the 1970s, the CMA financially supported "annual meetings with state medical schools" and paid expenses for "traveling faculty where medical school faculty would present evening sessions in rural hospitals not near a medical school."[27]

The AMA began questioning the role of the state and county medical societies in CME as the number of courses offered by the medical schools increased. Glenn Shepherd, MD, assistant secretary of the Council on Medical Education and Hospitals, wrote: "By 1946, the Council on Medical Education and Hospitals had changed its ideas from those of 12 years previously when it had stated that postgraduate medical education was a responsibility primarily for medical societies." In its report to the 95th Annual Session of the AMA House of Delegates, the Council stated: "More important than mere numbers of courses is the fact that more of these courses are of longer duration, more are being offered by universities and medical schools, and the geographic distribution is more extensive."[28]

Development of the CME Accreditation System

Appreciating both an increasing role of medical schools in CME and the desire of physicians to access CME locally, the AMA House of Delegates approved establishment of a formal survey and accreditation program in 1964. The AMA Council on Medical Education formally began accrediting providers of CME programs for physicians in 1967. By 1971, due to the increasing number of survey requests, the AMA Council on Medical Education limited accreditation surveys to institutions and organizations "national or regional in influence, attracting physicians in appreciable number from three or more states or territories, with recurring continuing medical education activities." At the same time, the "Council [on Medical Education] affirmed that state medical associations should be encouraged to consider the establishment of an accreditation program, approved by and periodically reviewed by the Advisory Committee and Council" for the accreditation of local hospitals, medical organizations without a national audience, and local units of voluntary health associations.[29] Rutledge Howard, MD, and C. H. William Ruhe, MD, of the AMA staff, were pioneers in the effort to accredit major national specialty societies and leading medical schools as CME providers and in developing state medical society accreditation programs.

The role of state medical societies in CME accreditation is interconnected with development of the AMA Physician's Recognition Award (PRA), formalization of AMA Category 1 credit, and implementation of the AMA Council on Medical Education accreditation program. In December 1968, the AMA House of Delegates approved a proposal for the AMA PRA, an award provided to physicians earning at least 150 hours of CME in a three-year period. Credit required for earning the award included participation in courses listed in an AMA annual listing of continuing education courses for physicians. In June 1971, the advisory committee on CME recommended including only courses offered by organizations accredited by the AMA Council on Medical Education in the AMA annual listing of CME activities. The council acted upon the recommendation beginning with the 1972 annual listing. According to the January 30, 1975, AMA Council on Medical Education meeting of CME survey team members, "This also meant that only the courses of accredited institutions would be eligible for Category 1 credit for the Physician's Recognition Award."[30] Increasing attention of state legislatures to the CME of physicians intensified the push for larger numbers of accredited organizations sanctioned to provide Category 1 credit.

Mandatory CME and Increased Demand for CME and the AMA PRA

In 1947, the American Academy of General Practice, now the American Academy of Family Physicians (AAFP), required members to participate in 150 hours of CME every three years. Twenty years later, the Oregon Medical Association (OMA) followed by approving CME as a requirement for membership. The elaborate plan established three criteria: CME must (1) be relevant to the practicing physician's needs, (2) have practical application, and (3) be effective as measured by available methods. Standards for participation and credit requirements were developed. The plan was pilot tested, surveys and reports were completed, and written materials were developed and distributed to the members. At the end of the first reporting year, the OMA received an increased number of objections and questions from its members regarding the new requirements. Many components of the program were simplified and options for meeting the CME requirement developed. In reciprocity agreements, members of the OMA who met the AAFP CME requirements or earned the AMA PRA also met the requirements for membership in the OMA.[31]

During the 1970s, the call to make participation in CME mandatory for medical relicensure was generally viewed as an infringement by state medical societies, and an increasing number were considering mandatory CME as a membership requirement to ward off state mandates. The strategy for addressing increasing demands from state legislators was laid out in a February 1976 AMA memorandum from Clarke W. Mangun, Jr., MD, assistant director, Department of Physicians Credentials and Qualifications, to presidents and executive directors of state medical associations. The subject line read: "A state medical association strategy for dealing with state legislative proposals advocating continuing medical education as a requirement for re-registration of the license to practice medicine." The memo advocated use of the AMA PRA to fulfill mandatory CME requirements. The experiences of two state medical societies were cited: An Illinois bill mandating CME for medical relicensure became law, despite the Illinois State Medical Society attempts to avoid the legislation by citing the number of Illinois physicians earning the AMA PRA; and the ongoing initiatives of the Ohio State Medical Society to maintain responsibility for overseeing the CME of physicians through documentation of physicians earning the AMA PRA. By 1972, according to an AMA survey, 22 state medical societies reported "action, resolution or recommendation" for CME as a requirement for membership in the society.[32]

The experiences of many state societies concerning mandatory participation in CME are reflected in a June 6, 1979, letter from Kinloch Nelson, MD, CME coordinator at the MSV. Nelson states, "As far back as 1967 members of the [Virginia] State Board of Medicine began to discuss the desirability of some kind of formal program of required CME." He describes the 1972 MSV House of Delegates endorsement of the MSV "Commission on CME and its development of accredited CME, first under the AMA and now under the LCCME [Liaison Committee for Continuing Medical Education]," which "served to slow down the movement toward required CME for relicensure." He notes that "further effort to stay this action was the decision in July 1977 to make CME mandatory for continued membership [in the MSV], beginning January 1, 1979."[33] Requirements for society membership included 90 hours of CME over a three-year period, with at least one-third of the hours qualifying as AMA PRA Category 1 hours. In 1973, the Virginia Physicians Recognition Award (VPRA) was developed. With the new membership requirement, physicians earning the VPRA or the AMA PRA also met the requirements for society membership. The number of states mandating CME for relicensure continued to climb and, by 2009, 62 boards required CME for license renewal and 43 state boards accepted the AMA PRA certification or application as equivalent for license re-registration.[34]

Virginia successfully held off formal consideration of mandatory participation in CME for licensure renewal until 1996 when the Virginia General Assembly directed the Virginia Board of Medicine to study the need for requiring CME. Findings were to be submitted in one year. In 1997, the commonwealth of Virginia passed a law to "ensure the continued competency of practitioners licensed by the [Virginia] Board of Medicine." It directed the Virginia board to include in its regulations continuing education, testing, and/or any other requirement that would address the following: (a) the need to promote ethical practice, (b) an appropriate standard of care, (c) patient safety, (d) application of new medical technology, (e) appropriate communication with patients, and (f) knowledge of the changing health-care system. The Virginia board of medicine developed a continuing competency and assessment form. Form completion was mandatory for renewal of a Virginia active medical license, requiring practitioners to participate in 60 hours of continued learning once every two years, with at least 30 hours in Type 1 CME, defined as:

[activities] offered by an accredited sponsor or organization which is sanctioned by the profession and which provides documentation of hours to the practitioners (For example: American Medical Association PRA category 1; American Osteopathic Association category 1; American College of Obstetricians and Gynecologists Cognates; American Academy of Family Physicians Prescribed credit; American Academy of Pediatrics credit hours toward the PREP educational award).[35]

Practitioners were required to complete the form, listing the (a) learning activities, resources, strategies, and experiences; (b) knowledge or skills maintained or developed; (c) outcomes in terms of whether a change will be made or if a need exists for additional information, and finally, to reflect on and identify problems or questions to be addressed in the next two-year period of medical license renewal.[36] Prior to implementation, parts b and c were made optional by the Virginia Board of Medicine.

In 1967, prior to the major movement for mandatory participation in CME, the AMA began formal accreditation of institutions and organizations offering CME. By January 1975, more than 440 providers of CME were accredited by the AMA Council on Medical Education. Categories of organizations approved by the AMA included medical schools, specialty medical societies, state medical associations, voluntary health organizations, hospitals, and other organizations with recurring CME activities attracting physicians from three or more states or territories. In addition, the AMA Council on Medical Education approved 33 state medical associations to conduct accreditation surveys in their states.[37] According to the 1971 AMA *Guidelines for State Medical Association Accreditation of Programs of Continuing Medical Education,* a larger than expected number of organizations sought accreditation and "it seemed logistically impossible [for the AMA Council on Medical Education] to carry out appropriate surveys unless the task could be decentralized and

delegated to or shared with local or regional organizations such as the state medical associations."[38] On March 12, 1971, the AMA Council on Medical Education recommended:

that state medical associations plan and implement their own programs, where feasible, of accreditation under a procedure approved and periodically reviewed by the AMA Council. Accreditation by a state medical association will give essentially the same status to an educational institution or organization as would accreditation by the AMA at the national level. This means that local institutions accredited under a state association plan acceptable to the AMA Council on Medical Education, will be considered to be fully accredited by AMA standards and will be included in the annual list of AMA accredited institutions.[39]

AMA Recognition of State Medical Societies in CME Accreditation

During the 1970s, state medical societies were encouraged to develop their own state-level accreditation program largely under the leadership of Howard, associate director of the AMA Department of Continuing Medical Education. Several letters dated December 1973 through December 1974 from Howard to the MSV Committee on Continuing Education show the willingness of the AMA to provide the state societies encouragement, advice, and support in developing state accreditation programs.[40] State medical societies were seeking approval from the AMA, while standards for accreditation were developing. The 1971 AMA *Guidelines for State Medical Association Accreditation of Programs in Continuing Medical Education* state the purpose as one "to help state medical associations establish their own programs of survey for accreditation in continuing medical education." The document provides suggested steps in planning an accreditation program at the state association level and asserts that:

The details of how individual [CME] programs will be reviewed may vary from state to state. . . . The guidelines are not intended to serve as a text or re-strictive advisory document, but rather one which will encourage diversity of approach and experimentation in continuing medical education at the community hospital and any other local educational institution or organization.[41]

A memorandum dated July 8, 1974, from Howard to all state medical associations and societies with approved programs of accreditation in CME included a new set of standards and procedures proposed by the California Medical Association (CMA). In the memo, Howard states: "You may wish to consider using their thoughts and procedures in your own accreditation program, particularly in view of the fact that the proposal was submitted by the CMA to the AMA Advisory Committee and Council and was approved by both bodies."[42]

Liaison Committee on Continuing Medical Education and AMA Withdrawal

Beginning July 1, 1977, the Liaison Committee on Continuing Medical Education (LCCME) assumed the accreditation role previously held by the AMA Council on Medical Education. The members of the LCCME included the five members of the Coordinating Council on Medical Education: the American Board of Medical Specialties (ABMS), American Medical Association (AMA), American Hospital Association (AHA), Association of American Medical Colleges (AAMC), and the Council of Medical Specialty Societies (CMSS), plus the Association for Hospital Medical Education (AHME) and the Federation of State Medical Boards (FSMB).[43] On July 25, 1979, the AMA House of Delegates voted to withdraw as a participating member of the LCCME and authorized the Council on Medical Education to resume its previous role in accreditation as the Council on Accreditation of Continuing Medical Education. According to the AMA, "The concept of the LCCME as a partnership which the AMA

had originally proposed to share its aims and interest in the further development of continuing medical education for the betterment of all physicians was not realized because of multiple problems that developed related to the organization of the LCCME and its contested function."[44] The remaining six members decided to continue as parent organizations of the LCCME. Concern was raised that a lone organization would not be considered an acceptable accrediting agency by some state medical boards, medical schools, and specialty societies and that allowing one medical organization to control accreditation "would raise questions of conflict of interest and could jeopardize the current voluntary accrediting system, perhaps resulting in government intervention in the process."[45] Reaction from the state medical associations was mixed. The Texas and Illinois delegations to the AMA Interim Meeting of December 19, 1979, submitted resolutions advocating reconciliation and a single system of accreditation. In a 1980 report to the MSV Council regarding the "AMA-LCCME Situation," Nelson states:

Dr. Russell S. Fisher, Chairman of the Council on Medical Education, seems to sum up the views of several AMA officials who urged . . . rejection for the Illinois and Texas resolutions when he asked delegates: would you rather have accreditation carried out by an organization you are familiar with and have some control over [the AMA] or by an organization in which the AMA participates freely but has only one of five controlling votes? CME is one of our children, and we ought to continue to raise it rather than turn it out into the street for five parents to supervise.[46]

Some state associations expressed concern that the LCCME would not clearly recognize them to accredit intrastate providers of CME as reflected in a November 22, 1978, memo from George H. Ladyman, MD, chairman of the Missouri State Medical Association (MSMA) Commission on Continuing Education and Health Manpower, to the state societies' CME chairmen.

The memo states: "The MSMA believes that the authority to accredit a particular organization or institution lies within the State Association, rather than having the State Association recommend accreditation and be required to wait a considerable time for LCCME approval."[47] According to the timeline compiled by Nelson—from November 9, 1979, to December 14, 1979—Pennsylvania, Delaware, New Jersey, Georgia, and Indiana expressed support for the AMA position and approval from the AMA. Other state societies continued deliberating whether the intrastate CME providers were accredited by the AMA, LCCME, or both.

A resolution introduced by the Massachusetts Delegation at the December 1979 AMA annual meeting called for "the state medical societies to be given the power to accredit intrastate continuing medical education program with quality control and standards for the state society accreditation activities to be maintained through the American Medical Association Council on Medical Education and through regular periodic review of each state society's standards and accreditation procedures."[48] In a follow-up to the resolution, the AMA conducted an in-depth analysis and developed a report adopted by the AMA House of Delegates during the July 1980 AMA interim meeting. Among other findings, the report concluded: "Intra-state accreditation by state societies must be assured" and "AMA's role must be assured and the basic purpose of accreditation must be maintained."[49]

Formation of the Accreditation Council for Continuing Medical Education

In 1980, the AMA announced plans to join the LCCME in forming a new organization: the Accreditation Council for Continuing Medical Education (ACCME). ACCME became the accreditor of national CME providers beginning in January 1981 and also recognized state societies as accreditors of intrastate CME providers. At the September 1982 State/ACCME Conference, partici-

pants developed a draft document titled "Protocol for the Recognition of State Medical Societies to Accredit Intrastate Continuing Medical Education." The protocol indicated:

One of [ACCME's] purposes, as specified in the Bylaws, is "to promote, develop and encourage the development of principles, policies, and standards for continuing medical education." To implement this purpose, one of the functions of the ACCME, also stated in the Bylaws, is to "develop standards by which state medical societies (or state accrediting bodies in states where medical societies do not accredit alone) will accredit local institutions and organizations and be responsible for assuring compliance with these standards."[50]

The preamble notes, "Achieving state-to-state uniformity will require periodic review of the standards and procedures which the various state societies use in accrediting intrastate continuing education providers." The protocol identifies the Committee on Review and Recognition of State Medical Societies as Accreditors of Continuing Education Providers (CRR) and states: "The findings, decisions and recommendations will be forwarded by the Chairman to the next meeting of the ACCME following the meeting of the CRR." The protocol lists five criteria for recognizing the quality of the state medical societies' accreditation programs.[51] On June 7, 1984, the CRR held its first meeting, in which it determined the final text for the "rerecognition data questionnaires and survey report forms." Additionally, a survey schedule and procedures for reviewing state society accreditation programs were discussed.[52]

Autonomy of State Medical Society Accreditation Programs

With initiatives in 1971 to recognize state medical societies as accreditors of local CME programs, the AMA provided encouragement, support, and advice on how the state societies might manage their accreditation programs. For example, in a December 14, 1975, letter to the MSV, the MSV was "approved to conduct its own program of accreditation, aimed at institutions and organizations of local scope and focus in the field of continuing medical education." The MSV was instructed, "Once accrediting action is taken, you simply need advise Mrs. Etheridge, in this office, of the name of the institution surveyed, its mailing address, and the accrediting action. We do not need to have a copy of your survey report."[53] From inception of the LCCME in 1977, to AMA withdrawal from the LCCME in 1979, through formation of the ACCME in 1981, and recognition surveys of state medical society accreditation programs beginning in 1984, the medical societies continued accrediting local providers of CME with little oversight from an outside organization. On January 1, 1984, the new *ACCME Essentials and Guidelines* and the *ACCME Accreditation: Procedural and Administrative Information* became effective. During the same year, the ACCME Committee on Review and Recognition began surveying the accreditation programs of state medical societies, requiring submission of an application for continuing recognition and conducting an on-site visit of the state society accreditation program.

Equivalency in CME Accreditation

The five ACCME criteria for recognizing the quality of the state medical societies' accreditation programs have expanded considerably since their introduction in 1982. Later referred to as the decision-making elements, the five criteria served as the basis for recognition decisions by the ACCME through its Committee on Review and Recognition until 2009. Mounting concerns regarding rising health-care costs, uneven quality of care in the United States, and the influence of commercial interests in CME have resulted in greater focus on CME and the accreditation system. In September 2006, in an effort to link CME to quality improvement in health care, the ACCME introduced updated criteria for the accreditation of providers of CME. The updated criteria apply to both national providers of CME accredited by the ACCME and intrastate providers of CME accredited by state medical societies. With the increased attention, greater need for an equivalent CME accreditation program was recognized. At a 2007 meeting of the ACCME board of directors, the CRR reported "a newly developed construct for recognition in the context of 'equivalency' among and between state medical society accreditors and the ACCME." In 2010, state medical societies began to be surveyed using the ACCME's new recognition requirements in rules, process, interpretation, accreditation outcomes, and evolution/process improvement, referred to as the ACCME Markers of Equivalency.[54]

With increased costs associated with accreditation activities and recognition initiatives of the ACCME, fees for national providers of CME are increasing along with the per intrastate provider annual fee charged to state accreditors. Reactions from state medical societies are mixed. Some are concerned that the 2011 fee increase will impede intrastate providers from continuing their accreditation. Others indicate that they are uncertain of the effect increased fees will have on retention. In addition, some have expressed support for an equivalent accreditation system and suggest that an organization withdrawing from accreditation because of the fee increase may not have the commitment to CME necessary to be an accredited provider.[55]

During the June 2009 AMA annual meeting, the AMA House of Delegates passed two resolutions related to accreditation programs of state and territorial medical associations. Resolution 312, introduced by the New Jersey, Louisiana, and Oklahoma delegations, asked the AMA to strongly urge ACCME to reconsider the proposed annual fee increase for intrastate accreditation fees and "if the ACCME refuses to reconsider the proposed fee increase" for the AMA "to investigate and recommend ways physicians may receive appropriate, accredited continuing medical education other than through ACCME-accredited activities."[56] Resolution 302, introduced by the Illinois delegation, called for the AMA to "study and report back at the 2009 interim meeting on the system of intrastate accreditation, including the ACCME fee structure for state accreditors and their providers, the concept of equivalency, and the new criteria for compliance and the impact these changes will have on state accreditors and their providers."[57] At its November 2009 interim meeting, the AMA Council on Medical Education submitted an informational report to the House of Delegates and indicated plans to prepare a more extensive report for the 2010 AMA annual meeting. On June 15, 2010, an executive summary was submitted to the AMA House of Delegates with recommendations based, in part, on historical documents and information collected from state medical societies, intrastate accredited CME providers, and from the ACCME.[58] Final recommendations passed by the AMA House of Delegates included that the AMA continue working with the ACCME to reduce the financial burden of institutional accreditation and state recognition; reduce bureaucracy in these processes; improve continuing medical education; and encourage the ACCME to show that the updated accreditation criteria improve patient care. In addition, the AMA agreed to work with the ACCME to mandate meaningful involvement of state medical societies in policies that affect recognition and to reconsider the fee increases to be paid by the state-accredited providers to the ACCME. Finally, the Council on Medical Education was required to monitor results of the recommendations and to report back to the House of Delegates at the 2011 annual meeting.[59]

The AMA continues to play a central role in the US CME accreditation system and in its development. As of 2009, the number of accredited organizations providing CME in the United States totaled 2,225. Of that number, ACCME accredited 707 and state medical associations accredited 1,518.[60] Only those organizations accredited by ACCME or through an ACCME-recognized state or territory association may certify CME activities for AMA Category 1 Credit.

Conclusion

Early on, physicians formed associations to exchange medical information, to regulate the practice of medicine and to develop medicine as a profession. In 1781, the MMS became the first state medical society to successfully petition its legislature for incorporation, but prior to that time several medical associations already had formed. Some disappeared, others reemerged, and today 50 state medical associations, in addition to a larger number of local component societies, exist.[61]

Following the 1960s, federal agencies, private insurers, and managed care organizations sought to limit health-care spending. Increasingly, the medical societies found themselves in the role of advocating for physicians against growing regulations and, at the same time, assisting their members in managing third-party payer issues and coding, billing, and other regulatory compliance concerns. The perceived value of intrastate accreditation as a member benefit decreased. According to the ACCME, from 1982 to 2009, nine state medical societies discontinued their intrastate accreditation programs, including the Medical Society of Delaware (1987), Vermont Medical Society (1992), Guam Medical Society (1999), Montana Medical Association (1999), Virgin Islands Medical Society (2004), Tennessee Medical Association (2005), Medical Society of the District of Columbia (2005), the Arkansas Medical Society (2008), and the Wyoming Medical Society (2009).[62] In an effort to continue their existence, many state medical societies began to increase accreditation fees by shifting expenses to the intrastate accredited providers.

Escalating health-care costs and quality of care concerns have resulted in closer scrutiny of CME. At the same time, the value of traditional CME, accreditation, and AMA Category 1 Credit are all being questioned.[63] The continuing education of health-care professional teams is being considered as one method to help reduce rising costs and to improve the quality of care in the United States. The future of national and intrastate accreditation and the direction of CME will be determined by the characteristics of medical education deemed necessary by private and public entities with a vested interest in the future of health care.

Notes

1. Peter D. Hall, ed., "Documentary History of Philanthropy and Voluntarism in the United States, 1600–1900. Section 12. Voluntary Associations and the Rise of the Profession. Hauser Center on Nonprofit Organizations," John F. Kennedy School of Government, Harvard University Web site, http://ksghome.harvard.edu/~phall/doc histcontents.html (accessed October 19, 2009).

2. Ibid.

3. Ibid.

4. Richard Aghababian and Henry Tulgan, "The Evolution of Continuing Medical Education: The Massachusetts Experience," Berkshire Medical Journal 12 (2004): 3–7.

5. Thomas Hunt and others, A History of the County of Berkshire, Massachusetts in Two Parts: The First Part Being a General View of the County; The Second, an Account of the Several Towns (Pittsfield, Mass.: Samuel W. Bush, 1829), 171.

6. William Lincoln, History of Worcester, Massachusetts. From Its Earliest Settlement to September, 1839: with Various Notices Relating to the History of Worcester County (Worcester: Moses D. Phillips and Co., 1837), 323–324.

7. Aghababian and Tulgan, "Evolution of Continuing Medical Education," 3–7.

8. Hall, "Documentary History of Philanthropy"; "MedChi," Maryland Medical Society Web site, http://www.medchi.org/ (accessed May 10, 2010).

9. Abraham Flexner, Medical Education in the United States and Canada: A Report to the Carnegie Foundation for the Advancement of Teaching (Washington, DC: Science and Health Publication Inc., 1910); P. G. Altbach and others, eds., American Higher Education in the Twenty-First Century: Social, Political, and Economic Challenges, 2nd ed. (Baltimore: Johns Hopkins University Press, 2005), 264.

10. James B. Bruce, "Postgraduate Education in Michigan," Journal of the Michigan State Medical Society 36 (1937): 372.

11. Ira C. Clark, The Development of Physician Continuation Education (Iowa City: University of Iowa Press, 1966), 24.

12. Clark, The Development, 24–26; "Postgraduate Course: Suggested Course of Study for Use by County Societies," Journal of the American Medical Association 49 (1907): 1043.

13. American Medical Association Council on Medical Education and Hospitals, "Extension Work in Graduate Medical Education," Virginia Medical Monthly 55, no. 3 (1928): 201; Clark, The Development, 28–32.

14. N. P. Colwell, "Extension Work in Graduate Medical Education," American Medical Association Bulletin (1927).

15. AMA Council, "Extension Work," 205; G. B. Zehmer and G. W. Eutsler, Post-Graduate Medical Education in Virginia, vol. 14 (Charlottesville: University of Virginia Extension Series, 1930), 11.

16. Zehmer and Eutsler, Post-Graduate Medical Education, 14:11–12.

17. Ibid., 13–15.

18. Bruce, "Postgraduate Education," 373.

19. J. A. Hodges, "Foreword," in Zehmer and Eutsler, Post-Graduate Medical Education, vol. 14.

20. J. W. Preston, "Exhibit B: Letter to Members of the Medical Society of Virginia," in Zehmer and Eutsler, Post-Graduate Medical Education in Virginia, 14:44.

21. Zehmer and Eutsler, Post-Graduate Medical Education, 14:25.

22. Ibid., 7.

23. Ibid., 7–8

24. Ibid.

25. American Medical Association Council on Medical Education and Hospitals, "Medical Education in the United States and Canada," Journal of the American Medical Association 111 (1938): 801, 809.

26. Ibid.

27. P. R. Manning, letter to Pam Mazmanian, May 24, 2010.

28. Glen R. Shepherd, "History of Continuation Medical Education in the United States since 1930," Journal of Medical Education 35 (1960): 748.

29. American Medical Association Council on Medical Education, Report from Meeting of Continuing Medical Education Survey Team Members (Chicago, January 30, 1975).

30. Ibid.

31. C. L. Marshall, "Quality Assurance and the Continuing Education of Physicians," Journal of Community Health 2, no. 4 (1977): 287; R. Boissoneau, Continuing Education in the Health Professions (Rockville, Md.: Aspen Systems Corporation, 1980), 206–213.

32. Clark W. Mangun, Jr., "Subject: A state medical association strategy for dealing with state legislative proposals advocating continuing medical education as a requirement for re-registration of the license to practice medicine," memorandum to all presidents and executive directors of state medical associations, 1976; "Table E," in *Survey of Medical Education Activities, State Medical and Medical Specialty Societies* (Chicago: American Medical Association Department of CME, 1972), 9(b).

33. Kinloch Nelson, letter to Donald M. Switz, June 6, 1979.

34. Charles L. Crockett and Kinloch Nelson, "History, Objectives, and Procedure of the MSV Continuing Medical Education Program," *Virginia Medical* 106 (1979): 783–786; *State Medical Licensure Requirements and Statistics* (Chicago: American Medical Association, (2009): 53–56.

35. "The Virginia Board of Medicine Continued Competency and Assessment Form," Virginia Department of Health Professions Web site, http://www.dhp.state.va.us/Forms/medicine/ContinuingComp/PhysicianCE_form.doc (accessed July 12, 2010).

36. "The Virginia Board of Medicine Continued Competency and Assessment Form, 2000," Virginia Board of Medicine Web site, http://www.dhp.virginia.gov/Forms/medicine/ContinuingComp/PhysicianCE_form.doc (accessed October 19, 2009).

37. 1975 AMA Information Sheet, referring to the Advisory Committee on Continuing Medical Education, October 24, 1972, and the Council on Medical Education, November 24–26, 1972, decisions; "Meeting of Continuing Medical Education Survey Team Members" (American Medical Association, Council on Medical Education, January 30, 1975), 3.

38. American Medical Association, *Guidelines for State Medical Associations Accreditation of Programs in Continuing Medical Education* (1971), 2.

39. Ibid.

40. Rutledge W. Howard, letter to George Carroll, November 13, 1973; ibid., December 4, 1973; Rutledge W. Howard, correspondence to David S. Walthall, December 19, 1974.

41. American Medical Association, *Guidelines for State Medical Associations*, 2.

42. Rutledge W. Howard, memorandum to all state medical associations and societies with approved programs of accreditation in continuing medical education, July 8, 1974.

43. S. V. Lawrence, "The Alphabet Soup Boils Over, LCCME continues despite AMA pullout: AMA plans own CME accreditation," *American College of Physicians Forum on Medicine* (October 1979): 674–675; P. R. Manning, "Continuing Medical Education in Midpassage (Medical Education)," *Western Journal of Medicine* 128 (1978): 260–265.

44. American Medical Association Council on Medical Education, *Future Directions for Medical Education* (1979), 24–25.

45. Lawrence, "Alphabet Soup Boils Over," 674–675; Manning, "Continuing Medical Education," 260–265.

46. Kinloch Nelson, *Committee on Education Report to and Questions for Council* (Medical Society of Virginia, February 2, 1980).

47. George H. Ladyman, memo to chairman of state continuing medical education, November 22, 1978.

48. Massachusetts Medical Society, *Resolution No. 66* (American Medical Association Annual Meeting, December 2–5, 1979).

49. American Medical Association Board of Trustees-II, JJ, *Review of Mechanisms for Accrediting Medical Education, Reference Committee C* (AMA Interim Meeting, July 22–26, 1980), 72.

50. *Protocol for the Recognition of State Medical Societies to Accredit Intrastate Continuing Medical Education, Draft II* (Accreditation Council for Continuing Medical Education, 1982).

51. Ibid.

52. *Actions and Items under Discussion which May be of Interest* (Accreditation Council for Continuing Medical Education meeting, June 8, 1984).

53. Rutledge W. Howard, letter to David B. Walthall, December 19, 1974.

54. *Executive Summary* (meetings of the ACCME Board of Directors, November 2007), http://www.accme.org/dir_docs/whats_new/aa64ed0e-fbbc-44fd-abad-550a6da7edef_uploadfile.pdf (accessed October 2009).

55. Administrators of the state medical society CME intrastate accreditation programs, e-mail messages "Re: ACCME Plans to Charge Annual Fees to State-Accredited Providers," November 3, 2008.

56. Illinois Delegation, *Resolution 302, Subject: Opposition to Increase CME Provider Fees* (American Medical Association House of Delegates, 2009).

57. New Jersey, Louisiana, and Oklahoma Delegation, *Resolution 312, Subject: Proposed Fee Increase by the Accreditation Council for Continuing Medical Education* (American Medical Association House of Delegates, 2009).

58. American Medical Association, Report of the Council on Medical Education (A-10), Opposition to Increased CME Provider Fees, CME Report 14-A-10.

59. Jeanette Harmon, e-mail message to state medical societies CME accreditors, July 13, 2010.

60. 2009 Annual Report Data, Accreditation Council for Continuing Medical Education Web site, http://

www.accme.org/dir_docs/doc_upload/f2e89864-
b4c1-428f-8ebe-1ba197a31928_uploaddocument.pdf
(accessed July 12, 2010).

61. "State Medical Society Websites," American Medical Association Web site, http://www.ama-assn.org/ama/pub/about-ama/our-people/the-federation -medicine/state-medical-society-websites.shtml (accessed October 19, 2009).

62. Mary Martin Lowe, e-mail message to Pamela Mazmanian "Re: Question on SMS," October 9, 2009; Sharon P. Nordling, telephone conversation with Pamela Mazmanian, May 6, 2010.

63. Suzanne W. Fletcher, *Continuing Education in the Health Professions: Improving Healthcare through Lifelong Learning* (conference proceedings, Josiah Macy, Jr. Foundation, 2008): 13–23.

Marcia Jackson, Theresa Kanya,
and Bruce Spivey

CHAPTER 9

Medical Specialty Societies: Innovation in Meeting Physician Member Needs

The adage "birds of a feather flock together" holds true for specialty societies. As medicine became differentiated in the late 1800s and early 1900s, physicians began to coalesce around common areas of interest, and specialty societies were formed. Among the mission of almost every specialty society is its role as a CME provider for members. The Accreditation Council for Continuing Medical Education (ACCME) reported that 265 nonprofit physician membership organizations were accredited as continuing medical education (CME) providers in 2009.[1] Each of these societies has a unique pathway to its current CME activities, and no single source can provide a collective history, although some common threads weave through the tapestry of most specialty society CME programs.

The earliest education of specialists occurred through travel and tutorials. As word spread of new procedures, new findings, and new technologies, physicians interested in expanding their practice to incorporate these procedures, findings, and/or technologies traveled to work directly with the pioneers who were the inventors or discoverers. Specialists in the last half of the nineteenth century and first half of the twentieth century often trained in Europe and returned to the United States where they hung their shingle as a specialist. Since anyone could declare oneself to be a specialist—regardless of whether one had

been trained—those who had been trained became determined to establish quality standards that differentiated the two groups. This gave rise not only to the formation of specialty societies but also, over time, to the creation of certifying boards.

The primary education activity for almost all specialty societies is the annual meeting. This event updates members on new scientific advances, reinforces retention of specialty core content, serves as a forum for social networking, and sets the culture of the organization for new members. Many societies publish journals to deliver research findings and scientific advances in the field. Members typically reference the journal as one of the most important elements of a society's education program, which has been acknowledged by the addition of journal-based CME to the American Medical Association (AMA) Physician's Recognition Award and credit system. Live programs continue to be the bedrock of specialty society education: in 2009 the ACCME reported that societies directly sponsored more than 5,000 courses. As time demands increasingly hinder member presence at these courses and member familiarity with technology increases, societies have increased the amount of education that is available through electronic delivery. ACCME reported that in 1998 the specialty societies provided a total of 62 Internet-based live activities and enduring materials, whereas in 2009 these activities had increased to more than 2,800 in number.[2]

This chapter does not provide a history of CME in all specialty societies. Rather it presents the story of CME in three selected societies. The American Academy of Ophthalmology (AAO), a surgical specialty, is one of the oldest specialty societies. The American Academy of Ophthalmology and Otolaryngology was established in 1896. The two specialties separated in 1976 into the AAO and the American Academy of Otolaryngology (AAO-Head and Neck Surgery). The American College of Physicians (ACP), incorporated in 1915, is one of the largest societies, with more than 126,000 members worldwide. The new kid on the block is the American College of Cardiology (ACC), a subspecialty of internal medicine that was incorporated in 1949 by a small group of immigrant physicians.

The American Academy of Ophthalmology

It can be said of all specialties in medicine that their early evolution was gradual and that the 1920s was a period of transition, when organized medicine and academic medicine began taking a critical look at the educational requirements for specialty practice. The American Board of Ophthalmology (ABO) was becoming accepted as a standard of achievement, and an increasing percentage of medical graduates decided to specialize in ophthalmology. By 1930, 30 percent of medical graduates were entering specialty practice and, amazingly, 13 percent were specializing in eye, ear, nose, and throat.[3] By 1940, 73 institutions afforded opportunities for about 123 new ophthalmic residents per year.

The AAO, referred to as "the Academy" by ophthalmologists, develops programs for all levels of the medical education curriculum, but the AAO started its educational programming by directing it toward this expanding number of residents. The initial AAO education activity designed to serve this audience was the annual meeting, which spawned the publication *Transactions of the Annual Meeting* from 1903 until 1975, when it evolved into the journal *Ophthalmology*. Synopses of courses presented at the AAO annual meeting began in 1931. After World War II, there was a rush to improve the science of the specialty as well as the quality of education in the residencies, at which time the AAO began to focus the annual meeting on CME for practicing physicians as well as for resident education.

During the 1940s, the AAO began to publish "Home Study Courses for Residents," a series of questions in basic and clinical topics that were answered in "blue books" and evaluated by faculty. Heretofore, there existed little basic science education, no organized approach to teach basic science, no clear outline of what needed to be covered in a residency program, nor any knowledge of how best to organize such education. The AAO home study courses, as well as the ABO test outline, filled these voids.

The home study courses were recognized as "a stop gap to fill the period of here, where we have inadequate instruction, to where all institutions are giving the proper type of instructions to their residents."[4] As the home study courses gained in popularity and maturity, the AAO moved forward in the arena of CME and began developing and disseminating monographs (1938–1986), manuals (1946–1986), atlases, and even a motion picture titled *Embryology of the Eye* (1950). The demand for duplicates of slides that were used in the atlases of pathology and in pathology courses resulted in their availability for rental from the AAO during the 1950s through the 1970s.

The AAO formed an office of education in 1969, and AAO education was officially launched in 1970. The home study courses were modified to become the AAO Basic and Clinical Science Course (BCSC), where basic information was compiled in small books. The initial eight BCSC books were relatively thin and included basic and clinical sciences; members were expected to complete the series of books in two years. Today the series comprises thick compendiums of 13 books that are the gold standard of curriculum for ophthalmology resident education nationally and internationally. In 1972, the AAO established a self-education program for practitioners by sending a scoring examination to all AAO members, which was eventually merged into the BCSC to serve both residents and practitioners.

The AAO has expanded its emphasis markedly on resident and continuing education for ophthalmologists since the mid-1970s. The BCSC continued to meet member needs both nationally and internationally. The AAO developed and delivered regional courses, but these did not prove popular and were disbanded. The AAO began to publish modules on specific clinical topics, and a series called "Focal Points" with practitioner-friendly educational tips has flourished. As clinical guidelines moved into prominence, the AAO began to develop preferred practice patterns. These serve as the basis of clinical practice in 20 specific conditions treated by the ophthalmologist.

The AAO worked collaboratively with the ABO to establish the scope of the specialty and thereby set the parameters for the AAO educational programming and the ABO examination blueprint for the maintenance of certification (MOC) program. Using nine subspecialty panels of 10 members each drawn from practice and academia, the AAO defined the core, comprehensive, and subspecialty ophthalmology knowledge base. The AAO and the ABO are the first specialty board and society to achieve this milestone. The AAO has created an educational knowledge-based program based on this curriculum.

Over the past six years, an AAO major educational endeavor has been the creation of the Web-based program Ophthalmic News & Education (O.N.E.™) Network. Launched in November 2007, the O.N.E. Network combines clinically relevant content, news, and tools derived from a wide variety of vetted resources. The O.N.E. Network has unique interactive features that allow the learner to tailor his or her experience, including customizable subspecialty news, the delivery of a vast array of clinical content via video, cases and podcasts, and tools designed to help ophthalmologists stay abreast of current advances in the specialty. Ophthalmologists can create a custom learning plan with interactive self-assessments and real-time evaluation, supported by an online curriculum to prepare for recertification. The curriculum, which includes a suite of MOC tools as well as access to the MOC Exam Study Kit and the BCSC, is likely to be the dominant Web-based educational program in ophthalmology throughout the world.

Many sources have guided the development of the AAO CME programs, including experience gained from existing programs, strong individual advocates for new programs, and qualitative and quantitative data suggesting areas of members' learning needs. Each of these sources is essential and has contributed to the current robust CME program of the AAO.

The American College of Physicians

Ralph Waldo Emerson said, "An institution is the lengthened shadow of one man." For the ACP, that man was Heinrich Stern, MD, a German-born American internist who proposed the idea of an American college of physicians in 1913.[5] Stern was determined to have an organization in North America devoted to "promoting the science of medicine through regular scientific meetings and recognition of prominent internists."[6] At first he received little encouragement for his idea, but he persevered in convincing his colleagues. His vision was realized when the ACP, also referred to as the College, was incorporated on May 11, 1915, as a nonprofit scientific organization for internists.

The early leaders of the ACP strived to institute high standards for admission to fellowship, similar to the Royal College of Physicians, which required passing a rigorous examination. In 1934 the ACP Committee on Examinations recommended creation of an American Board of Internal Medicine (ABIM) to certify internists and to be financed by the ACP until fees could be collected. Through the combined efforts of the ACP and AMA, the ABIM was established in 1936. College historian W. G. Morgan noted in 1940 that the formation of ABIM may be regarded as one of the "most significant and enduring accomplishments" of the ACP in its first quarter century.[7]

The initial role of CME is embodied in the early constitution and by-laws of the ACP:

> to uphold and maintain high standards in medical education and practice; to encourage research, especially in clinical medicine; to foster measures for the prevention of diseases and for improving public health . . . and to maintain the dignity of [the] profession in its relationship with patients.[8]

The ACP held its first Scientific Session in December 1916. The three-day program of lectures and discussion represented a new standard for scientific work and laid the foundation for future CME activities for internists.[9] Since 1916, the ACP has held a scientific meeting every year. Early programs comprised formal papers delivered in general sessions and numerous clinics held in various hospitals, laboratories, and medical schools. Later programs added special lectures and round table discussions on selected subjects.

Within a few years after its founding in 1927, the *Annals of Internal Medicine* began publishing summaries of addresses and clinics presented at the annual scientific meeting. These summaries were intended as an important educational resource for ACP fellows who could not attend the meeting and a permanent reference for those who could. The summaries complemented the journal's articles on new advances and discoveries in the field of internal medicine for practicing physicians, reviews, case reports, editorials, and book reviews.[10] From the start, the journal was one of the most important activities of the ACP and a major CME publication for internists, and it remains so today.

The introduction of certification for internal medicine in 1936 created a need for new educa-tional initiatives to help internists certify.[11] In 1938, the ACP initiated postgraduate courses in various branches of internal medicine at or close to the time of the annual meeting in the city where the meeting was held and in nearby medical centers. Organized for fellows and associates, the courses became so popular that nonmembers were admitted only if space in the facilities permitted. Within a decade, the program was expanded to offer courses in the spring and fall to meet high demand. Expansion of the program continued for several years to accommodate the steadily increasing number of participants.

The ACP took pride in these early educational activities, which have evolved through the years and are a mainstay of the ACP CME program today. The three-day annual scientific meeting now offers more than 250 sessions. Many sessions—like "Clinical Pearls," which attracts up to 1,000 physicians per session—use an audience response system to involve learners. Other educational offerings make use of facilitated group discussion or hands-on workshops to actively engage participants in the educational process. The Herbert S. Waxman Clinical Skills Center uses standardized patients, expert faculty, simulators (like Harvey, the cardiopulmonary patient), and computer stations to promote interactive learning.

The Medical Knowledge Self-Assessment Program (MKSAP) defined a new era of CME for the ACP. A rich history of MKSAP abounds in published articles, board of regents minutes, and committee reports. It starts in 1965 when the Educational Activities Committee of the ACP recognized a widening gap between the increase of knowledge in the biological, physical, and chemical sciences and the application of this knowledge to clinical practice.[12] The ACP had offered a number of high quality educational programs, but the ACP felt it was necessary to do more to bridge the gap between what was being discovered and what was being applied in practice.[13] The president of the ACP appointed an ad hoc committee to examine the current status of CME. Through a survey to inform its work, the committee discovered that the missing element in CME was that no one knew what physicians did not know, including the physicians themselves. In other words, for physicians to correct their deficiencies they had to evaluate themselves to identify gaps in their knowledge.[14] Thus, MKSAP was conceived.

The committee proposed a voluntary self-evaluation program for members of the ACP, consisting of multiple-choice questions and following strict guidelines. While physicians would want to know their own informational deficiencies, receive guidance for further CME, and increase their professional competence, the committee believed it was critical to guard the anonymity of an individual's test scores (and knowledge deficiencies) for this pioneer program to be successful.[15] The board of regents accepted the committee's proposal for a self-evaluation program but only after overcoming its doubt that most physicians would not use the program and it would, therefore, have a high chance of failure.[16]

MKSAP I was issued in January 1968. The program comprised a total of 720 clinically oriented multiple-choice questions in nine content areas of internal medicine. Physicians would know what medical educators thought should be known and how to apply this knowledge to diagnosis and patient care.[17] They could submit their answers to the questions for computer scoring or self-score their answers and compare their results to group norms. MKSAP III, released in 1974, added a syllabus with key references and emphasized information appearing in journals or other publications within the previous five years that was useful to practicing physicians. More than 29,000 physicians subscribed.

MKSAP is one of the most important and successful programs developed for CME.[18] Since its inception, the program has been published every three years, and, in recent years, on average more than 40,000 physicians worldwide subscribe to each English-language edition. The program is available in print, conversational audio, and digital formats; offers online updates of multiple-

choice questions between editions; has a *Board Basics* book for certification preparation; is used to earn credit towards MOC; is translated into Spanish and Japanese; and led to *MKSAP for Students* in its fourth edition and *Internal Medicine Essentials for Clerkship Students* in its second edition. Its bank of multiple-choice questions is an important resource for other ACP activities. In a class of its own and approaching the 16th edition, MKSAP truly remains the flagship self-assessment program for ACP and internal medicine. MKSAP-like products are now being created by many other specialty societies.

During strategic planning in 2001, the idea was conceived for a program that would address the gap between current and ideal practice for conditions that are common to internal medicine practice. Closing-the-Gap was launched in 2002, informed by the Institute of Medicine (IOM) report *Crossing the Quality Chasm*.[19] The program set a new direction for CME focused on practice performance and quality improvement and new interactive platforms for delivering CME. It also established how staff from the CME, quality improvement, and software development departments of the ACP would work together as a cohesive team in support of the CME Program. Since its inception, Closing-the-Gap has grown substantially and expanded through new programs that ACP believes are making a measurable difference in health outcomes.

Closing-the-Gap trains teams of physicians, nurses, or other allied health professionals and office administrators on how to improve the quality of their care for patients with chronic disease. With coaching from expert faculty, the team collects practice data (1) at the start of the program; (2) after participating in educational sessions on specific evidence-based clinical content, improvement strategies, and systems change; and (3) after completing the program to measure the success of implemented changes. Closing-the-Gap evolved from a live meeting, to an Internet-based program that uses a state-of-the-art technical platform for managing projects, submitting abstracted patient data, accessing interactive educational resources and improvement tools, and viewing customized feedback and reports. The reports compare team data with national standards and other teams in the program. Physicians who participate in this program can receive credit towards the practice improvement component of MOC as well as CME credit. Closing-the-Gap inspired the creation of the clinical care guide *ACP Diabetes Care Guide: A Team-Based Practice Manual and Self-Assessment Program*—published in print and electronic formats by ACP (2007)—that integrates self-assessment and clinical assessment and also offers CME credit. The guide emphasizes team-based care and quality improvement, using Closing-the-Gap content and clinical assessment tools as well as self-assessment questions modeled after MKSAP but targeted to the team.

The extensive resources and references, for both patients and clinicians, from these new programs are presented on the ACP Web portal by specific clinical condition. They are updated regularly and include interactive practice tools, content from ACP publications and educational products, high quality outside resources from other not-for-profit publishers, multimedia presentations of content delivered during live meetings, and patient handouts.

Looking ahead, ACP expects to expand this new line of programs to all IOM priority areas[20] relevant to internal medicine practice, informed by the extensive research underway to measure their effectiveness in closing practice gaps, as envisioned almost a decade ago.

American College of Cardiology

As of 2009, the American College of Cardiology (ACC) had more than 25,000 board-certified cardiologists as members who are supported by a diverse and multi-faceted program of CME presented through the American College of Cardiology Foundation. This growth in membership and CME programming is remarkable in that the ACC was chartered as a national organization with 14 members in 1949. The history of CME at the ACC has been shaped by each of the following factors: (1) a small group of immigrant practitioner cardiologists who settled in New York City were excluded from positions of influence in the New York Heart Association and the American Heart Association (AHA), (2) the AHA was reorganized in 1948 to become a voluntary health organization whose physician members were primarily from academic settings; (3) cardiovascular disease became increasingly prevalent among the US population; (4) rapid advances occurred in pharmaceutical treatments and clinical technology relating to cardiovascular disease; and (5) technologies emerged to support the distance delivery of CME.[21]

Cardiology emerged as a specialty field of practice in the early 1900s, and in 1925 the inaugural issue of the *American Heart Journal* was published to meet the demand for a periodical that addressed this field of practice. The first annual meeting of the AHA—the only organization for specialists in cardiology during this period—was held in 1925.

The 1940s created the circumstances that gave rise to the ACC as an organization and also created the focus for its CME program that continues to the present day. A small group of immigrant physicians specializing in diseases of the heart migrated to New York City, where they tried to join their US peers in the New York Cardiological Society and the AHA. Excluded from any leadership positions in these organizations, these physicians became determined to found their own organization. In 1949, they succeeded in this effort and the ACC was chartered. From the outset, the ACC's foremost mission was professional education directed to practicing cardiologists rather than the academic cardiologists who led the AHA. The latter organization, facing financial constraints when it served only physician members, had been reorganized in the late 1940s to become a voluntary health organization. This transformation expanded AHA membership to include allied health professionals, scientists, and the public, thereby reducing the role of physicians in the organization. Unlike the AHA, the ACC had an initial agenda that emphasized education of the practicing cardiologist and made no mention of public health programs.

Meetings constituted the initial CME activities of the ACC. The first scientific meeting was held in 1951 on the topic of coronary artery disease. It was followed closely in 1952 by the first annual meeting. The ACC continued to hold two national scientific meetings each year: an annual spring meeting and an interim fall meeting. Both consisted of single sessions on two or three major topics that emphasized recent developments of interest to clinicians. Many innovations were introduced into these meetings during the 1950s. Even at that time, experts decried passive learning and urged more interactivity in CME. The ACC introduced fireside sessions where small groups of attendees could hold an informal dialogue with leaders in the field; luncheon panels that included medical motion pictures were added to the annual meeting.

Cardiology as a specialty field expanded rapidly during the 1950s, which proved advantageous for the ACC. Practitioner cardiologists— the ACC's primary audience—struggled to stay abreast of new findings and new technical procedures. The CME provided by the ACC met those needs and the meetings flourished. The 1960 annual meeting realized a profit of $9,000, a fact that elicited applause from the trustees.[22]

The ACC constitution included a pledge to publish a journal, and in 1958 the *American Journal of Cardiology* debuted. From the outset, like the ACC itself, the journal was devoted to clinical cardiology and directed primarily to the practicing cardiologist and internist. Advertising revenues from the journal allowed the ACC to expand its CME activities. The journal was also instrumental in bringing academics into the ACC because it offered a publication outlet for research that was critical to a member's career path.

Academic cardiologists were critical to advanc-

ing the CME agenda because they led the educational activities. To meet the escalating costs and travel expenses of academicians—many of whom still did not consider the ACC to be a mainstream organization—ACC charged tuition fees to supplement the journal's advertising income.

Although the ACC became established as an organization with a growing membership by 1960, it continued to experiment with its education program. Clinical workshops held in teaching institutions during the late 1950s evolved into large national symposia that became a major part of the ACC CME program during the 1960s. International circuit courses were also introduced in the 1960s, where a panel of expert US cardiologists would spend a few days as visiting experts in other countries. Introduced in 1969, the audiotape journal *American College of Cardiology Extended Study Services*, also known as *ACCESS*, became an immediate success because it offered more flexibility than structured courses. Cardiologists could listen to educational sessions anywhere and any time.

The ACC experienced much transformation during the 1970s. Headquarters moved to a new building in Bethesda, Maryland, that featured a semi-circular classroom undergirded by state-of-the-art technology to support distance delivery of programs. The new building was called Heart House and the classroom was known as the Learning Center. Each program attendee was assigned a large, comfortable captain's chair complete with controls for volume, positioning, talking, and listening. The intended plan was to disseminate information from the Learning Center using audiotapes, videotapes, slide sets, and manuals. This plan was implemented and expanded through the 1980s and 1990s until the Learning Center doors closed in the early 2000s.

Cardiology has always been a practice shaped by new technologies, but the invasive procedure of coronary angiography significantly changed the practice of cardiology and the profession. Cardiologists became invasive specialists, and ACC stepped up with its CME programming to help teach these new procedures. Newly emerging clinical technologies continue as the subject of many of the ACC CME activities.

The ACC was well established as an organization and as a CME provider by the 1990s. The Annual Scientific Session attracted large numbers of national and international registrants and exhibitors and was characterized by dozens of sessions led by hundreds of academic and practitioner cardiologists. The annual meeting featured scientific reports and updates but maintained its primary mission to meet the learning needs of the practicing, clinical cardiologist. A robust series of small programs were held yearly at the Learning Center and throughout the United States.

The ACC distance delivery library expanded significantly in the 1990s with the entrance and rapid growth of self-assessment learning products. The Adult Clinical Cardiology Self Assessment Program (ACCSAP), modeled after the highly successful MKSAP of the ACP, evolved with every edition and was soon joined by self-assessment products developed for cardiology subspecialty areas. These products were distributed initially in print format, but gradually this was supplemented by electronic delivery.

The ACC leaders invested in two products during the late 1990s that began to see fruition in the 2000s: a Web site for education—Cardiosource—and the development of data registries—the National Cardiovascular Data Registry™ (NCDR). Cardiosource has grown rapidly and served as a primary CME and information resource for most cardiologists by 2009. The NCDR collects information from more than 2,400 participating hospitals on patient risk factors, procedures, devices, and clinical outcomes. These data support the performance improvement activities of physicians who participate in the registry.

Whereas education technology shaped the ACC CME activities from the 1970s through the 1990s, the call for transformation in CME during the 2000s emerged from national and regulatory agencies. As public safety became an increasingly paramount issue, the certifying boards introduced MOC requirements for board-certified diplomates. In 1990, American Board of Internal Medicine certificates in cardiovascular disease switched from time-limited to 10 years. Activities to support MOC began to appear in every delivery venue of the ACC. Sessions were introduced during the annual meeting, the self-assessment products became approved for MOC credit, and stand-alone programs were planned for cardiologists wishing to gain credit for recertification.

The Future of Specialty Society CME

Many forces shape the CME activities of specialty societies. The public call for patient safety in medical care has given impetus to regulatory changes reflected by the certifying boards' mandated MOC programs and the review of licensing requirements underway by the Federation of State Medical Boards. The societies described in this chapter are moving quickly to provide education and support systems to assist their members in staying abreast of the specialty field and in maintaining core knowledge that is essential to meet the MOC activities.

Specialty societies are using the rapid expansion of distance delivery technologies to take CME activities to the members. Web-based education emerged in the 1990s and is used by specialty societies to deliver content through Webinars and blogs.

The fundamental mission of every society is to ensure the highest quality care of patients being treated by the members of the society. CME programming is directed to this end, and the emerging importance of physician review and improvement of practice aids the societies in achieving this mission. Societies create the guidelines for care in a specialty area and the performance measures to assess adherence to the guidelines, and they develop programming to fill consequent gaps in performance. Performance improvement CME that links society quality and education activities is rapidly expanding.

Specialty societies fulfill a unique and important role for physicians, and the education provided by the societies is specific to the practice of members. As member practice changes, so, too, does the society education portfolio. The future will likely bring education programming directed to team performance and patient care, enhanced implementation of guidelines in practice, and topics reflecting advances in science and technology. Whatever changes the future may bring, one thing is certain: patients will benefit from the CME activities provided by specialty societies.

Notes

1. "ACCME Annual Report Data 2009," Accreditation Council for Continuing Medical Education Web site, http://www.accme.org/dir_docs/doc_upload/f2e89864-b4c1-428f-8ebe-1ba197a31928_uploaddocument.pdf (accessed July 17, 2010).

2. Ibid.

3. S. A. Bryan, *Pioneering Specialists. History of the American Academy of Ophthalmology and Otolaryngology* (Rochester: American Academy of Ophthalmology, 1982).

4. H. S. Gradle, "Teachers' Section," *Bulletin of the American Academy of Ophthalmology and Otolaryngology* 8 (1939): 10–21.

5. W. G. Morgan, *The American College of Physicians: Its First Quarter Century* (Philadelphia: American College of Physicians, 1940).

6. Ibid.

7. Ibid.

8. Ibid.

9. Heinrich Stern and Edward E. Cornwall, eds., *Transactions of the American Congress on Internal Medicine: First Scientific Session, New York City, December 28–29, 1916* (New York: Burr Printing House, 1917).

10. Morgan, *American College of Physicians*.

11. B. R. Lemley, "The American College of Physicians: The First 75 Years," *Annals of Internal Medicine* 112, no. 11 (1990): 872–878.

12. F. D. Davidoff, "The American College of Physicians and the Medical Knowledge Self-Assessment Program Paradigm," *Journal of Continuing Education in the Health Professions* 9 (1989): 233–238.

13. "Self-Assessment of Medical Knowledge," *New England Journal of Medicine* 278, no. 17 (1968): 964.

14. Davidoff, "American College of Physicians," 233–238; "Self-Assessment," 964.

15. Ibid.

16. Davidoff, "American College of Physicians," 233–238.

17. H. R. Butt, "Self-Assessment of Medical Knowledge Programs," *New England Journal of Medicine* 291, no. 15 (1974): 791–793.

18. Davidoff, "American College of Physicians," 233–238.

19. Institute of Medicine, *Crossing the Quality Chasm: a New Health System for the 21st Century* (Washington, DC: National Academy Press, 2001).

20. Ibid.

21. W. Bruce Fye, *American Cardiology: The History of a Specialty and its College* (Baltimore: Johns Hopkins University Press, 1996).

22. Ibid.

PART III

Newer Institutions and Organizations in Continuing Medical Education

CHAPTER 10

The Accreditation of Continuing Medical Education: The Early Years

Continuing medical education (CME) has probably been around as long as doctors have been practicing medicine, but it was never formalized, accredited, or regulated in the United States until well after World War II.

Undergraduate medical education only began to be regulated in the early 20th century when it became obvious that scientific progress had finally reached the point when there was a marked difference in the patient's outcome from diagnosis and treatment by those who were well trained in medicine and those who were not. The first work in this line was begun by the American Medical Association (AMA) in 1904 when it established the Council on Medical Education and Hospitals. The council was concerned about medical education and sought out the Carnegie Foundation to fund a study that became known as the Flexner Report of 1910. The council became formalized by a partnership between the AMA and the Association of American Medical Colleges (AAMC) that would, in 1942, become the Liaison Committee on Medical Education (LCME). The partnership set up requirements and surveyed medical schools to certify adherence to these criteria. The result was fewer but far better medical schools.

The formalization and regulation of graduate medical education (GME) began with the formation of specialty societies and later the creation of specialty medical boards. By the 1930s, this resulted in the Advisory Board of Medical Specialties, which would, in 1970, become the American Board of Medical Specialties (ABMS). Before World War II most doctors were general practitioners and the pace of their learning of new methodologies and new medications was a slow one accomplished mainly through medical magazines such as the *Journal of the American Medical Association* (*JAMA*) or the *New England Medical Journal* (*NEJM*). Following World War II and with the aid of the G.I. Bill, specialty training expanded enormously.

Also after the war, the pace of development of new medications and treatment methods increased rapidly. The postwar period was the era of miracle drugs. No general practitioner could possibly keep up in all of the various fields; specialization became a necessity, not an option. Specialties and subspecialties proliferated. They resulted in more specialty societies and more specialty boards with more examinations. These required more residency programs, which were supervised by residency review committees (RRCs) composed of representatives from one or more specialty societies concerned with the discipline, the relevant ABMS board, and the AMA. In an effort to obtain uniformity and increased excellence, these various RRCs were coordinated and supervised by the Liaison Committee for Graduate Medical Education (LCGME). The LCGME had four representatives from the AMA, American Hospital Association (AHA), and AAMC and two from the ABMS and the Council of Medical Specialty Societies (CMSS) for a total of 16.

Furthermore, the development of so many new treatments for diseases meant a much greater opportunity to care in better ways for the American people. Unfortunately, information about these spectacular therapeutic innovations was not communicated as quickly from the laboratory to the practitioners as patients and payers desired.

When Medicare and Medicaid were being implemented following their passage in 1965, then Assistant Secretary of Health, Education, and Welfare Philip Randolph Lee, MD, lamented the gap from "bench to bedside." The era's wonderful scientific breakthroughs were not being put into use at the clinical level. This concept of speeding the flow of new medical knowledge from the research laboratory to patient therapy was attempted to be implemented within the Regional Medical Program (RMP), a partially federally funded initiative to wipe out heart disease, cancer, and stroke.

One part of the RMP was the provision that medical schools would take responsibility not only for undergraduate medical education and postgraduate residency training but also for the CME of practicing doctors. Each medical school would be responsible for educating practitioners in a specific geographic area. For instance, Stanford was given a number of central California counties for which it assumed responsibility for all physician CME regardless of where the physicians had been trained. Impractical and unsuccessful, the RMP was soon abandoned. However, the impetus to have mandatory CME so that practicing doctors would take advantage of all of the new developments in medical research continued.

At that time, the specialty boards had not yet engaged in periodic re-examinations for recertification to ensure continued knowledge of the specialty by allopathic practitioners. Therefore, an exploration was undertaken of the possibility of implementing an examination that practicing doctors would take in order to maintain licen-

sure. However, it became obvious, after a period of study by those of us working with the National Board of Medical Examiners (NBME), that no single examination could check the competency of all specialties.

But a push for a solution continued as many state legislatures began demanding physicians partake in a mandatory amount of CME. The answer was to require a given number of CME hours for relicensure. During the Medicare implementation era of the 1960s and early 1970s, the legislatures of the more populous states passed laws requiring CME for continued licensure and explored methods of ensuring that these programs were effective in improving the practice of medicine by the doctors who attended the programs. Organized medicine—especially state medical societies—was eager to guarantee that the control of CME did not pass from the profession to the politicians.

The problem then shifted to determining what kind of CME hours should count toward relicensure. What constituted meritorious CME? Who was responsible for deciding this? California was one leader in this effort. In the 1960s, the California Medical Association began a system of accrediting the state's CME programs. However, it proved to be difficult to ascertain which CME programs were truly of value for particular segments of the physician population. A program in gastroenterology was of little value to dermatologists, but hours spent in attendance could still result in meeting requirements of mandatory CME for licensure renewal.

At about the same time, a concern developed that undergraduate medical education, GME, and CME were going in separate directions. The perceived discontinuity in the lifetime acquisition of medical knowledge led to a demand for a continuum of medical education from the time one entered medical school until the time one retired from practice. This resulted in the establishment of the Coordinating Council for Medical Education (CCME), which oversaw medical education at all levels. Representatives from the AMA, AHA, AAMC, ABMS, and CMSS made up the CCME. The LCME, LCGME, and Liaison Committee on Continuing Medical Education (LCCME), which had oversight of CME, reported to the CCME. However, this attempt by the CCME to control all of medical education through a single organization proved far too cumbersome and the three accrediting liaison committees went their separate ways.

With state legislatures mandating CME for licensure renewal, the delivery of accredited CME became desirable or even necessary in order to attract attendees to the CME programs. Every organization—be it medical society, hospital, medical school, or commercial entity—wanted to offer accredited hours. The LCCME had the difficult task of coordinating the individual accreditation efforts of the different state societies, some of which (particularly the California Medical Association) had relatively sophisticated methods for assessing the value of the CME programs put on by local organizations (chiefly hospitals) within the state. However, too many other states had primitive or totally inadequate systems of evaluating local CME.

Moreover, organizations attracting doctors from multiple states did not wish to approach several state medical societies to obtain accreditation from each. The national medical societies, and particularly the specialty societies, had the desire to obtain accreditation at the national level. Obviously, obtaining one national seal of approval was infinitely superior to obtaining 50 approvals. The credit system developed by the AMA for its Physician Recognition Award proved helpful because most states accepted it as proof of CME.

There was an obvious need for a single national system of determining whether an individual program or series of programs given by an institution was of a sufficient quality to be accredited. Of further concern was the possibility that the private sector would fail at this task and state governments would instead implement their own systems. This led to the formation of the LCCME.

Initially, the LCCME was run from the AMA headquarters. C. H. William Ruhe, MD, of the AMA, had been a leader for years in CME and its measurement and regulation. He headed the overall medical education efforts of the AMA expertly and in a manner acceptable to the other organizations. Rutledge Howard, MD, of the AMA, developed some principles of CME that, though not written as strict rules, proved to be a useful guideline.

In those early years, however, the process of certifying the validity of the screening done by the individual states of the CME producers was haphazard and rather idiosyncratic. LCCME members and component society staff, some who like L. J. Carow of CMSS were competent in their own fields but neither physicians nor educators, would pore through documents sent to the AMA by the providers and second guess the accreditation done by, for instance, the state society CME committee. The process was, as is often the case when attempting something entirely new, rather erratic. It was also, at times, infuriating to the state societies when one of their decisions was overturned on a technicality.

Because the AMA began program accreditation, its leadership had a proprietary interest in the process and often did not see the presence of the other LCCME organizations as improving it.

To further complicate matters, during the mid- and late 1970s the staffing of the LCCME within the AMA was done by Leonard Fenninger, MD. Unfortunately, Fenninger and some of the representatives of the other organizations had many differences of opinion. In particular, Glen Leymaster, MD, the executive for ABMS, disagreed with Fenninger frequently and, occasionally, heatedly. Leymaster's fair complexion would turn a fiery red as they debated a point. AAMC president John A. D. Cooper, MD, and his representative on the LCCME Gus Swanson, MD, also had disagreements with the AMA policy in general and Fenninger in particular.

As mentioned, one area of disagreement was the accreditation of programs by state medical societies. The LCCME reviewed individual decisions made by the state societies and occasionally reversed them. Because the CME accrediting rules were at the very least somewhat vague and, at times, capricious, the state societies often lodged complaints with the AMA House of Delegates. The House of Delegates agreed and, in July 1979, AMA Executive Vice President James Sammons, MD, notified the LCCME that the AMA was withdrawing and the LCCME was to disband and unilaterally return CME accreditation to the AMA. Sammons did this by forming the AMA Committee on Accreditation of CME (CACME).

However, the other members of the LCCME met with AHA president J. Alexander McMahon and found that the departure of the AMA from the LCCME did not legally dissolve the LCCME as it would a partnership and that the LCCME could continue without the AMA. All of the remaining members voted to continue the LCCME and assigned the task of program administration to me as the CMSS executive vice president. Because CMSS was the junior member of the group, this assignment was not meant as an honor but as a serious responsibility and difficult mission.

It was a daunting task. Few files (most of which were held by the AMA) and few guidelines were available. The budget was minuscule. I served as the only staff member. Fortunately, I had recently hired a secretary—Francis Maitland, RN—for the CMSS who had been working for and was recommended by the chief executive officer of the Academy of Orthopaedic Surgeons. Maitland proved to be competent and a quick learner. She soon developed an understanding of CME that allowed her to organize the files and manage much of the CME accreditation side of CMSS business. Subsequently, Maitland developed into a leading player in CME accreditation.

We had a series of meetings around the country to distill the principles for accreditation into implementable essentials for accreditation. We also engaged in the recruitment of reviewers and the setting of standards for the reviews of the work of the local organizations. This, together with organizing meetings of the LCCME, determining lengths of time before resurveys, etc., plunged us into a maelstrom of activity.

We slowly developed standards and began accrediting organizations, chiefly the medical schools, specialty societies, other national organizations, and large hospitals that had multistate attendance. Separately, CACME accredited chiefly the state societies. However, many organizations, including state societies, sought accreditation from both CACME and LCCME. Some state legislatures specified LCCME accreditation while others cited the AMA as the body responsible for certifying the quality of CME within the state so that CME providers were forced to obtain dual accreditation in many states.

The onerous nature of having to be inspected twice, pay two sets of fees, and adhere to somewhat differing regulations made the situation totally unsatisfactory. It was also dangerous to the medical organizations because it encouraged various governmental bodies to consider setting their own standards and accrediting in their jurisdictions.

In addition, friction increased between the AMA and the other members of the accreditation of GME with a threatened splitting up of the Liaison Committee for Graduate Medical Education (LCGME).

Therefore, in 1981, the five leaders of the organizations—Cooper of AAMC, Leymaster of ABMS, McMahon of AHA, Sammons of AMA, and I of CMSS—met for two days. The first day was devoted to a reorganization of the LCGME and the residency review committees into the Accreditation Council for Graduate Medical Education (ACGME).

On the second day, representatives of the Federation of State Medical Boards (FSMB) and the Association for Hospital Medical Education (AHME) joined the five leaders. It was agreed that each of the original five organizations would have three representatives on the new body and that the two new member organizations—FSMB and AHME—would each have one. There would be a single set of essentials for accreditation and the management would continue to be by the CMSS. This meant that Maitland and I, joined by staff as time went on, acquired the CACME files and consolidated them with those of the LCCME. Sammons requested a name change to identify this as a new organization and thus the LCCME became the Accreditation Council for Continuing Medical Education (ACCME).

Fortunately, the representatives chosen by the member organizations were excellent and worked together in harmony. We developed the guiding principles, known as the essentials of accreditation, into a few easily understood sentences and insisted upon adherence to them. The adverse influence of funders, especially pharmaceutical firms and medical device manufacturers, on the content of programs was and still is a major concern. Principal requirements we set included that program decisions, such as the speakers and topics, be made by the accredited CME provider not the funder and that funds be given to the program without restrictions.

One of the significant events of the 1980s was the filing of a $400 million antitrust suit against the ACCME and its sponsors. The cost of hiring defense counsel severely affected the small annual ACCME budget of approximately $300,000. I attended law school in an effort to reduce these expenses without jeopardizing our legal position.

The suit concerned the ACCME withdrawal of accreditation from a medical school whose CME director, a salesman, had, unbeknownst to the school administration, given CME credit approval to the manufacturer of some low quality films to be shown to vacationing doctors on cruises. The manufacturer-distributor claimed that it would have grossed $400 million if ACCME had not removed its seal of approval. The suit questioned the legal right of the ACCME to decide what CME was appropriate for state licensing boards to use as a basis for granting or denying licensure renewal. It alleged that for monetary reasons the ACCME favored programs put on by the AHA member hospitals, AMA and its state societies, CMSS member specialty societies, and AAMC medical schools and, therefore, was an antitrust violation. The suit further crystallized a need for rigid adherence to high and defensible standards. The suit itself was groundless; the plaintiffs were being sued by the Internal Revenue Service and were using the suit and its allegations to ward off the government. When the suit finally came to trial five years later, it was summarily dismissed. However, it left ACCME as *the* organization to accredit CME in the United States.

Throughout the first decade of the ACCME, we continued to refine the essentials of accreditation, keeping them brief, straightforward, and implementable. We also worked hard to keep the process simple and economical. The number of accredited institutions increased rapidly and the acceptance of the ACCME as a control of the quality of CME satisfied the legislatures' requirements that doctors in their states were gaining knowledge of new developments. Control of the quality of CME was confirmed as belonging in the hands of the profession and medical educators. The underlying fundamentals of what constituted meaningful and valuable continuing education were firmly established and implemented.

The LCCME began the 1980s as one of two small, floundering, ill-regarded competing bodies. The ACCME ended the decade as the single nationally respected authority on the assurance of quality in CME programming. The fundamental policies that still are used to accredit CME were developed and implemented in those years through the efforts of pioneers in this new and previously uncharted field. Thanks to the efforts of a dedicated group of CME leaders from around the country, doctors would no longer attend programs that did not offer accredited CME.

Maitland and I continued to work together at the ACCME until I left CMSS in January 1991. She continued as executive secretary until the administration of the ACCME was turned over to the AMA in 1994.

Murray Kopelow, Kate Regnier,
and Tamar Hosansky

CHAPTER 11

Instituting National Standards for Continuing Medical Education: The Accreditation Council for Continuing Medical Education

The Accreditation Council for Continuing Medical Education (ACCME®) was founded in January 1981 in order to create a national accreditation system. The ACCME purpose is to oversee a voluntary, self-regulatory process for the accreditation of institutions that provide continuing medical education (CME) and develop rigorous standards to ensure that CME activities across the country are independent, free from commercial bias, based on valid content, and effective in meeting physicians' learning and practice needs.

The ACCME was created as the successor to the Liaison Committee for Continuing Medical Education (LCCME) and the American Medical Association (AMA) Committee on Accreditation of Continuing Medical Education. A not-for-profit organization based in Chicago, the ACCME is governed by its board of directors, which sets the strategic direction for the organization. Seven member organizations make up the ACCME: the American Board of Medical Specialties (ABMS), the American Hospital Association (AHA), the AMA, the Association for Hospital Medical Education (AHME), the Association of American Medical Colleges (AAMC), the Council of Medical Specialty Societies (CMSS), and the Federation of State Medical Boards (FSMB) of the United States. Each of the member

organizations nominates individuals to serve on the ACCME board of directors. Representatives from the federal government and the public also serve on the board.

The ACCME mission is to identify, develop, and promote national standards for quality CME that improve physician performance and medical care for patients and their communities. Throughout its almost 30-year history, the ACCME has been resolute in its commitment to carry out its mission, ensure compliance with its standards, and maintain a relevant and responsive accreditation system that supports CME as a strategic asset to US health-care quality and safety initiatives.

Establishing Accreditation Requirements

In 1982, the ACCME proposed and its member organizations ratified guidelines for accreditation that are referred to as the Seven Essentials. The guidelines outlined the approach CME providers should take to program management and education development. The guidelines were developed originally by Rutledge Howard, MD, with the AMA Committee on Accreditation of CME. By instituting the Seven Essentials, the ACCME began to articulate its philosophy regarding accredited CME. The ACCME believed that providers should use a curriculum planning model to create CME activities.

To be eligible for accreditation, CME providers had to create a written continuing medical education mission statement, describing the goals and scope of the program, characteristics of potential participants and an overview of the activities and services provided; use a needs assessment process to plan educational activities; develop educational objectives for each activity, and communicate those objectives to prospective participants; design and implement activities that met physician needs and the educational objectives; evaluate the effectiveness of their overall CME programs and use these evaluations in future planning; establish and document an organizational structure that was effective in fulfilling its CME mission; and accept responsibility for meeting the requirements of the Essentials when jointly sponsoring an activity with a non-accredited organization.

The Seven Essentials laid the foundation for creating a highly respected national accreditation system. Beginning with the Essentials, the ACCME initiated the process of assuring physicians and the public that accredited CME activities met accepted standards of education. By granting accreditation to institutions based on their compliance with the Essentials, the ACCME encouraged CME providers to improve their programs, thus raising the quality of CME across the country.

Empowering the State Accreditation System

Since the AMA Physician's Recognition Award had been established, medical societies in the United States and its territories had been accrediting CME providers. These intra-state accredited providers offered CME primarily to learners from their state or contiguous states as opposed to a national or international audience.

In 1983, the ACCME created its Committee for Review and Recognition (CRR) to oversee the accreditation of intra-state providers. Rather than take over the role of accrediting local providers, the ACCME decided to recognize the states

and territorial medical societies as accreditors through the CRR. This recognition process formalized an infrastructure, made up of the partnership of the ACCME and the state/territory medical societies, that was able to review and accredit more than 2,000 intra-state accredited providers.

Howard Madigan, MD, who chaired the CRR for its first seven years, faced significant challenges. When the CRR surveyors (ACCME-trained volunteers who monitored and evaluated the accreditation process) began visiting the states, they discovered a good deal of variation in practice. Most of the challenges were process issues, inconsistencies with appeals and accreditation decisions, as well as vagueness about the criteria required for the establishment of state medical society CME accreditation programs. By applying the guidelines set by the new recognition process, these issues were successfully addressed through the joint efforts of the ACCME and state medical society volunteers.

The recognition process empowered the state system while advancing the ACCME aim of creating consistent, high standards for CME accreditation across the country.

Standards for Commercial Support: Safeguarding CME's Independence

With the accreditation system firmly established at the national level and state levels, the ACCME took on the challenge of developing guidelines that would set boundaries between accredited providers and pharmaceutical and medical device companies. Increasingly, CME programs were being subsidized by industry grants, generating concern and debate within the health-care system, the government, and the public. In addition, fueled by the provisions of the 1980 Bayh-Dole Act, there was, as there is today, a complex web of interrelationships between health-care professionals and industry. Many of these same professionals also served as CME faculty or on CME committees, raising concerns about conflicts of interest. (Also known as the University and Small Business Patent Procedures Act, the Bayh-Dole Act gave universities, small businesses and non-profit organizations intellectual property control of discoveries and inventions that resulted from research funded by the federal government, including the right to patent and license discoveries. This legislation opened the way for greater partnerships between medical institutions and the pharmaceutical industry.)

While pharmaceutical and medical device companies were regulated by the Food and Drug Administration and other government agencies, there were no specific guidelines regarding CME funding. Taking a leadership role to safeguard CME's independence from commercial influence, in 1987, the ACCME issued its eight-point Guidelines for Commercial Support of Continuing Medical Education. These guidelines were the starting point for a series of requirements limiting—and eventually severing—commercial supporters' influence over CME content or faculty. Just as the Seven Essentials created the framework for developing high quality education, the commercial support guidelines laid the foundation for managing conflicts of interest in accredited CME programs.

In 1990, the US Senate Labor and Human Resources Committee held hearings on the marketing practices of pharmaceutical companies, including their funding of CME. The ACCME and its member organizations testified at the hearing, explaining that the ACCME guidelines established firm boundaries between industry funders and CME providers.

The hearings drew more national attention to the potential for conflicts of interest within CME. In response to the changing environment, to make sure that CME continued to be a self-regulated enterprise and to demonstrate its accountability to the public, the ACCME decided to strengthen its guidelines. An ACCME committee, chaired by J. S. "Dutch" Reinschmidt, MD, spearheaded the development of the ACCME Standards for Commercial Support of Continuing Medical Educa-

tion ("the Standards"), with input from stakeholders. The Standards were adopted in March 1992. While recognizing that commercial support could contribute significantly to the quality of CME activities, the ACCME stated in the Standards that CME providers were responsible for ensuring that activities were designed to improve physicians' care of patients—and must be based on scientific evidence. The Standards included the following requirements: accredited providers (1) are responsible for the content, quality, and scientific integrity of activities and (2) must have policies requiring faculty members and sponsors to disclose significant financial relationships with the manufacturers of products that are discussed in educational activities.

In addition, the Standards stipulated that providers must have signed agreements with commercial supporters and that arrangements for commercial exhibits should not influence the planning or interfere with the presentation of CME activities. While the Standards allowed providers to use commercial support to pay reasonable honoraria for faculty, they prohibited providers from using commercial support to pay for travel, registration, or other expenses for non-faculty attendees.

The Standards set the national model for boundaries between CME providers and commercial supporters and gained the respect of legislators, other accrediting institutions, and CME stakeholders, ensuring that CME remained a self-regulated profession. The American Academy of Family Physicians subsequently adopted the Standards for application within its own CME accreditation system, and the Pharmaceutical Manufacturers Association (now called the Pharmaceutical Research and Manufacturers of America) took action to endorse the document.

Strategic Planning: The Second Decade

To fulfill its responsibilities as the national accreditation standard bearer and to meet the needs of the growing CME enterprise, the ACCME needed to expand its staffing and administrative structure.

Up until 1994, CMSS provided ACCME with office space, part-time executive staff, and administrative services. In 1992, the AMA proposed to the other ACCME member organizations that the ACCME should expand its administrative operations to a size appropriate to a national accrediting body. In 1994, the ACCME accepted the AMA offer to become the ACCME vendor of administrative services. In 1994, the ACCME relocated its offices to the AMA Headquarters in Chicago in order to accommodate a larger staff and provide more resources to the CME provider community. The AMA provided large annual donations of services and operating funds to support this transition, on the condition that the ACCME become self supporting.

The ACCME undertook a national search for a new full-time executive director who was a physician. Richard Wilbur, MD, had been the first ACCME executive (1981–1991), followed by Frances Maitland (1991–1993), both of whom split their time between the ACCME and the CMSS. Mitchell Rhodes, MD, was the first full time executive director (1993–1994). When Rhodes left the ACCME in 1994, Sue Ann Capizzi, MBA, was recruited as executive administrator.

On August 1, 1995, Murray Kopelow, MD, a Canadian pediatrician, was appointed ACCME executive director and secretary. In addition to his other academic credentials in clinical medicine, medical education, and educational assessment, Kopelow had worked with physicians in such serious need of individualized educational support that their ability to continue to practice medicine was in jeopardy. The ACCME considered this concern for the individual learner a key attribute that would enable the ACCME to meet physicians' evolving continuing professional development needs. With the accelerating pace of medical breakthroughs, it was critical that CME provide physicians with the knowledge and skills they needed to maintain their competence and improve their practice. The ACCME needed to focus on the learner in order to demonstrate its accountability to the public. Appointing a full-time executive director—who was a physician—sent a strong message about the ACCMEs credibility and value. With the appointment of Kopelow, the ACCME began the process of building its staff, growing from four to 11 staff members over the next decade.

Elevating Accreditation Requirements

In the early 1990s, the CME community called for the ACCME to simplify its requirements. Supported by the AMA administrative structure and with a physician executive director at the helm, the ACCME was positioned to take the accreditation system to a new level of excellence by revising the Seven Essentials. The ACCME, led by its 1994 Chair James Hallock, MD, decided that it was no longer enough for CME providers to demonstrate that their programs transmitted important knowledge to physicians. Providers needed to demonstrate the link between their activities and changes in physician performance. According to Charles Daschbach, MD, appointed by Hallock as chair of the ACCME Ad Hoc Committee to Review and Evaluate the Accreditation Process, the ACCME goal was to encourage providers to measure the outcomes of their activities and show that their programs contributed to improving physician competence, patient care, and public health, thus demonstrating CME's value to the wider health-care system.

The committee began by considering no fewer than 21 different educational models. Out of this research, the committee created draft discussion documents for CME stakeholders to review. The ACCME recognized that adopting a new system would be a challenge for CME providers. The committee stressed that the new accreditation system would be flexible and evolving. Institutions would not have to meet benchmarks immediately. Accredited providers would have the opportunity to grow into the new system as long as they demonstrated their strategies for improvement.

To inform the CME community personally about the proposed changes, Kopelow took to the road. Heeding the advice of a colleague who told him Americans do business face-to-face and as part of the ACCME commitment to accountability, he held a series of town hall forums with CME providers and state medical society accreditors around the country. Despite the ACCME assurances that it would adopt a flexible approach, Kopelow encountered quite a bit of resistance when he first shared the new concepts with CME providers.

Kopelow continued the sometimes difficult discussions, showing providers that the ACCME was genuinely interested in their input. The ACCME listened to the reports from the field and then acted on the input. For example, the ACCME had proposed a special competencies approach, where providers would receive a basic accreditation and then be separately accredited for specialized areas within CME, such as remedial CME programs or Internet CME. Providers responded that this approach seemed too complicated. Therefore, the ACCME did not go forward with that part of the proposal.

Through this collaboration, the ACCME developed the Essential Areas and their Elements, also known as System98. The streamlined guidelines consisted of three Essential Areas, each comprised of several Elements. The Essentials encouraged providers to move to a more advanced level and focus on CME that linked identified educational needs with desired results. Further, the Essentials asked providers to evaluate the effectiveness of their CME activities in meeting those educational needs. The ACCME developed criteria for each element in the Essential Areas to measure whether the accredited provider met the requirements of accreditation. Criteria and examples were developed for noncompliance, partial compliance, compliance, and exemplary compliance.

The ACCME Essential Areas and Their Elements encouraged providers to measure their effectiveness and improve their programs by re-warding them with Accreditation with Commendation (a six-year accreditation term instead of the usual four-year term) if they achieved exemplary compliance with certain Elements:

- Created a mission statement that included all of the basic components (CME purpose, content areas, target audience, type of activities provided, and expected results of the program) with a strong emphasis on assessment of results.
- Used innovative and creative planning processes consistently, documenting that educational needs contributed to appropriate methodology and desired results for the offered CME activities.
- Described the purpose or objectives of the activity in terms of physician performance or patient health and consistently communicated the objectives to the learner.
- Consistently evaluated educational activities for effectiveness in meeting identified educational needs, as measured by practice application and/or health status improvement.
- Applied innovative and creative mechanisms to measure the effectiveness of the overall CME program with evidence of improvements being made on a regular basis.
- Included a process to review and continually improve the organizational framework.

With the Essential Areas and Their Elements, the ACCME raised the credibility and visibility of CME within the wider field of medical education and the broader health-care system.

In 1998, graduate medical education institutions and the specialty certification boards were also beginning a move toward requiring that physicians participate in life-long learning based on self-assessment and practice-based performance measurements. The new ACCME emphasis on measuring educational effectiveness provided an excellent complement to these expectations. The ACCME was now poised to assist its providers in incorporating the concept of physician mainte-nance of certification (MOC™) into CME, and in demonstrating the actual linkage between CME and changes in physician behavior.

In November 1998, the ACCME adopted its new system for accreditation. After unanimous approval by the seven member organizations, the Essential Areas and Their Elements were put into place in January 1999. The ACCME made the first accreditation decisions under the new guide-lines in July 2000. State medical society accredi-tors completed their transition to the new system in December 2001.

The ACCME implemented a broad-based edu-cational program to ease the transition to the new system, with ACCME staff conducting more than 50 presentations, including sessions at national meetings of the Alliance for CME, the Society for Academic CME, the Association for Hospital Medical Education, and the American Medical Association. In 1999 and 2000, Understand-ing ACCME Accreditation workshops and the ACCME State Medical Society Annual Confer-ence focused on helping providers understand the new Essentials.

Clinical Content Validation

As the ACCME approached its 20th anniversary, it continued to respond to the needs of a changing health-care education environment. Increasingly, health-care leaders, legislators, and the public de-manded that the medical system be held account-able for providing effective and safe patient care. Although ACCME guidelines had always stipu-lated that CME should be based on valid content, the wider health-care system expressed concerns that some CME activities focused on unproven therapies and did not rely on scientific evidence. Responding to those concerns, the ACCME de-cided to issue specific requirements to further safeguard the accuracy and reliability of the CME activities, which physicians used to maintain their licensure and credentialing privileges.

In December 2000, Thomas Kirksey, MD,

chair of the ACCME board of directors, assigned a task force to study the issues involved with ac-creditation and content validation. In November 2001, the task force issued a draft proposal with new content validation requirements and a call for comment. The proposal called on CME pro-viders to evaluate the content of each CME ac-tivity to make sure it was evidence-based. Re-sponses to the proposal were mixed, with an almost equal split between those favoring and op-posing the new proposal.

Upon reviewing the responses, the ACCME narrowed the content validation focus. Rather than including the full spectrum of CME activi-ties, which, for example, encompass new research results and emerging breakthroughs, the policy ap-plied only to content that included patient care rec-ommendations. The ACCME adopted an action plan in July 2002 to educate providers about the issues involved in content validation and issued the following three clinical content value state-ments: (1) all recommendations involving clinical medicine and CME activities must be based on evidence that is accepted within the profession of medicine; (2) all scientific research used to sup-port patient care recommendations must con-form to generally accepted standards of experi-mental design, data connection, and analysis; and (3) providers will be ineligible for ACCME ac-creditation or reaccreditation if their activities promote treatments that are known to have risks or dangers that outweigh the benefits or are known to be ineffective in patient treatment. These statements reinforced ACCME account-ability and value, further protected the integrity of CME, and demonstrated to the wider health-care system that CME contributed to physicians' maintenance of competence and to the quality and safety of patient care.

Revising the Standards for Commercial Support

At the same time, concern increased regarding the influence of pharmaceutical companies and device manufacturers. They began describing accredited CME as one of their marketing tactics, and grants to CME providers often came out of companies' marketing budgets. Companies produced promotional meetings and events to showcase drugs and devices, hiring physicians as speakers. Many of these same speakers subsequently became involved in accredited CME.

The US Food and Drug Administration (FDA) looked to the ACCME to manage conflicts of interest between FDA-regulated companies and accredited CME providers, and national leadership organizations in the field of medicine in the United States asked ACCME to consider the need for changes. The ACCME believed it was essential to respond by broadening the scope of the Standards for Commercial Support. It was time to "brighten the line" between the educational and promotional activities produced by industry and ACCME providers' independent CME.

The process for updating the Standards for Commercial Support began in December 2001 with the creation of the Standards for Commercial Support Task Force. Chaired by Norman Kahn, MD, the task force recommended changes to further ensure that CME was independent and free of influence from FDA-regulated companies.

The ACCME issued a draft of the revised Standards for Commercial Support in January 2003, calling for comment from the CME enterprise. Recognizing that the economic interests of CME providers or their agents are sometimes substantial enough to be in conflict with the public interest, the draft Standards stated that the disclosure rules in the 1992 Standards might not always be enough to ensure the separation of promotion from education. The proposal suggested excluding people and organizations with a conflict of interest with a commercial interest from controlling the content of CME, for example, from serving as a planning committee manager or teacher.

The recommended restriction created great concern among CME providers, who said that many of the most renowned and highly qualified faculty had financial relationships with industry.

Under the draft guidelines they would be forced to exclude these high quality experts from participating in their CME activities. The ACCME clarified that it did not intend to block all physicians who received any remuneration from pharmaceutical or medical device companies from participating as planners or teachers in CME activities that might be related to their conflicts of interest. Rather, the ACCME goal was to articulate clear, reasonable, and practical safeguards to ensure the resolution of conflict of interest without excluding experts.

ACCME took the comments and concerns into account when revising the draft. In November 2004, the ACCME released a new version. The 2004 Standards for Commercial Support: Standards to Ensure the Independence of CME Activities are designed to make certain that CME activities are independent, free of commercial bias, and beyond the control of persons or organizations with an economic interest in influencing the content of CME. The new document comprised six standards: independence, resolution of personal conflicts of interest, appropriate use of commercial support, appropriate management of associated commercial promotion, content and format without commercial bias, and disclosures relevant to potential commercial bias. The revised Standards included the following new elements:

- CME providers must ensure that CME planning decisions are made free of the control of a commercial interest, including the selection of all persons and organizations that will be in a position to control CME content.
- A commercial interest cannot take the role of non-accredited partner in a joint sponsorship relationship.
- Providers must be able to show that everyone who is in a position to control the content of educational activities has disclosed to the provider all relevant financial relationships with any commercial interest.

- Those who refuse to disclose relevant financial relationships are disqualified from participation.
- Providers must implement a mechanism to identify and resolve all conflicts of interest.
- The provider must have written policies and procedures governing honoraria for planners, teachers, and authors.

When making decisions about implementing the Standards for Commercial Support, ACCME said that CME providers must be guided by what is in the best interest of the public and must always defer to independence from commercial interests, transparency, and separating CME from product promotion. In other words, the interest of CME in the health and well-being of the public is more important than any economic interest.

The CME community was informed about the adoption of the 2004 Standards, and the ACCME provided documents with frequently asked questions, explanations of expectations, and compliance examples on its Web site to assist providers. Staff made numerous presentations and worked directly with many providers at major CME organizations to make sure they received accurate information to address their concerns. The ACCME did not make accreditation decisions based on the revised Standards until late in 2006, giving providers time to implement them and the ACCME time to assist providers.

The 2004 Standards received a great deal of media attention. An Associated Press news article about them ran in more than 120 newspapers in the United States and several drug and device industry newsletters.

The 2004 Standards for Commercial Support were widely accepted as a major enhancement to the CME system. They were immediately accepted by the American Academy of Family Physicians and subsequently by the Accreditation Council for Pharmacy Education and the American Nurses Credentialing Center. They were referenced by government representatives as the basis for the development of independent CME.

Representatives from industry actually asked other health-care professions to consider adopting the ACCME Standards to provide a basis for their interactions. The Standards continue to be viewed as a model system.

Updating the Accreditation Criteria

With the 2004 Standards establishing a bright line of demarcation between independent, accredited CME and promotion, the ACCME took steps to support a new and expanded role for CME providers in contributing to physicians' lifelong learning.

The 1998 ACCME accreditation model, the Essential Areas and Their Elements, had served well for almost a decade, with medical education literature showing that the CME enterprise had been effective in providing educational opportunities and helping physicians improve patient care. The Essential Areas and their Elements rewarded providers that designed educational activities aimed at improving physician performance or patient health and/or measured the effectiveness of their activities in achieving those goals. However, the ACCME compliance data showed that only 5 to 10 percent of providers were reaching that level, while the rest designed activities with the objective of changing participants' knowledge or increasing their satisfaction with CME. These objectives were no longer enough to meet the expectations of the health-care system.

The government, the public, and organized medicine called on the CME system to be even more accountable in facilitating and demonstrating physician practice improvement. The ACCME was asked by its member organizations and others to assist in repositioning the CME enterprise as a strategic asset to the quality improvement and patient safety imperatives of the US health-care system, such as addressing health-care disparities, the prevention and treatment of chronic disease, and the reduction of medical errors. The Institute of Medicine reports "To Err Is

Human: Building a Safer Health System, Crossing the Quality Chasm" and "Health Professions Education: A Bridge to Quality" identified critical factors for improving the quality of care. The ACCME decided to identify ways for the accreditation system to step up and help achieve these goals.

The ACCME Task Force on Competency and the Continuum received oral and written testimonies from a wide representation of organizations within the CME enterprise as well as other organizations interested in physician education. Its final report released in April 2004 stated, "To meet the needs of the 21st century physician, CME will provide support for the physicians' professional development based on continuous improvement in the knowledge, strategies and performance of practice necessary to provide optimal patient care."[1]

Toward that end, in September 2006, the ACCME released its updated accreditation criteria. They were based on a learner-centered, quality improvement model of CME, rather than the 1990 and 1998 curriculum planning model, which would provide educational support for physicians in the real world in which they practiced. The criteria push CME providers to not just give information to physicians but to empower them to address obstacles to improving their practice and make greater contributions to the overall health-care system. The 22 criteria call for CME to be practice-based learning; derived from physicians' professional practice gaps; designed to change physician competence, performance, or patient outcomes; evaluated for its effectiveness in changing competence, performance, or patient outcomes; and representative of the desirable physician attributes now widely utilized in medicine.

The revised model represents a change in emphasis. Learning and change are the goals—both for the learners and providers, as described in the article "Accreditation for Learning and Change: Quality and Improvement as the Outcome," by

ACCME Deputy Chief Executive Kate Regnier, et al., in the *Journal of Continuing Education in the Health Professions,* September 2005. Under the 2006 Accreditation Criteria, all providers must develop activities designed to change competence, performance, or patient outcomes, and must analyze changes in learners. They must also analyze their own effectiveness at meeting their mission and identify plans for improvement.

The 2006 Accreditation Criteria foster leadership, collaboration, and system-wide change by rewarding CME providers with Accreditation with Commendation, if, among other requirements, they act as a strategic partner in quality and safety initiatives within their institution, health system, or community through collaborative alliances. Such providers must have mechanisms in place to identify and overcome barriers to physician change and to integrate CME into wider health-care improvement initiatives. Achieving Accreditation with Commendation elevates the value, visibility, and credibility of CME within the health-care and wider communities.

Reaction from CME providers was mixed as to the content and process the ACCME chose to update its requirements. Some providers responded that the criteria were timely and offered the opportunity to measure change in physician performance and patient outcomes, and aligned well with the learners' need for CME to meet MOC™ and maintenance of licensure requirements. Some felt that the emphasis on change and improvement was appropriate.

On the other hand, some providers were perturbed because the criteria were implemented without consultation or a call for comment; they felt that the criteria represented too much change too fast. They were concerned that the criteria made demands on providers that went beyond their current abilities, presenting insurmountable challenges to certain provider groups.

In a series of communications with providers, ACCME executives explained that the process was actually initiated in 2001 by the Task Force on

Competency and the Continuum. It chose not to distribute the draft document for comment because it was necessary to move quickly to position CME as a strategic partner in maintenance of licensure and certification and to align CME with the quality and safety initiatives underway in the United States, including the work of the Institute of Medicine and the Agency for Healthcare Research and Quality.

To facilitate compliance with the criteria, ACCME staff conducted trainings for surveyors, CME providers, and recognized state accreditors at the annual meeting of the Alliance for CME and other conferences. In addition, ACCME accreditation workshops covered the new criteria, and the ACCME developed training webinars and a toolkit. CME as a Bridge to Quality, a call to action booklet, was published by the ACCME to help providers demonstrate the value of accredited CME to their stakeholders and to encourage collaborative efforts to improve patient care—steps that would help them achieve Accreditation with Commendation.

The 2006 Accreditation Criteria elevated the perception of CME's value with organizations such as the American Board of Medical Specialties and its member boards, as well as the FSMB and its member boards.

"The new accreditation elements will prove to be valuable in the national initiatives to ensure competence of physicians. This level of activity is just what is needed to place the continuing medical education community at the forefront of improving quality and the practice of medicine," said James Thompson, MD, who was then president and CEO of the FSMB.[2]

In 2006, the 24 boards that are members of the American Board of Medical Specialties (ABMS) adopted the ABMS Maintenance of Certification (MOC™) process for board-certified physicians. The process includes lifelong learning, self-assessment, and practice performance assessment, components that are directly supported by the ACCME 2006 Accreditation Criteria.

Through the criteria, ACCME encourages providers to take an innovative and thoughtful approach to not only understanding the health-care environment in which their physicians practice but to seek solutions beyond their own boundaries to identify and remove obstacles that stand between current care and the best care for patients.

The accreditation review process that the ACCME has honed over the years works well to support the principles of learning and change embodied in the 2006 Accreditation Criteria. During the accreditation process, providers complete a self study report, which provides them an opportunity to analyze their program's current practices, identify areas for improvement that reflect the vision and values of the program, and determine future directions.

After the self study report has been submitted, providers are interviewed by volunteer surveyors, experienced CME professionals, who ask questions and listen carefully to providers' descriptions about their program. Surveyors are particularly eager to hear about creative strategies that providers have implemented to achieve their goals, as well as plans for future improvements. Surveyors make their report and recommendations to the Accreditation Review Committee. The committee decides whether providers have met the criteria or not, and what the appropriate accreditation outcome should be. The Decision Committee of the ACCME Board of Directors then must approve those decisions.

As time went on, providers grew more receptive to the criteria. The most talked about challenge continued to be how to effectively measure the results of activities and programs. To assist CME providers further, ACCME released a document containing real world examples of compliance extracted from the accreditation decisions, and included ACCME commentary.

Through this process, the ACCME ensures that providers adhere to its high standards, and fosters an environment where providers are motivated to continuously improve their programs and activities.

Encouraging Team-Focused Continuing Education

The ACCME also strives to embody the model of broader health system collaboration described in the 2006 Accreditation Criteria. In June 2002, the Institute of Medicine produced the report Health Professions Education: a Bridge to Quality, which set forth five competencies that all health professions must incorporate into their curricula in order to bridge the quality chasm in the health-care delivery system. One of those is working in interdisciplinary teams. The IOM report said that health professionals needed to "cooperate, communicate, and integrate care in teams to ensure that care is continuous and reliable."[3]

Embracing that goal, in March 2009, the ACCME joined with two other national accrediting bodies, the Accreditation Council for Pharmacy Education, which accredits continuing education for pharmacists, and the American Nurses Credentialing Center Accreditation Program, which accredits CE programs for nurses, to develop "Accreditation of Continuing Education Planned by the Team for the Team." The purpose of this joint accreditation is to support health-care, team-focused education that improves patient care, and to streamline the accreditation processes. The joint accreditation is available for organizations already accredited by at least two of the three organizations. To qualify, 25 percent or more of the provider's education must address the professional practice gaps of the health-care team, and the planning process must reflect input from health-care professionals who make up the team.

This joint accreditation builds on the ACCME's long-standing, ongoing collaboration with the ANCC and ACPE. Earlier, the three groups developed a combined application for providers seeking initial accreditation and then moved on to create shared values, definitions, and terms. Through this collaboration, the ACCME aims to support providers who are educating not only physicians but other health professionals. By aligning standards, accreditation processes, and values, the ACCME, the ACPE, and the ANCC assure the public that health-care teams receive education that is independent, free from commercial bias, based on valid content, and effective in improving the quality and safety of care delivered by the team.

Creating Uniformity in the State System

Building on the state medical society recognition system created in 1983, the ACCME and the Recognized State Medical Societies worked together to address a top priority: establishing a construct of equivalency for the accreditation process across the nation. The purpose in moving toward uniformity in accreditation was to help assure physicians, state legislatures, CME providers, and the public that all CME programs are held to the same high standards. Created in 2007, the Advisory Committee on Equivalency (ACE), an ad hoc group comprised of state medical society leaders from across the country, was brought together to develop and refine the concepts of equivalency. ACE members were given blinded data that showed the variance of accreditation decision outcomes among state medical societies in areas such as compliance rates, accreditation terms, criteria for progress reports, and due dates. In some cases, states did not offer Accreditation with Commendation as an option. The variation was due to differences in process, including data collection, as well as differences in how state medical societies interpreted the data. Convinced by the data describing the wide variation in accreditation outcomes, the entire state-based system agreed on the importance of implementing a new framework for equivalency, which ACE and the ACCME drew from the data to create. In 2008, the ACCME adopted the Markers of Equivalency, which will serve as the foundation for Recognition decisions beginning in 2010. There are five markers: equivalency of rules, process, interpretation, accreditation outcome, and evolution or process improvement. Working with the recognized state medical society accreditors to implement these markers is a high priority for the ACCME.

International CME

On the international front, the ACCME has also taken a leading role in developing the concept of equivalency of accreditation with other systems. Countries around the world are in various stages of developing CME standards and processes. In this era of globalization, more and more health professionals cross borders for their education and career development, and it is increasingly important to set high standards for CME around the world.

Toward that end, in 2002, the ACCME and the Committee for the Accreditation of Continuing Medical Education of the Association of Canadian Medical Colleges created "A Framework for Establishing Substantial Equivalency between Continuing Medical Education Accreditation Organizations," a document designed to facilitate discussion about strategies for improving CME across national boundaries.

In 2005, the ACCME joined other organizations from Bulgaria, Canada, France, Germany, Italy, Spain, the United Kingdom, and the European Union to develop a consensus on basic values and responsibilities underlying substantial equivalency of CME and continuing professional development (CPD) systems. (See http://www.bmj.com/cgi/content/extract/328/7451/1279-b.) The goal is to facilitate the free movement of learners between the various nations' CME or CPD systems and to build a foundation that will lead to mutual recognition and reciprocity while maintaining each nation's cultural and historical identity.

The ACCME is viewed by countries around the world as an accreditation leader. In 2003, the ACCME was invited by the government of Italy to participate with the Italian CME community in discussions on the development of a CME accreditation system. Throughout the years, the ACCME has participated in CME initiatives with the European Accreditation Council for Continuing Medical Education in Brussels, and with government, health system, and CME representatives from a wide range of countries including Spain, Ireland, France, Japan, Jordan, India, South Africa, New Zealand, Singapore, Sudan, and the United Arab Emirates. Currently, Kopelow is a member of the International Rome Group on Harmonization of CME/CPD credit.

By advancing equivalency of CME systems on a global level, the ACCME builds toward a future where patients—regardless of where they are treated or the nationality of their physician—will be assured that their doctors maintain their competence by participating in CME that meets consistent and high standards.

Expanded Education and Outreach

To support CME providers in their own continuing professional development and to nurture CME leadership, the ACCME strategic imperatives going forward include expanded education and outreach to the community of accredited providers, recognized state medical societies, state accredited providers, and volunteers and staff. In 2009, the ACCME launched a series of regional forums for state medical societies, locally accredited providers, volunteers, and staff to educate them about compliance with the 2006 Accreditation Criteria and also to help advance their leadership skills within their organizations and communities, positioning CME as a strategic partner in public health initiatives.

In 2008, the ACCME went through its second major expansion, increasing its office space 100 percent to improve services and resources offered to providers, volunteers, leadership, and staff. In 2009, the ACCME hosted a series of town hall forums at its offices for specific provider groups, including medical education and communication companies, hospitals, medical specialty societies, and medical schools. These forums facilitated dialogue between the ACCME and providers, allowing providers to voice their concerns and challenges.

Launched in 2009, the Education and Training Web pages at the ACCME Web site offer providers a variety of resources. Video FAQs answer providers' most pressing questions about compliance with accreditation requirements, and video tutorials offer step-by-step guidance for planning and implementing CME activities. The Perspectives section features video interviews with CME and other health-care system leaders who share their approach to planning effective education, including strategies they use to overcome challenges and build bridges with other health-care stakeholders. The Education and Training Web pages are continually updated in response to providers' needs.

Greater Transparency and Accountability

The ACCME continues to insist on the separation between accredited CME and commercial support, making certain that CME is by the profession, for the profession. To be eligible for initial accreditation or reaccreditation, providers must submit evidence that demonstrates their compliance with Standards for Commercial Support, as well as the other accreditation requirements. Accredited providers that are found out of compliance may be put on probation. They are given the opportunity to correct the problem and asked to submit progress reports to demonstrate improvement. Should they fail to do so, their accreditation status will be discontinued. In 2009, the ACCME accelerated its enforcement process. CME providers that are out of compliance with the Standards for Commercial Support must now submit an improvement plan within weeks of the findings and a demonstration of compliance within six or 12 months.

To continue to promote the validity of the CME enterprise, the ACCME is also taking steps to make its system increasingly transparent. Beginning in August 2009, the ACCME provider list on its Web site featured more information than it had in the past, including providers' current accreditation status, whether providers accept commercial support, whether providers receive advertising and exhibit revenue, and the numbers and types of activities produced and the number of participants. This increased transparency empowers all stakeholders in the system, including physician learners, licensing and certification bodies, and the public to assess an individual provider's funding structure and the independence and scope of the accredited CME enterprise in the United States.

Testifying before the US Senate Special Committee on Aging during a July 2009 hearing addressing conflicts of interest in CME, Kopelow detailed the new monitoring and enforcement measures, assuring the committee that the ACCME was an effective firewall between pharmaceutical industry marketing and independent continuing education.

Summary

The ACCME is a different organization from the one founded in 1981. The ACCME is now recognized by federal and state government agencies as the national standard bearer for CME accreditation. Several states have incorporated ACCME requirements into laws protecting the independence of CME. Federal legislators have turned to the ACCME to gain an understanding of how the Standards for Commercial Support safeguard CME from commercial influence. On the international front, the ACCME has gained a reputation as an accreditation leader, as evidenced by the numerous requests for guidance that the ACCME has received from health-care organizations and governments around the world.

ACCME accreditation aims to assure the public and the medical community that CME provides physicians with relevant education in support of closing the quality gap in US health care and that such education is designed to be free of commercial bias and based on valid content. Building on its long-standing relationships with the ABMS and the FSMB, the ACCME has created an accreditation system that serves as an essential link between physicians' lifelong learning and physician licensure and maintenance of certification requirements.

Initially staffed by a few part-time personnel, ACCME now has more than 20 employees. As it has since its inception, the ACCME continues to rely on its network of dedicated volunteers. Currently, approximately 150 volunteers serve on the national level as surveyors and ACCME Board and committee members; thousands of volunteers serve at the state level. Taking into account national-level volunteers, Recognized State Medical Society accreditation volunteers, and CME committee volunteers serving ACCME-accredited and state-accredited providers, perhaps more than 20,000 people across the country support the system. Initially aided by member organizations' administrative support and development funds, as well as provider fees, the ACCME achieved financial independence in 1999 and now is supported solely by provider fees and workshop registration fees.

There are currently more than 700 ACCME directly-accredited organizations, including medical schools; nonprofit physician membership organizations, such as medical specialty and state medical societies; hospitals and health-care delivery systems; publishing and education companies; government and military organizations; and insurance and managed care companies. The ACCME recognizes approximately 45 state and territory medical societies as accreditors for local organizations, such as community hospitals, offering CME. In total, ACCME accredits approximately 2,200 CME providers.

The CME enterprise continues to grow. According to the 2009 ACCME annual data report, total income for CME programs was $2.2 billion. That figure represents an increase of 146 percent since 1998, the year ACCME first issued its annual data report, when providers' total income was $889 million. The number of participants has grown steadily over the years. CME activities drew more than 10.7 million physician participants in 2009, a 24 percent increase in a two-year period. In addition, CME providers reported that 6.7 million nonphysician health-care practitioners attended activities in 2009, bringing total participation to more than 17 million.[4]

Approaching its thirtieth year, the ACCME remains committed to continuously improving the accreditation process to meet the challenges of the evolving health-care system. Recognizing that US health care is at a crossroads, the ACCME is dedicated to ensuring that accredited CME provides solutions that will help close health-care quality gaps and effectively address current and emerging public-health concerns.

Notes

1. "Competency and the Continuum: A Report from the ACCME Task Force," Accreditation Council for Continuing Medical Education Web site, http://www.accme.org/dir_docs/doc_upload/41849588-561a-4ca4-bf16-d823da6f7157_uploaddocument.pdf (accessed July 19, 2010).

2. James Thompson, letter to the ACCME, August 30, 2006.

3. "Health Professions Education: A Bridge to Quality," The National Academies Press Web site, http://www.nap.edu/catalog.php?record_id=10681 (accessed July 19, 2010).

4. "ACCME Annual Report Data 2009," Accreditation Council for Continuing Medical Education Web site, http://www.accme.org/dir_docs/doc_upload/f2e89864-b4c1-428f-8ebe-1ba197a31928_uploaddocument.pdf (accessed July 19, 2010).

CHAPTER 12

Evolution of the Society of Medical College Directors of Continuing Medical Education into the Society for Academic Continuing Medical Education

In 1990, James Leist, president of the Society for Medical College Directors of CME (known today as the Society for Academic CME "[SACME]"), persuaded Richard Caplan, MD, to accept the task of recounting the history of SACME. That history, reprinted in part within the section of this chapter titled "The First 12 Years: 1976–1988" was first published in 1996.[1] The second section of this chapter, titled "The Next 20 Years: 1989–2009," continues SACME's history and is written by Paul Lambiase. Both sections approach the history not in a chronological manner but a thematic one.

The First 12 Years: 1976–1988

The Association of American Medical Colleges (AAMC) formed a committee on continuing medical education (CME) in 1950, though by 1960 only 18 medical schools had an identifiable CME program. That number grew rapidly, stimulated by state legislative decisions that required CME for re-registration of the medical license, by specialty societies (pioneered in 1947 by the American Academy of General Practice) that required CME for continued membership, and by the federally funded Heart, Stroke, and Cancer Program (better known as the Regional Medical Program), which provided financial support for developing many medical college CME pro-

grams. During the 1950s and 1960s, many medical schools took the initiative to develop their own CME programs. Such developments were probably major stimuli that prompted W. Albert Sullivan Jr., MD, of the University of Minnesota, to convene a meeting in 1960 to which all medical colleges with identifiable CME programs were invited. Its theme, "How to Get Medical Schools Involved in CME," was followed later that year by a meeting in Albany, New York, convened by Frank Woolsey, Jr., MD.

In 1967, Jesse Rising, MD, CME director at the University of Kansas, called together a highly informal group in a retreat-like venue to discuss their shared problems and activities regarding CME programming. The retreat was so well received that it became an annual event hosted by other medical schools.

In 1969, the AAMC committee on CME recommended that the AAMC place CME among its primary concerns, that it urge its member schools to recognize CME among their major responsibilities, and that the AAMC establish an administrative unit to support CME activities arising within its component medical schools. These recommendations were not accepted and the AAMC in 1971 discharged its CME committee. In 1974, the steering committee of the AAMC Group on Medical Education, responding to growing CME pressures, agreed to expand its interests to include "the continuum of medical education," thus seeming to include CME in its administrative and programmatic purview. By then, the Group on Medical Education contained so many component interests that the administrative leaders of medical school CME seldom felt their needs to be adequately met within the group.

A second annual gathering, rather more focused on research issues than the retreats, was convened by Phil Manning, MD, CME director at the University of Southern California, in 1971 in Palm Springs, California. The need for organization, self-help, and recognition (even from many medical college deans and other faculty members) coupled with the too-little-too-late response of the AAMC (which might have seemed the natural base for such a group of academic professionals functioning in the world of CME) finally led the activists to form an independent organization.

Birth

At one of the Palm Springs meetings, interest in forming an independent organization began to crystallize. When it was learned, via help from the American Medical Association (AMA) legal office, that incorporation was not required, Manning and others felt that an opportunity for decision-making should be extended to all schools. That invitation led to a well attended discussion during the November 1975 AAMC meeting in Washington, DC, which generated much enthusiasm for forming an independent organization. Manning was chosen as the interim president of the fledgling organization. All schools were invited to attend the next Palm Springs meeting (as they were called) in April 1976. Robert Combs, MD, head of CME for the University of California at Irvine, presented a draft constitution and bylaws, which were adopted on April 2, 1976. SACME was now off and running, with Manning elected as its first president.

Childhood

The original constitution, adopted April 2, 1976, was amended in 1978, 1980, 1984, 1986, and 1987. The most important modifications involved members, officers, and committees. Categories of membership expanded from regular and honorary life members to include associate members, continuing members (no longer eligible for membership because of a change in professional activities but wishing to continue the affiliation), emeritus members, corresponding members, and, by 1994, student members.

The founding constitution specified only three committees: executive, nominating, and finance. Later versions added committees for program, membership, and research. Throughout the several modifications, the purposes of SACME remained constant: "to establish the national forum for The Society of Medical College Directors of Continuing Medical Education, and to improve patient care through Continuing Medical Education." Thus the CME goal to provide education and produce better care for patients was present from the outset. This concern for payoff in health outcomes indeed represented the adopting of a new posture.

Throughout the 1960s and 1970s the rapid expansion of CME increased the sense of need for standards, accreditation, and other measures of quality. In 1968, the AMA activated a voluntary program to acknowledge individual CME participation called the AMA Physician's Recognition Award. Other events, in tandem with the beginning of SACME, produced other CME organizations. By 1988, most of the US and Canadian allopathic medical schools were represented among the voting members of SACME. Beyond the factors already mentioned that stimulated CME growth lay the movement toward obligatory CME for renewal of certification by many specialty certifying boards and the development of the Accreditation Council for CME (ACCME), a relatively independent organization that provided a standard of quality and prestige. These developments may be contrasted with the situation in 1967, when Rising convened the first retreat group, consisting of 36 persons, who attended with invitations extended by hearsay and word-of-mouth. At its 1987 meeting, SACME celebrated the first retreat with a special 20th anniversary program honoring that early effort.

Although always related to medical schools, SACME members were individuals, never institutions, even though each voting member had to be certified by the respective collegiate dean as the individual in charge of that school's CME program. Thus the voting membership could never exceed the number of existing allopathic medical schools. The category called associate membership—persons acknowledged by the voting member as an important contributor to the school's CME effort—could potentially rise to several times that number of members.

Adolescence

The organization recognized its need to become a 501(c)(3) tax-exempt organization in the eyes of the Internal Revenue Service (IRS). This would permit tax-exempted charitable donations and liberate the organization from the hazard of federal tax intrusion into its treasury. The lengthy process was completed in 1982.

The evolution of a satisfactory logo and appropriate stationery helped the organization's sense of identity. The process proved surprisingly difficult, however, and consumed an extraordinary amount of discussion time at meetings for the first few years. Part of the difficulty related to the name of the organization (then SMCDCME), which many people sought to reduce in length and simultaneously to produce a pleasing acronym. Those efforts failed utterly, but a logo was adopted.

Almost from its outset, the young organization found itself relating (or failing to relate) to cognate organizations, particularly the AAMC, AMA, ACCME, Association for Hospital Medical Education (AHME), Alliance for Continuing

Medical Education (ACME), and publishers of the journal *Mobius*. The relationship to the AAMC was rocky in the early days. Once the SACME was firmly established, however, its officers began to assess the possibility of relating to the AAMC for obviously appropriate connections. Yet, out of a feeling of youthful vigor and independence, perhaps mixed with a little spitefulness, the officers wanted to run no risk of losing the newly earned status of an independent organization. When the administration of the AAMC was contacted, its chairman John Gronlund, MD, and vice president John Sherman, MD, suggested that because the voting members of SACME were all faculty members at medical schools, the organization might seek membership in the AAMC component known as the Council of Academic Societies (CAS). The posture of Gronlund and Sherman seemed welcoming in that regard, and so SACME began a lengthy process to make itself appropriately constituted to meet the requirements for admission to the CAS. But the submitted application was rejected, largely on grounds that SACME's members were functioning as administrative officers rather than as faculty of a clearly defined discipline. (Becoming a clearly defined discipline was one of the most important developments of the early years.) This frustrating sequence once again kindled angry feelings in many of the members who had lived through the organizational years. A reapplication ultimately was accepted, however, in 1989.

In the mid-1970s, the AAMC assigned Emanuel Suter, MD, a liaison role in which he attended SACME meetings and performed constructive liaison functions. Gradually, however, the AAMC Group on Education, which had earlier chosen to include CME within its spectrum of medical education, began conversations with SACME, leading ultimately to joint symposia and colloquia at the AAMC annual meetings. After the retirement of Suter and a brief hiatus, Louis Kettell, MD, formerly dean of the medical school at the University of Arizona, who had become a senior AAMC administrator, sought to smooth the

AAMC-SACME relationship. He did that well for just short of two years, until his premature death in 1992.

In its early years, SACME had little direct contact with the AMA, though a few SACME members were relatively active because of some other role they filled. Once the AMA established a medical school component in 1977, many SACME members were named by their respective medical school deans to attend AMA meetings. This seemed a constructive step. In 1988, Dennis Wentz, MD, then associate dean and director of CME at Vanderbilt University School of Medicine, became full-time director of the AMA Division of CME. Because Wentz had served as president of SACME, this linkage was highly fortuitous. One of the specific benefits was Wentz's ability to give more visibility to CME concerns within the AMA.

Because it set standards for and judged the quality of institutions that wished to be accredited for CME, the ACCME was always important to SACME. The medical schools themselves, by the operating procedures of the ACCME, were always to receive their accreditation directly from the ACCME. Whenever that organization changed its philosophy, rules, or procedures, the medical schools felt highly interested and occasionally unhappy or threatened. Although SACME was not a parent organization for the ACCME, some SACME members had served as ACCME members or review committee members or had participated in ACCME site visits. Although indirect, relationships always seemed cordial. The small staff of the ACCME was cooperative in making presentations at SACME meetings, and SACME members cooperated with various ACCME tasks.

AHME had a small overlap in membership with SACME, but the activities of the organizations were distinct. Occasional inquiries explored whether the AHME and the ACME might wish to hold meetings jointly with the Society to facilitate scheduling and reduce expenses for persons who were members of both organizations. The ACME interests were allied to SACME, but its mem-

bership was far less narrowly restricted. Many SACME members were also actively involved with the ACME. Occasional conversations looked toward merging SACME with AHME or ACME or both, but the members of the respective organizations seemed to feel that the missions and activities were distinct enough that an actual merger would be inappropriate. After a moderate amount of jockeying, however, SACME joined with the ACME and AHME to sponsor the *Journal of Continuing Education in the Health Professions* (*JCEHP*). This move not only increased the sense of kinship, at least among the leaders of the organizations, but also provided practical support to the *JCEHP* editors and publishers. In the early years of SACME, several committees sought to draft documents that were felt to be important in assisting members or helping outsiders identify the role and the importance of SACME and of CME. Malcolm Watts, MD, had called on members informally in evolving "The Anatomy of CME," published in the first edition of *Mobius* (1981). The *Essentials for Medical College CME* and the *Society Goals for the 80s* were both adopted on May 19, 1981. At the annual meeting the following year (May 18, 1982) the organization adopted *Guidelines for Excellence of Medical College CME*. These documents, meant to assist individual members in their personal work and the work of their respective schools, were seen as major progressive steps regarding the quality of CME, which in turn was viewed by the organization as making a significant contribution to the health and well-being of the nation. These documents and the processes that led to their appearance assisted the organization and its members to an expanded consciousness of their work as an independent discipline and an altruistic force in society.

From its early days, the organization believed in the value of sharing information with the members. The spirit of the retreat groups, so important to the founding of' SACME, served this purpose. A more quantitative mechanism to understand the medical colleges' CME behavior took the form of an annual member survey. For the early years, the questionnaire arose at the University of Nebraska and was subsequently shepherded by R. Van Harrison, PhD, at the University of Michigan. Results from the sometimes complicated questionnaires were ultimately shared with the members. Because of the remarkable variation in the origins and operations of medical school CME units, it was difficult to pose the survey questions so as to draw forth answers from which generalizations could be made. Despite such difficulty, the members welcomed the annual surveys as a means to suggest new ideas or soothe concerns about how closely one's own organization and its activities lay near the mainstream of medical college CME.

Once SACME had become securely established, the desire arose to attempt collective research, especially prompted by the vision and impetus of George Race, MD, during his presidency (1982–1983). Reminding the members that research was an activity especially available to and expected of academic faculties, he predicted that SACME's status, recognition, credibility, and respect could be assisted by performing high quality research. Apart from a sense of obligation, self-seeking, or curiosity, the world of CME needed well-performed research to answer many practical concerns. The nature of SACME with its broad representation from medical schools not only allowed but invited certain kinds of research that would have been difficult to impossible for individual persons or institutions.

Race appointed a research committee headed by Harold Paul, MD, of Rush Medical School as chairman. An emphasis on research also allowed a fuller participation by a number of associate members who had special interest and talents in educational research, an expertise not as clearly present in most of the more senior, clinically oriented voting members. Those especially active and interested in such research included Robert Fox, EdD, Paul Mazmanian, PhD, David Guillion, MD, Nancy Bennett, PhD, Wayne Putnam, MD, Jocelyn Lockyer, PhD, and David Davis, MD,

among many others. A particularly important contribution was the nationwide study of factors that produce change in the knowledge, attitudes, and behavior of physicians. It ultimately found publication as the 1989 monograph *Changing and Learning in the Lives of Physicians* (edited by Fox, Mazmanian, and Putnam). This extensive study, a data-based analysis of the factors that lead physicians to change their patient care procedures, emphasized the value of research to the world of CME and modified much of the subsequent thinking about the environment, methods, and expected outcomes from CME effort. A related activity was a forum that focused on the process and outcomes of Research in CME (RICME). The several RICME conferences were held in alternate years beginning in 1986 in Montreal, organized by Dale Dauphinee and Dave Davis, and again in 1988 in Los Angeles, organized by Phil Manning. The conferences provided a forum for members to illustrate and disseminate their work, plus opportunities to acquire inspiration and methodological finesse from other members. Preparing such conferences and guiding collaborative research under the aegis of SACME are complicated processes, slow to mature; yet the results can be unique, obtainable in no other way, and gratifying to those who have been active in the projects.

The organization's growth continued. The treasurer eventually drew attention to a sobering possibility: the IRS might not look kindly on a supposedly educational/charitable organization with its residual funds and its income exceeding approximately one year's annual expenses. The organization's treasury was not in great hazard of exceeding that amount, but there was a certain pleasant conundrum in reaching the place where such matters needed to be thought about. The use of funds eventually to attract other support to a research-and-development fund remained a pleasing future prospect.

A major purpose of the organization from the outset was to provide professional development opportunities for its members, that is, continuing education for the continuing educators. The programs, therefore, have always dealt with topics of practical importance and attempted to sensitize members to evolving trends and issues. An appropriate mixture of guest and member resource persons, panel discussions, and small group meetings were important modes. Some members wryly observed on occasion that in spite of our andragogic utterances, our format was quite conventional, resembling most other contemporary CME programs, and that, somehow, we should be more oriented to individualized work and problem solving. These considerations, valid though they seemed, made little change in the structure of the programs.

The retreat, which had been so important in catalyzing SACME's formation, continued as an appendage to the regular meetings but subsequently gained a more integral status. The sponsorship of the RICME meetings provided impetus and example as well as techniques and results for all the members but particularly for those with research interests.

Throughout the first 12 years, SACME was able to maintain and secure further its sense of independence while holding discussions about cooperative activities with other organizations, each having its own perspective and needs in the face of considerable overlap of members and functions.

In these early years, SACME was committed to creating a greater visibility and influence for the discipline of CME and also for its members. Before long the organization was serving not only as an ego-booster but also a clearinghouse for information about jobs, career opportunities, status (individually and collectively), and matters dealing with fees and operating budgets. Many problems, in the early years, attracted major attention from the executive committee and the members at general meetings. These involved, for example, accreditation; budgeting (of CME shops, fees for conferences and courses); status and prestige and how these could be obtained by individual CME directors and their offices at their respective schools; adjudicating the proper relationship and loyalty of medical school teachers to the programs of their own institutions; the prestige of the profession of CME in the eyes of faculty colleagues and other organizations; the proper posture of CME toward industry and the appropriate, ethical use of its financial support; and the relationship to other closely allied professional societies.

Among the special task forces or committees established to address timely issues was the important committee charged to study the appropriate relationship between CME purveyors and the potentially conflicting interests of pharmaceutical and manufacturing companies whose attitudes and budgets proved important to the operation of many CME units. SACME members varied in their sensitivity to these potential or direct conflicts of interests. President Race first appointed a group to explore these problematic relationships. By the late 1980s, consciousness of this problem had blossomed fully and the concern spread not only to other medical organizations engaged in CME but became a hot issue in the halls of the Food and Drug Administration (FDA) and even in Congress.

A phenomenon apparent by 1988 was the gradual transition from the relative elitism of members who were directors of medical school CME organizations to a more egalitarian participation of all members. Along with this shift, and partly because of it, the membership quickly grew and changed. The election of associate members, many of whom were not physicians, as officers and directors became prominent. Another gradual change away from CME directors being physician faculty members, led to greater participation and leadership by persons more trained in education, educational research, and administration. Many had extensive work experience in CME and were knowledgeable about operating a medical school CME unit and the relevant persons and procedures needed. This development produced an organization that increasingly exhibited the professional characteristics associated with the broad arena of continuing education. Thus, educational theory and methods, research techniques, learning and behavioral outcomes, leadership and management, and ethical considerations all received increasing attention.

Furthermore, the often transitory trajectories of individuals working in medical school CME became more conspicuous as the 1980s progressed. This evolution and transience is evident, in part, by new members assuming responsibilities; of the 36 persons who attended the 1967 retreat meeting, 18 (50%) were no longer active in this sort of work 20 years later. Many other persons had entered and left the CME arena and SACME in those years. The deaths, retirements, and career changes that accounted for such attrition were accompanied by the previously mentioned greater conspicuousness of persons whose background lay not in medicine but in educational administration, psychology, social work, testing, and marketing.

A mark of maturity appeared in the late 1980s when SACME began to bestow honorary membership on individuals felt deserving of that distinction. The first recipient of such an award was Professor Cyril O. Houle, marking SACME's recognition of outstanding contributions by persons in the general fields of continuing education or in medical education and more specifically in CME.

Throughout SACME's existence, matters of communication and publication have been highly important. Initially, messages to the members consisted of letters. Such mailings contained mainly announcements and arrangements for forthcoming meetings; however, agendas and minutes for both executive committee meetings and general membership meetings were included. At variable intervals a membership directory appeared. By 1987, the newsletter format became transformed into the more formal bulletin *Intercom,* first edited by Harold Paul and assisted by Dene Murray. It contained news items, announcements, information about research, personal items about members, editorial com-

ments, etc. SACME members, acting alone or in small groups, also published articles and editorials in various journals.

In 1981, a journal appeared that was dedicated to "lifelong continuous learning in the health sciences professions." Its title was *Mobius.* Edited by Lucy Ann Geiselman, it was supported and published by the University of California at San Francisco. In 1988, *Mobius* was renamed *Journal of Continuing Education in the Health Professions.* Published commercially, it later became the official journal of SACME, ACME, and AHME. Several SACME members have served on its editorial board.

In 1990, President Robert Cullen established an informal advisory group of the organization's past-presidents. Its official functions were nil: simply meet for breakfast or lunch during the regular meetings and reflect on activities of the organization. Its unofficial function would be to offer reactions and counsel to the current president. This group first convened in San Antonio on the morning following an evening of socializing at a nearby ranch where armadillos and armadillo racing entertained guests. One of the past-presidents suggested the group be called the Armadillo Society, out of regard for the relative sluggishness and unimportance of its members. The aptness of that name found immediate approval, and the group has enjoyed continued existence. Although having no formal status, no authority, and no documented evidence of effectiveness, the anecdotal self-testimony to its diffuse benefit continues to cheer the aging members.

Maturity

The passage of time plus vigorous activity led to a sense of security and accomplishment. Many of the issues that occurred during SACME's period of adolescence continued into a period that might be called *maturity.* But SACME, like any other organization that aspires to continuing life, must continually infuse energy into its being.

The Next 20 Years: 1989–2009

From 1989 through 2009, SACME faced a number of challenging issues. Should SACME open its ranks to those not in medical school CME offices? How could SACME encourage more educational research by its membership? Can SACME engage with the many talented and productive educational researchers working in its respective institutions but not aligned with its CME offices? What can, or even should, be done to more clearly differentiate SACME from the ACME? The then rapidly increasing size of the ACME and the growing sophistication of its annual meeting offered ample opportunity for many CME basics to be learned there. Would this allow SACME meetings to focus on more academically oriented CME pursuits such as researching and developing more effective educational processes, delivery formats, and evaluation mechanisms of CME? (The term *outcomes measurements* was not yet in vogue.) What effect would such a shift in focus have on the current membership, not all of whom had the resources, the mandate, or in some cases the desire to engage in educational research?

SACME's Identity

By the late 1980s and early 1990s, a number of pressures were occurring within SACME that prompted a serious look at how it was perceived and what it represented. Issues of incorporation, changes in membership categories, a name change, bylaws changes, and the need for a more permanent administrative home were being addressed during a series of presidential terms.

The identity of an organization, its interests, membership, and even its reason for being are often communicated through its name and its logo. SACME's original name—the Society for Medical College Directors of Continuing Medical Education—and its acronym—SMCDCME—did not easily roll off the tongue or readily lend itself

to development of a simple, easy-to-identify logo. Numerous unsuccessful efforts were made to develop a satisfactory logo.

While SACME had been granted 501(c)(3) status by the IRS in 1982, it did not benefit from the additional protections offered to a corporation. With plans to develop an endowment and the gradual building of its financial resources as membership and projects expanded, the board decided to seek the safeguards of corporate status for SACME. Following discussions at SACME meetings, advice of counsel, and the guidance of Vice President George Smith, MD, articles of incorporation were filed on May 6, 1992, in Alabama. Alabama was selected because Smith was then dean for CME at the University of Alabama, Birmingham, and, notably, the state offered one of the less complex incorporation processes. President Martin Kantrowitz signed the resolution making the SACME incorporation official as of July 1, 1992.

SACME membership has steadily evolved. Membership was originally composed almost exclusively of deans and directors in medical school CME offices; most were physician-faculty members. Society bylaws were originally adopted to permit membership only to those in medical school CME offices. But over the next decade, there was a gradual shift in membership composition as a new generation of medical school CME leaders was evolving. By the early 1990s, a majority of SACME members were nonphysicians. These were a mix of educators and administrators, sometimes with little or no medical background, hired to manage a nationally accredited CME program.

In 1995, the ACCME developed more-comprehensive accreditation requirements, most of which were, at least initially, organizational or administrative in nature. The administrative demands of the new accreditation standards and the growing perception that CME was becoming a business may have made these roles less attractive to physicians wishing to also maintain a clinical practice, and fewer physicians were stepping into medical school CME leadership.

Gradually, as ACCME accreditation standards grew increasingly sophisticated, more effectively integrating educational methodology with clinical content, and the perspective of physician lifelong learning, this membership tide turned again and more physicians began taking active roles as CME leaders. SACME initiatives and meetings began to focus more on ways to improve CME effectiveness. CME research was starting to move from an interest of a subset of the membership to a primary focus of the organization. Early adaptors in this movement included Barbara Barnes, MD, at the University of Pittsburgh; Ellen Cosgrove, MD, at the University of New Mexico; and Luanne Thorndyke, MD, at Pennsylvania State University. These physicians had decided to make CME, in its more sophisticated sense, a significant part of their careers. As SACME became visible as a more academically oriented organization, nontraditional applications for membership began to arrive. Many of these were from outside the medical school CME Office. The talents and interests of these individuals meshed readily with SACME's evolving direction, but the organizational structure did not permit full membership. New membership categories were needed.

The other major national CME professional organization is the ACME. With the ACME capably handling regular educational and operational needs of CME providers, the SACME leadership struggled to better define itself, its mission, and its focus. One solution gaining support was for SACME meetings to limit operational types of programming and focus on improving the quality and educational outcomes of CME. This movement, towards CME research, required by Canadian medical schools, was only slowly becoming part of the CME consciousness in the United States. A number of US medical schools had already moved ahead in this area, including the University of Pittsburgh and the University of Michigan. Others expressed concerns that they did not have the expertise or resources, or in some cases the desire, to make such change. Gaining acceptance from some members, perhaps not skilled or interested in educational research, was still to come.

A discussion began on how to change the organization's name to more accurately represent this direction. In 1997, President Dave Davis appointed an ad hoc committee to study the issue of a name change. A recommendation was made to change the organization's name to the Society for Academic Continuing Medical Education (SACME), and it was approved in April 1998. The switch from SMCDCME to SACME became official on July 20, 1998.

From its inception, SACME's business affairs were conducted through its board, relying on the secretary-treasurer. As the organization grew, this position required more attention than could reasonably be expected by volunteer effort from an already busy CME professional. However, SACME's resources were not adequate to engage a full-time executive secretariat. In 1988, SACME President Dale Dauphinee's goal was to "take the routine burdens of running a society away from our volunteer officers so that we may spend our efforts . . . seeking new horizons." Through the efforts of Dauphinee and Wentz, SACME accepted a proposal for the AMA to become SACME's first permanent executive secretariat, effective July 1, 1990. The AMA gradually took on duties including support for the executive committee, membership and mailing services, support to the secretary-treasurer, fall meeting registration duties, and assisting Murray with *Intercom*. This continued through mid 1992.

SACME's application for membership in the AAMC CAS was finally approved in 1989. President-elect James Leist and Past President Dauphinee were SACME's first CAS representatives. In 1991, SACME sought to strengthen its position as an academic organization and President Jack Mason negotiated a move of the executive secretariat to the AAMC. Starting on July 1,

1992, SACME's second permanent secretariat was operated from the AAMC Office of Educational Affairs under the guidance of M. Brownell Anderson. Anderson's open, supportive, and cooperative style enabled SACME to further develop its AAMC relationships at multiple levels. Unfortunately, this relationship was not to last, as the AAMC was undergoing internal restructuring. SACME President Meryl Haber was informed that effective the end of 1998 the AAMC would no longer be able to serve as secretariat. Immediate alternate arrangements were needed.

With board approval, the author, then SACME vice president, would house an interim secretariat at the University of Rochester and conduct the search for a new permanent secretariat. With the help of John Boothby of Virginia Commonwealth University, a request for proposal was distributed, and in spring 1999 the board contracted with Prime Management Services (PMS) of Birmingham, Alabama, to be the new executive secretariat. PMS remains our secretariat today under the competent eye of James Ranieri.

The board also charged the interim secretariat to develop a new SACME logo that would include the word *society*, a caduceus, and the name of the organization. The approved logo, still in use today, incorporates a strong, full-bodied S, making it stand out on letterhead and newsletters. Originally adopted in a bright red color, the logo color has shifted to blue. While academic medical centers are generally seen as more liberal, that shift does not appear to have been politically motivated.

Although SACME changed its name, membership was still limited to those in medical school CME offices. There was vigorous debate over just how open membership should be to individuals from nonmedical school CME environments.

Some felt SACME should accept into membership those with interest in academic CME pursuits, regardless as to whether they were from a medical school. The synergies and cross-fertilization of ideas possible with a more diverse membership seemed appropriate to the evolving focus on CME research. Barbara Barnes made a convincing argument in her inaugural *Intercom* article as society president in spring 2001:

> It is . . . evident that we need to establish a vision for our organization, understanding how we can contribute to the development of a new model of continuing professional development for physicians.
>
> SACME has spent a lot of time in the last few years talking about who we are and how we relate to other constituencies in CME. The decision to change our organization's name . . . was based on the realization that we are defined not by where we work but rather by what we do and how we think about our work. What does it mean to be "academic" CME professionals? Certainly this involves more than just providing CME activities and credits. The characteristics of scholarship offer a mechanism for understanding how we might describe our roles and chart our future.

Barnes defined characteristics of scholarship to include discovery, integration, application, teaching, dissemination, reflection and critical evaluation, and commitment to professional standards. She continued:

> Must every SACME member practice all elements of scholarship? Not necessarily. What is needed is a commitment to these principles as well as participation in the areas that are consistent with the strategic interests of one's institution, available resources, and personal areas of expertise. . . . Our future success will be determined by our ability to attract a membership diverse in expertise but united in the commitment to the scholarly practice of CME. . . .

Many equally sincere members felt that such an opening of membership criteria would dilute the original intention and collegial value of the organization. From its inception, SACME was a closely knit organization. Total membership averaged fewer than 150. But the active portion of the membership was considerably smaller; that portion averaged 40 to 60. It was this cadre that regularly attended meetings, staffed committees, and provided the leadership that allowed SACME to develop and prosper. Discussions on redefining membership criteria were held between 1999 and 2001. Throughout this time the membership committee, chaired by Susan (Duncan) Tyler worked with the bylaws committee to develop new membership criteria that were acceptable to the majority of the membership. The following bylaws changes were approved at the fall 2001 meeting:

- A change in membership classification from institutional memberships, with one vote per institution, to individual memberships; eliminating the category of associate membership and permitting an unlimited number of voting members
- Opening membership to interested individuals from any medical college or faculty of medicine accredited by the Liaison Committee for Medical Education (LCME) or branch campus of such an institution
- Opening membership to individuals at academic medical centers, medical specialty organizations, or government agencies whose interests in research and education are consistent with the SACME mission

These changes did not flood SACME with new members. Nor did they result in measurable departure of existing members. The opportunity had been created to move SACME in a new direction. Over the next several years, encouraged by the efforts of SACME presidents Barbara Barnes, Nancy Davis, and Jocelyn Lockyer, membership ranks expanded to include many interested in the scholarly practice of CME as enunciated by Barnes.

While building upon this sophisticated sense of CME, SACME leadership was increasingly approached for perspective on evolving issues and input into policies affecting the national CME environment. Today, SACME leaders are represented in most national CME policy discussions, and the membership is regularly polled to provide grassroots operational perspective.

Leadership and Communications

While SACME's bylaws provide a framework for its operation, its growth, and leadership rotation, there was a need for policies that could provide operational consistency. In the first 11 years of its existence the bylaws were modified five times. Changing bylaws is a cumbersome and inefficient method for what was needed.

Recognizing this need, Past-President R. Van Harrison developed SACME's first policy handbook. Originally released in 1994, the handbook spelled out SACME's growing web of relationships, delineated officer and board member responsibilities, and provided a much needed framework for operational stability and consistency. The policy handbook was updated in 2005 and is now an online resource for all members.

As defined in the original bylaws, the secretary-treasurer was SACME's primary business manager. By the late 1980s, it had become clear that more help was needed, even with some assistance being provided through an executive secretariat. At the spring 1992 meeting, the role of secretary-treasurer was divided into two separate positions: secretary and treasurer.

The 1992 bylaws changes also included a number of other proposals to restructure the leadership track. The new four-year leadership track was defined as vice president, president-elect, president, and immediate past president. Only the vice president position would be voted on each year, with individuals progressing through the track. In addition, the nominating committee would be required to identify *at least one candidate* for each vacant position, paralleling nominating procedures in other organizations. This has evolved so the vice president position has a single nominee each year.

The complexion of an organization with officers in place for a fixed period will often shift, sometimes dramatically, with the issues of the day and the characteristics of those in leadership roles. Though lasting only a single year, every presidential term has its own pressures, with decisions and consequences driven by the personality of the incumbent. The intent of a more clearly defined leadership track was to try to minimize significant policy shifts, as well as to be a training ground for subsequent presidents. At its October 31, 1997, meeting, President-Elect Haber presented a draft resolution to the board that suggested restricted eligibility criteria for CME accreditation and asked for the board's endorsement. The board declined to endorse the resolution but appointed a task force, to be chaired by Haber, to revise and resubmit for further consideration. This resolution or white paper, as it would become known, would go through several revisions. During the next two years, it created such strife within SACME and placed pressures on its leadership to the point of dividing the membership and stifling progress on other important initiatives. The nine signatories of the original white paper, all SACME members, challenged the ACCME position regarding eligibility for accreditation. It was their opinion that:

the ACCME must adopt minimal standards of eligibility and limit accreditation to the medical institutions licensed by the state and responsible for undergraduate medical education and postgraduate resident training, as well as the specialty societies and state medical societies that comprise the medical profession.

Risks and benefits of endorsement were laid out in a letter to the membership by President John Parboosingh, MD, in June 1999. Ultimately, SACME leadership would not formally endorse the white paper but suggested that each member pursue whatever actions his or her own conscience and individual school would approve.

In 1997, Deborah Danoff, MD, joined the AAMC as assistant vice president in the division of medical education with responsibility to define

CME within medical education. As the AAMC moved to incorporate aspects of CME within is structure, Danoff would become an advocate of CME and advisor to SACME's leadership. With the SACME objective to align itself within the academic community, the invitation from the AAMC to formally participate in the Group on Educational Affairs (GEA) presented a great opportunity. The first step was to define the CME section and how it would relate to the GEA. Nancy Bennett was elected the first chair of the newly formed CME section of the AAMC GEA.

The broad range of issues facing SACME was more than could be meaningfully covered during the normal board meetings. Time was needed for greater reflection and long range planning. Thus an annual SACME leadership retreat was begun in 1998.

Strategic Planning

SACME had evolved from informal small group meetings to a national organization espousing standard setting, professional development, and CME research. Periodic strategic planning reviews were needed for SACME to remain viable. One goal of President Robert Cullen, MD, was to involve the membership in every phase of the strategic planning process:

Our Society has grown and changed. . . . It is now time to re-examine the organization, its mission and our expectations. . . . Is the Society still in "sync" with the environment? . . . We must make sense of our past if we hope to manage our future.

In 1987, a strategic planning exercise was initiated by George Smith, and on October 1, 1989, the Report of the Strategic Planning Committee was published. The report included seven goals, each with implementation objectives. Its recommendations helped guide the next decade of SACME growth.

In 1995, under President Gloria Allington, University of Miami, SACME published "Future Directions for Medical College Continuing Medical Education." This report set a vision for medical college CME that included the following concepts: CME leaders who are scholar-practitioners; alliances that are working linkages; contributions to undergraduate and graduate curricula; enhancement of CME's role with biomedical research.

Under Van Harrison, the board created a task force on CME and health-care reform and charged it with bringing together national organizations involved with future CME policy. The task force produced a position paper titled "The Connection between CME and Health Care Reform." Special recognition went to Stephen Jay, MD, William Easterling, MD, and Allington. The task force on CME and health-care reform was stewarded through various committees of the AAMC, AMA, and ACCME. It also became the basis for resolutions in multiple states to incorporate support for CME "as central to the provision (of) patient care of the highest possible quality."

This task force drafted a set of principles to define educational essentials that would foster quality, nurture innovation, and emphasize flexibility while requiring observance of ethical standards. The final proposal also suggested reaccreditation by self-study. The proposal was well received by the AAMC and the ACCME, and the effort helped to strengthen relationships with colleagues at ACME and AHME.

Communications

The evolution of *JCEHP* has been mentioned earlier in this article. In 1998, Mazmanian became the editor. Lockyer started a movement in 1992 to include *JCEHP* into Index Medicus and, in 2001, the National Library of Medicine recommended *JCEHP* be included. In 2006, *JCEHP* was accepted by the International Science Index (ISI) for coverage in Current Contents/Clinical Medicine. ISI is the recognized authority for evaluating journals providing systematic, objective means to evaluate impact on the global research community. Under Mazmanian's editorial leadership, an electronic version of *JCEHP* became available in 2002.

The *Intercom* is a key SACME publication. Past President Harold Paul completed a five-year tenure as *Intercom* editor in spring 1992. Then Rosalie Lammle, of the University of Utah, became editor, supported by Lockyer and Deborah Jones. Their era took the newsletter from four to 12 pages per issue. This "troika" was succeeded as *Intercom* editors in 1994 by Jean Bryan, of the University of Tennessee, and Carol Malone, of the University of Alabama at Huntsville. In 2001, following a short term by Mark Gelula, of the University of Illinois at Chicago, Joyce Fried, of UCLA, became editor, and in 2002 *Intercom* production responsibility shifted to the SACME executive secretariat. Melinda Steele, Texas Tech UHSC, became editor in 2005, followed in 2007 by David Pieper, Wayne State University, and in 2009 by Melissa Newcomb, University of Rochester. The *Intercom* has continued to be a high quality newsletter, available in both print and electronic formats, providing timely news and event information. Much appreciation goes to www.CMEinfo.com for their long-term grant support of *Intercom*, enabling production of the print version.

In 1995 under the leadership of Robert Bollinger, PhD, Wayne State University, SACME first initiated its Internet Listserv. The Listserv remains at Wayne State, currently administered by David Pieper, PhD. In 2000, a SACME Web site took shape under the leadership of Bollinger. It was designed to have both a public section to enhance the organization's image and a members only section for more confidential materials. Substantial development and attention were provided to the Web site for several years on a volunteer basis by Anne Taylor-Vaisey, MLS. She was awarded an honorary SACME membership in 2001 for her longstanding efforts. Since 2004, Listserv administration has been assisted by the executive secretariat. With leadership from Joyce Fried and Taylor-Vaisey, SACME opened its new content management system Web site in 2007.

In 2000, Vice President Jack Kues assembled a task force to better coordinate the various communication vehicles and examine SACME's information needs. This task force, in 2002, formally became the SACME Communications Committee.

SACME Awards

In 1990, an awards committee was appointed to recognize members with long-standing history of contributions to the organization. In 1991, Malcolm Watts was presented with SACME's First Distinguished Service Award: "Dr. Watts was greatly instrumental in the formation of SMCDCME and served as President of the Society and in many other capacities, particularly in its formative years."

Phil Manning retired on June 30, 2002. Because he was the first president of SACME, a mentor to many, and an inspiration to three generations of CME professionals, SACME recognized Manning's contributions by creating the Manning Award for Research in CME, first awarded in 2001. Subsequent years would see other awards, such as Lifelong Advisor Awards.

SACME Finances and Development of the Research Endowment

In 1990, under President Leist, a development and endowment committee was formalized. Originally established by President Wentz in 1987, it was intended to help meet the research committee's request for resources to support CME research.

In 1993, President Harrison directed treasurer Lambiase to develop five separate funds to administer SACME's growing resources. These included the audio digest endowment (funded by $30,000 from the Audio Digest Foundation) to support spring meeting speakers; the CME congress account to manage and provide seed funds for CME congresses; the research committee fund for funds from or for research committee activities; the reserve fund to develop strategic operating reserves; and a donor restricted research endowment to fund CME research grants. Initial contributors to this fund included Abbott Laboratories; Ciba Geigy Corporation; Genentech,

Inc.; Glaxo Wellcome; Hoechst Marion Roussel; Merck & Company; and Pharmacia and Upjohn, Inc. All contributions were invested to provide resources for funding CME research initiatives.

Professional Meetings

SACME traditionally organizes two annual meetings: fall and spring. The fall meeting is held in conjunction with the AAMC annual meeting because some SACME members hold various positions in their medical schools having involvement with undergraduate and residency training, as well as CME.

This collaboration has had advantages and challenges. On the positive side, convening with the AAMC offers the opportunity to meet with multiple professional groups during the same trip; provides a broader understanding of multifaceted issues facing medical education in general; allows access to prominent national speakers, often beyond the means of a small society; and permits interaction with our deans on professional levels away from our schools.

These advantages are offset by our small society group being overwhelmed by AAMC attendance, which is in the thousands. The logistics of finding nonconflicting meeting times and space also force SACME to meet in advance of the AAMC. Meeting times are often limited, constraining content. And, there are two conference registration fees, as the AAMC requires that attendees of all affiliated convening meetings pay the AAMC fee. As expressed by more than one member, "The meeting was too big, and too much was going on without time for reflection." While this has occasionally been a contentious issue, SACME leadership has consistently decided to follow this tradition, as the advantages of integrating SACME and its members into the broader environment of academic medical education are very valuable.

The spring SACME meeting has traditionally been the time when our membership has focused on its own needs. Meeting schedules are more leisurely, allowing much needed time for reflection and dialoging with colleagues. The various committees and task forces are given adequate time to grapple with their current issues face-to-face, after communicating much of the rest of the year by phone, electronic, or other means. This is the time for the all-important relationship building and camaraderie that in so many ways is responsible for the close-knit sense and easy sharing of ideas that permeates and adds much value to SACME.

CME Congresses

The first CME congress, which combined with the third RICME, was organized in 1988 with the guiding influence of Manning. In addition to SACME, the congress was mounted in cooperation with seven other participating sponsors: the ACCME, ACME, AMA Council on Medical Education, AHME, the Council of Medical Specialty Societies, and RICME. The thinking behind the congress was to bring together all the organizations active in CME. This was patterned after Digestive Disease Week, an annual coming together of various organizations in gastroenterology. Subsequent congresses have also been organized with multiple (although not always the same) sponsors.

Davis captured some of the essence of this meeting in an *Intercom* article shortly after the first congress.

The dichotomy in CME was probably best reflected in the wide variety of learning and teaching experiences provided by the Congress. At one point, I found myself writing notes, medical school style, about high-tech video discs and artificial intelligence. And there were, of course, lectures to 50 or 300 people about how individual physicians learn and change, and personal continuing education programs.

A major flavor of the Congress was the emergence into the realm of possibility of competency-assessment measures introduced regularly and in a mandatory way into physicians' lives, and subsequent, targeted remedial CME, forged in the nursery in

adult-learning theory, that the physician must himself determine his own learning needs and seek ways to meet them.

The reality . . . is that these conflicting approaches will remain . . . (I)t is this tension, and the intense commitment to excellence, which the Congress represented, that will push CME forward . . . towards full professional recognition, maturity, and the 21st century.

The question of how frequently to hold CME congresses was raised by President Dauphinee immediately after the first congress. The conflicting needs and meeting schedules of various sponsoring organizations, including our own, would generate much debate. Based on rapid advances in CME and frequent changes in accreditation and regulatory constraints, a decision was made to organize a CME congress every four years.

Cooperation with Industry Conferences

On August 28, 1987, members of the SACME Committee on Cooperation with Industry met in New Orleans with representatives of several commercial companies. As stated by meeting chair and Past President Gail Bank, MD:

The purpose of the meeting is to provide a forum where key officers of selected pharmaceutical companies and selected members of the Society can exchange information on particular operating and business characteristics and continuing medical education objectives. We hope in this way that we can identify and enhance opportunities for mutual cooperation.

In 1989, the SACME Committee on Cooperation with Industry, chaired by Martin Shickman, MD, of UCLA, with assistance from Joseph D'Angelo, of Tulane; Lee Yerkes, of Marion Merrill Dow; and Ruth Glotzer, of Tufts, among many others, initiated a discussion to promote understanding between CME providers and the pharmaceutical industry. In the early 1990s, the FDA began to express concerns about drug promotion under the guise of CME. This led to a national conference on Industry/CME Collaboration, jointly sponsored by SACME, AMA, and AAMC. The ACCME and ACME were co-sponsors.

Called a landmark conference and themed "Relationships in Transition," it was held in August 1990 and devoted to developing a consensus on standards that would help govern future activities. SACME members Shickman and Cullen, working directly with the AMA, were instrumental in this effort. This would give SACME national prominence as it provided a platform for these discussions, broader ethics in CME, and related accreditation issues.

The task force on CME provider and industry collaboration was born at this conference, with members of the SACME Committee on Cooperation with Industry forming the core of the task force, and Past Presidents Wentz and Cullen serving as co-chairmen. As reported by Cullen, this collaboration of CME providers and the pharmaceutical industry soon resulted in recommendations to the ACCME, eventually leading to new guidelines for commercial support of CME. Said Cullen, "Our Society has played a major role in this accomplishment." The issue of industry support, in various forms and stoked by different organizations, has remained a hot point through the first decade of the 21st century, and the annual conferences continue to be held each fall hosted by the AMA.

Directly or indirectly, SACME has been involved with numerous other meetings and activities related to CME. Such involvement has been substantial, as with the Mayo Consensus Conference and the Conjoint Committee on CME. Special SACME efforts include the summer research institutes organized by the SACME research committee and, beginning in 2010, a summer leadership institute.

The Tri-Group
In the late 1980s, SACME leaders began meetings with counterparts from the ACME and AHME to explore initiatives of mutual interest. It was orig-inally established as an informal group to oversee the *JCEHP* administrative board. Oversight of the recurring CME congresses was added to the Tri-Group's expanding role. Leadership rotated annually between the three organizations. SACME continued to administer the CME congress fund, as it had originated as just a SACME venture. Ultimately, this fund was discontinued and the balance divided between the Tri-Group members. Tri-Group meetings continue as a means for these groups to exchange ideas.

Research Initiatives
SACME's Canadian members have been consistently more involved with CME research because it is part of the accreditation requirements and mission of their medical schools. The past two decades, however, have seen considerable increase in CME research in US medical schools. SACME's role has been instrumental in this change. Research was one of the committees named in the early SACME bylaws. Although this acknowledged SACME founders' recognition of its importance and potential value, CME research efforts were often limited to a small number of schools with deans or directors possessing the interest, training, and/or resources to implement such efforts.

In 1988, one of President Dauphinee's goals was to encourage SACME and its members to develop new research initiatives in CME. Agreement was reached for SACME to initiate and publish the Change Study: *Changing and Learning in the Lives of Physicians.* Royalties from sale of this volume were donated to SACME, placed in a research committee fund, and used to help underwrite other SACME research projects including the periodic summer research institutes.

Research Endowment Council
By 1994 the research endowment fund was established and the research endowment council was formed to administer this fund. It was initially chaired by Brian O'Toole. By 1996, the coun-

cil had developed its procedures and generated enough funds through its investments to start making awards.

Research Grants and Fellowships

Proposals were solicited beginning in winter 1996. The first two $5,000 awards were announced at the Richmond meeting. These went to Stephen Jay and a combined award to Lisa Cariaga-Lo, MD, and James Leist. In 1997, the first fellowship in CME research was awarded to David Bailey from Marshall University.

Two awards in honor of long-standing members continue. The Phil R. Manning Award offers $50,000 for a two-year CME research project. One award is given every other year. The Robert Fox Award is given to the best abstract presented at the periodic RICME meetings. The first Manning Award was given in 2001 to Yvonne Coyle, MD, University of Texas, Southwestern Medical Center. The first winner of the Fox Award was Michael Allen, MD, Dalhousie University.

Summer Research Institutes

Every second year, research institutes are sponsored by the SACME research committee. Generally hosted at one of the Canadian medical schools, these five-day retreats provide a comprehensive opportunity to obtain a practical foundation in CME research skills and utilize them in the design of a CME research project. Curriculum includes framing research questions, experimental design, critical appraisal of literature, designing questionnaires, integration of qualitative and quantitative data, and other areas. Participants are encouraged to present their completed projects at an upcoming CME congress.

Special Research Projects

In October 1992, SACME received a professional services contract from the Center for Health Statistics to develop a CME instructional module for certifying the cause of death. This death certificate project, initiated by Leist and spearheaded

by O'Toole, would help place SACME on the national stage.

In 1997, President Davis reported that the Robert Wood Johnson organization had funded a $450,000 grant to assess CME needs in the managed care environment. The project was jointly sponsored by SACME and the Medical Group Management Association. The research committee would administer the program and identify 10 medical schools to participate.

Summary

The increasingly complex CME regulatory environment has created challenges and opportunities for SACME. Members continue to be well represented on ACCME committees and as reviewers, as well as involved in national policy discussions. Although some members have decided to leave the CME field altogether, voicing frustrations with the evolving state of affairs, others have risen to the challenge, becoming immersed in outcomes methodologies and, like Past President Nancy Davis, helping to pave the way for a new CME world. Many others are working hard to understand and meet accreditation standards, while also struggling to integrate these standards within their own institutions.

A significant part of the changing CME environment is the movement to restrict, or even eliminate, the use, and therefore ostensibly the influence, of industry funding of CME. While not a direct influence on SACME itself, such a change would have a potentially dramatic effect on individual members, constraining operations and discretionary resources, the type of resources used to participate in professional society meetings and supporting activities.

The effects of broadening the membership have been positive, adding depth and sophistication to the organization. The leadership track has continued to function as designed, minimizing, though not eliminating, organizational policy shifts. Personalities strong enough to achieve senior leadership positions are often also able and willing to move in independent directions, not always with totally positive results. SACME continues to weather such fluctuations and grow.

Over the past several years, there has been a substantial shift in how SACME is viewed nationally. From its inception, its members have been active on the national scene and have participated in countless initiatives to move the field of CME forward. These efforts were generally due to the talents or interests of the individuals. And, although they were SACME members, each acted independently, representing only themselves, or perhaps their institution's perspectives. More recently, SACME has been called upon as an organization to provide perspectives representative of its membership. Such recognition is a significant compliment to the esteem in which the Society is held. It is also an obligation—to be sure that its leadership's responses are indeed representative.

CME is both a social and an intellectual good with a strong humanistic heritage. SACME members are individually and through the auspices of their institutions responsible in considerable measure for protecting and transmitting that legacy. This they have done and with guidance and effort will continue to do.

Note

1. R. M. Caplan, "History of the Society of Medical College Directors of Continuing Medical Education (SMCDCME): The First Twelve Years," *Journal of Continuing Education in the Health Professions* 16 (1996): 14–24.

The Alliance content authored by Harry A. Gallis;
AHME content authored by Robert K. Richards,
David R. Pieper, Thomas C. Gentile, Jr., Robert
L. Tupper, and Brian W. Little; CACHE content
authored by Jill Donahue and Bernard A. Marlow

CHAPTER 13

Organizations of Continuing Medical Education Professionals: The Alliance for Continuing Medical Education, the Association for Hospital Medical Education, and the Canadian Association for Continuing Health Education

This chapter highlights the role and development of three of the key organizations that support and foster continuing medical education (CME) in the United States and Canada. The history of the fourth—the Society for Academic CME, the sponsoring organization behind this book—is found in chapter 12. Within these four organizations, individuals committed to fostering the field of CME have found homes for their professional growth and development. Their individual stories are important to understand the foundations of CME in the United States and Canada.

The Alliance for Continuing Medical Education

The Alliance for Continuing Medical Education (the Alliance) is the largest membership organization for continuing medical education (CME) professionals in the world (2,465 individuals in 2009), with the majority of members from the United States and Canada.[1] The Alliance continues to have an open membership to all persons working in CME and related fields, including those in the pharmaceutical industry. Throughout the years, the Alliance annual conference has begun to approach and occasionally exceed 2,000 registrants and is easily the largest CME-focused

meeting, offering a forum for education for all persons interacting within the CME field.[2]

In 1994, on the occasion of its 20-year anniversary, the board of directors of the Alliance commissioned internist William Campbell Felch, MD, to write a personal history and to conduct a series of interviews with the key players in the early history of the Alliance. This is well chronicled in the 1996 publication *The Alliance for Continuing Medical Education: The First 20 Years* and the accompanying series of audiotape interviews conducted by Felch. Other than touching on a few of these highlights, this chapter focuses on a 15-year period beginning in 1995.

Key Events in the History of the Alliance and Their Impact on CME

The Alliance originated on December 12, 1974, at the Princeton Club of New York with organization and support provided by Lewis Miller of Miller and Fink Corporation, publisher of the magazine *Patient Care*. This initial invitational meeting included 36 individuals from academia, industry, medical practice, the government, and organized medicine to function as somewhat of a think tank for the nascent field of CME. The format was small group round table discussions followed by reporting in plenary sessions and consensus building. This group developed a specific charge for the new organization: "To identify, and promote the implementation of, a rational, pluralistic, and coordinated system of CME, for the purpose of enabling practicing physicians to be optimally effective in the delivery of patient care."[3] Following this initial meeting, a steering committee representing the major stakeholders was formed and included Felch; Joseph Gonella of Jefferson Medical College; Michael Goran of the Bureau of Quality Assurance, US Department of Health, Education, and Welfare; Miller; Tom Stern, American Academy of Family Practice (representative for specialty societies); and Dick Wilbur of Baxter Laboratories. This degree of representation continues to this day and is one of the essential characteristics of the Alliance as well as the concept that the Alliance should act as a catalyst for stimulating change and advancement within the field. Each member of the steering committee served as chair of the following six task forces: defining needs (Gonella), financing (Wilbur), coordination and planning (Miller), structuring programs (Felch), methods of evaluation (Goran), and methods of motivation (Stern).

The reports of these task forces formed the core for the first annual conference and invitational held in Atlanta from February 29 through March 1, 1976. One hundred three people attended and the core activity for the participants resulted in the development of the following six priorities for action: research linking CME to physician competence and to patient care; competence-based core curricula by specialty; uniform standards for program accreditation; establishment of a clearinghouse for CME materials and courses; development of a CME systems model; and research into physician nonparticipation in CME.

In 1978, the steering committee made the decision to convert the organization into a dues paying membership organization with approxi-

mately 100 initial members. This step led to a philosophic change in the intent of the organization, moving more in the direction of supporting and educating CME practitioners, resulting in the drifting away of a substantial number of the original group. Felch was appointed the first executive vice president, a part-time paid position, followed by Frances Maitland in 1991 in a full-time capacity. These executives provided substantial administrative support to the organization and its board and officers while overseeing the planning and implementation of annual conferences and other educational activities. Malcolm Watts, MD, University of California at San Francisco, was elected as the first president of the Alliance in 1979, which apparently was concurrent with his presidency of the Society of Medical College Directors of CME (now known as the Society for Academic CME [SACME]). It should be noted that, in the history of CME in North America, the work and influence of these two organizations is highly overlapping because of overlapping memberships and that many individuals have served as board members and officers of both organizations.

The concept of collaboration among the three CME membership organizations in the United States—the Alliance, SACME, and the Association for Hospital Medical Education (AHME)—was pushed forward originally by Robert Richards, PhD, the Alliance's second president. The three organizations continue to meet as the Tri-Group and have long partnered in sponsoring CME congresses and, most productively, as co-owners of the *Journal of Continuing Education in the Health Professions* (*JCEHP*), which was founded in 1981 and originally called *Mobius*. Watts became editor in 1985 and the journal's name changed in 1988. Watts authored the lead article in *Mobius* in 1981, the report of a SACME task force titled "An Anatomy of Continuing Medical Education," which delineated a possible body of knowledge for the field of CME. The journal has assumed a position of prominence in continuing education spheres and is, to this day, the preferred publication modality for CME professionals as well as those providing continuing education to other health professionals.

While the journal has the broad focus of continuing education in the health professions, the Alliance has continued, not without substantial debate, to focus on continuing medical education, even as medical practice has become a more interdisciplinary venture. Throughout the years of its existence, the Alliance has contemplated on numerous occasions an expansion into nursing, pharmacy, dentistry, allied health, and even veterinary medicine. The prevailing sentiment, even in the interviews conducted by Felch in 1994 and 1995, has been to maintain a broad view of patient care issues but to focus primarily on physician education.

Two significant events occurred during the presidency of Jim Leist (1995–1996). The first Alliance history was published and Maitland retired as executive director. Following an extensive search, Bruce Bellande, PhD, was hired and served in this role for the ensuing 10 years, moving the Alliance offices to Birmingham, Alabama, and overseeing the first significant expansion of staff. Following the hiring of Bellande, the Alliance continued a steady increase in growth and influence in the field of CME during the presidencies of Joe Green, Mel Freeman, and Don Moore. Annual conferences through the 1990s and into the 21st century focused on many of the critical issues facing physicians and the evolution of CME, specifically (1) the rising role of quality improvement in medical practice and the necessity for the involvement of CME professionals in the process; (2) increased government scrutiny of industry funding of CME; (3) dramatic changes in the Accreditation Council for CME (ACCME) accreditation requirements; (4) challenges to CME providers to demonstrate the value and influence of CME within the broad structure of medical practice; and (5) the increasing requirements for physicians to participate in maintenance of licensure and maintenance of board certification through demonstration of performance in practice.

Beginning with the first annual meeting,

which was based on the six priorities for action, most of the Alliance annual conferences have had a topical focus and were structured around broad topic areas that later evolved into a competency-based structure. The Alliance has a long history of attempting to delineate a set of competencies that define the field of CME, beginning in the presidency of Kevin Bunnell in the late 1980s. This initial set of competencies was partially informed by a group of "quality elements for the health professions."[4] Topic areas operational at the time of the 2003 initiative consisted of strategic leadership, accreditation, needs assessment, objectives setting, educational activities design and delivery, evaluation, program management, personal skills, and health-care delivery systems.

In order to expand and update these areas, the Alliance launched a new multi-year effort initiated by Leist and a committee chaired by Ellen Cosgrove, who authored the current iteration of the competencies, followed by a task force led by Richard V. King, PhD, and Sterling North, supervised and moved forward by Bellande, to assess this new competency set and to make it most relevant to the current practice environment. Their initiative established numerous panels of individual experts in a variety of competency areas, and embarked on modified Delphi process to solicit, rank, establish, and validate what members of the profession regard as the principal work of CME. These eight competency areas, which debuted at the 2005 annual conference, are comprised of 48 specific competencies forming the backbone for the current content of Alliance activities. The following key competency areas can be found in detail on the Alliance Web site:[5]

- *Adult/Organizational Learning Principles:* Comprehend evidenced-based adult and organizational learning principles that improve the performance and outcomes of the physician learner and the organizations in which they work.
- *Educational Interventions:* Apply and improve educational interventions using evidence-

based adult and organizational learning principles in appropriate contexts (learners, content, and settings) that produce expected results for the physician learners and the organizations in which they work.

- *Performance Measurement:* Use appropriate data to assess two components: (1) educational—the success of learning interventions, especially physician performance (CME activities)—and (2) administrative—the performance of the CME program.
- *Systems Thinking:* Recognize that physicians and CME professionals are part of a complex healthcare system with processes, other health providers and patients that must be considered in providing learning interventions.
- *Partnering:* Identify and collaborate with key partners and stakeholders in accomplishing their CME mission.
- *Leadership:* Provide leadership for the CME program that emphasizes continuous improvement, professionalism, and appropriate ethical practice.
- *Administration/Management:* Manage office operations to meet personnel, finance, legal, logistical, and accreditation standards.
- *Self Assessment and Life Long Learning:* Continually assess individual and organizational performance and make improvements through relevant learning experiences.

Each of the competency areas is followed by a group of performance indicators and knowledge, skills, and attitudes that form the basis for self assessment (as predicted by Felch in 1996) and educational activity design and may be adapted for varying levels of experience and expertise. The Alliance annual meeting is structured around these competency areas. In addition, the Alliance continues to produce several offerings for persons new to CME and these are also structured around some of the core elements within the competencies.

In addition to issues in the external medical practice and political environment, the Alliance board, around the turn of the millennium, began to benchmark its governance structure with that of other not-for-profit organizations resulting in a revision of its by-laws and policies and procedures for operations. In 2007, with a change in executive leadership, the Alliance board made a decision to look outside of CME to the field of association management for its next executive director, and Paul Weber, MA, who had strong association experience with the New Jersey Medical Society and the California Medical Association, was hired as its third full-time executive director.

This change in leadership occurred at the conclusion of an in-depth strategic planning process in 2005 and 2006 during which the board selected nine major initiatives aimed at ensuring that the Alliance would continue to provide value to its membership. These initiatives were grouped into four strategic imperatives: (1) advancing CME as a profession, (2) transforming knowledge into practice, (3) creating connections among colleagues and stakeholders, and (4) allocating resources prudently and effectively.

In advancing CME as a profession, the board felt strongly that the term *CME professional* required more specificity, especially around issues of ethical practices in CME as well as the general standards defining the core competencies within the profession. Simultaneously, the independent group the Commission for Certification of CME Professionals promoted the concept of CME certification through a standardized examination. This issue has been at the heart of discussions by Alliance founders and subsequent leadership since the 1970s, always evoking impassioned arguments pro and con. At a crossroads again in 2007, the Alliance board made the decision to focus on defining the core competencies in CME, providing education around these competencies, and leaving certification examinations to others.

The two goal areas of the Alliance at the heart of the Alliance as an organization continued to be education and professional development and providing an arena for the exchange of ideas through "transforming knowledge into practice" and "creating connections among colleagues and stakeholders."[6] One of the long-standing issues in the board's discussions was that the organization had only two major sources of revenue: annual membership fees and the annual conference. Diversification of revenue streams was seen as crucial to the growth and strengthening of the association. At the core of diversifying and expanding the revenue base was the development and implementation of a competency based curriculum, making the Alliance the education home for CME professionals.

As part of the 2006 strategic plan and advancing CME as a profession, the Alliance established a procedure for the development and promotion of position statements on critical issues in CME as well as occasional situations arising within the broader medical education environment. For the first time in its history, a communication-media specialist was hired as a consultant. The first foray into this arena was a meeting on Capitol Hill of members of the executive committee with key staff of the Senate Finance Committee to discuss the issue of industry funding and influence in CME and to better position the Alliance as a knowledgeable source of information and expertise in such issues. This meeting was followed by the first of a national series of stakeholder meetings with staff and volunteer leadership of key organizations involved in the CME enterprise, initially leading to Alliance solidification of its stance on CME certification.

It should also be noted that members of the profession have always played a key role in devising and setting the standards for CME accreditation. With the strong ties of Wilbur and Maitland to the ACCME predecessor organization (the Liaison Committee for Continuing Medical Education), developing and meeting accreditation standards has made up a significant portion of the content of Alliance educational activities. In 1996, the Tri-Group published an extensive set of recommendations for a new group of accredita-

tion standards, which were heavily incorporated into System98.[7] It should also be noted, as outlined by Felch in the first Alliance history, that the concept of a new paradigm for CME was a substantial part of the Alliance annual conference in 1994, and the tenets of the article authored by Moore, Green, Leist, Maitland, and Stephen Jay, MD, are at the heart of the updated ACCME criteria of 2006.[8] CME practitioners, whether members of the Alliance, SACME, or AHME, are heavily involved in the board and committees of the ACCME and continue to influence accreditation policy, oversight, and regulation. Substantial portions of Alliance educational activities continue to be devoted to accreditation standards.

The major challenge to the new executive director and to the Alliance Professional Development Committee was to expand the educational business lines of the Alliance outside of the annual conference such that increased revenue generation could lead to an overall expansion of the variety of educational activities available to the membership, especially in the realm of electronic media. In 2005, the Alliance embarked on a series of educational Webinars highlighting topics such as grantsmanship and pharmaceutical educational grants, followed in 2007 by the updated ACCME accreditation criteria and the integration of CME and quality improvement. These types of activities have proven to be immensely popular with members, allowing groups to convene locally without the expense of travel and time away from work.

In addition to enhancements to the types of educational activities offered, Alliance leadership also embarked on an initiative to transform the annual conference from an abstract driven meeting to one that better meets the competency-based needs of the membership through more small group and participative learning workshops and intensives.

This leads to the issue of leadership in CME and, indeed, that of leadership in the entire field of medical education. From the beginning of the organization, physician and nonphysician leadership has been balanced within the Alliance and CME in general. During the last decade, with the evolution of medical practice in the clinical practice arena, hospitals, and medical schools, it has become more difficult for physicians to devote substantive time to administrative issues such as leading a large CME enterprise. Initially blamed on managed care in the early 1990s, physicians in academia, as well as in private practice, continue to be pressured by the demands to serve more patients in less time, leaving little opportunity for administrative roles—volunteer or paid. Recognizing these pressures in the most recent strategic plan, the Alliance created a physician's leadership task force to explore issues relating to physicians in the practice of CME and to determine what if anything could be done to recruit more physicians into leadership positions within the enterprise as well as into the Alliance itself. Chaired initially by Alejandro Aparicio, MD, of the American Medical Association (AMA), and subsequently by Harry Gallis, MD, the task force made a number of recommendations that were adopted by the Alliance board in 2009. The core elements of the recommendations were to identify mechanisms to ensure significant physician representation on the board; to identify and promote stronger linkages with physicians currently active in CME within specialty and state medical societies, many of whom do not belong to or participate within the Alliance; and to partner more strongly with others such as the Annenberg CME Leadership Initiative to explore ways to develop physician involvement and leadership in CME. The parallel decision by the Alliance to move from a two-year to a one-year presidency may possibly allow more physician board members to seek this leadership position as the time commitment will not be so onerous in the future.

Other Issues in the National CME Environment and Their Impact on the Alliance

Because the Alliance is a membership organization and has no regulatory authority, it is difficult for it as an organization to impact the geopolitical environment of medicine and health care. The organization may make consensus statements on issues such as industry funding in CME but, other than the influence and/or power of its individual members, it acts primarily as a reporter and convener in the environment. The breadth of its membership base is viewed by its leadership as both a strength and a weakness. The Alliance functions today much as it did when conceived by its founding members, as a convener of stakeholders and a forum where all voices can be heard. It adds value to the field by supporting an academic journal; helping to define, focus, and educate CME practitioners; and supporting the improved capacity of its members to positively affect physicians' practices and patient care.

The Association for Hospital Medical Education

The initial meeting of about 20 directors of medical education (DMEs) in conjunction with the 1956 AMA Congress on Medical Education and their decision to form a national organization (then, the Association of Hospital Directors of Medical Education) evolved from World War II and postwar changes affecting medical education. During World War II, medical schools accelerated their teaching programs to produce more physicians to meet wartime requirements, and graduates were inducted immediately into the military services rather than taking a rotating internship and entering general practice as had been common during the pre-war years. Once in the military, physicians were assigned to specialty-organized services and gained life-changing experience in caring for the wounded.

After 1945, thousands of physicians, whose training had been interrupted by the war, provided willing applicants for postwar specialty residencies. The AMA Council on Medical Education and the Association of American Medical Colleges (AAMC) urged medical schools and hospitals to establish new residencies and to expand existing ones. Patriotic motivation to meet physician-veterans' training needs, growth in hospital volume and services, and concern about physician shortages led many community hospitals to establish specialty residencies in addition to their rotating internships.

The number of hospitals approved for residency training doubled from 587 in 1940 to 1,079 in 1950, and available residency positions increased from 5,120 to 18,669 over the same decade. In 1947, the AMA Council suggested that residency positions be reduced after the postwar demand by physician-veterans subsided and that some newly developed residencies be retained to educate physicians from foreign countries who wanted advanced training in the United States. The Exchange-Visitor program began in 1949 as the AMA began to report a surplus of residency positions. However, specialty residencies continued to grow, stimulated by increased hospital service requirements, institutional prestige, the higher status and earnings of specialists and the NIH-powered growth of biomedical knowledge. By the late 1950s, graduate medical education (GME) had evolved from a process that, before the war, prepared a few elite specialists to one in which a majority of current graduates pursued specialty education for three to five years after earning their medical degree.

Community teaching hospitals were faced with actively recruiting allopathic graduates from US medical schools for their residencies, screening foreign graduates applying through the Exchange-Visitor program, and managing a growing medical education enterprise. That led some to appoint a new type of dean, the DME. Initially, DMEs were isolated and learning on the job, but the 1956 creation of the forerunner of the AHME provided an organizational focus for them. In 1965, AHME moved its annual meeting from the AMA Congress to an independent forum in Phoenix where AHME attendees could talk in depth about the problems community hospitals faced. Although most initial AHME members were from hospitals in the northeast, the membership was gradually expanded to cover a wide range of individuals interested in hospital medical education.

The initial mission of AHME was GME leadership; however, the expansion of medical education in the late 1960s and 1970s and the creation of community-based medical schools led many AHME-member hospitals to become clinical training sites for third and fourth year medical students or partners in community-based schools. Some early DMEs became deans or assistant deans at new medical schools, and the role of the hospital DME was extended to include oversight of clinical medical student rotations. AHME first became recognized as a voice for community teaching hospitals in GME in the 1970s when the Accreditation Council for Graduate Medical Education (ACGME) appointed two AHME leaders to the Transitional Year Review Committee (successor to the rotating internship).

In CME, AHME was invited to become a member of the ACCME and to recommend members to serve on its board of directors and review committee. AHME also had representation on the ACGME board (without vote) and the Educational Commission for Foreign Medical Graduates and had nominated members to the Federal Council on Graduate Medical Education, which later became the Graduate Medical Education National Advisory Committee.

These opportunities plus position papers and Congressional testimony put AHME in the mainstream of national discussions of medical education issues and gave the young organization credibility within the profession. Norman Stearns, MD, AHME president (1976–1978), described AHME as "the power base and voice of medical educators including DMEs, medical directors, service chiefs and others in hospitals that recognize the importance of a community hospital as a primary locus for education and training of physicians."

In addition to AHME's participation as a sponsoring member of the ACCME, DMEs were key players as their hospitals sought state medical society accreditation as CME providers in the late

1970s and early 1980s. This stretched the DME role from third-year medical students and residency administration to CME for area physicians and, often, necessitated adding support staff to offices of medical education.

As one of the seven member organizations of the ACCME, AHME was allotted two members on the ACCME board of directors and three members on the ACCME Accreditation Review Committee. AHME also applied for and was granted status as an ACCME-accredited provider and continued to offer an educational conference in conjunction with the annual fall AAMC meeting as well as its own spring conference.

As early as 1977, AHME sponsored workshops related to CME including one titled "CME in the Ambulatory Setting." In 1979, AHME sponsored a workshop on patient care evaluation for hospital CME leaders. AHME and the Alliance cosponsored and received national recognition for the 1980 conference "Continuing Medical Education: State of the Art." At that conference, 62 registrants were AHME members, and 30 were Alliance members.

Under the leadership of Robert Tupper, MD, AHME president from 1986 to 1988, AHME councils were established, initially for Transitional Year Program Directors and for Administrative Directors of Medical Education. The latter council addressed growing AHME membership by nonphysician administrators and educators.

Around this time, AHME helped forge the Tri-Group with the Alliance and SACME. Bob Richards received board of directors approval in May 1991 for continuation of AHME's active role in Tri-Group and to become a financially supporting organization for *JCEHP*. In 1995, a letter of agreement was signed enabling AHME, the Alliance, and SACME to become co-owners of *JCEHP*. The on-going development of *JCEHP* has been and is a commitment of AHME leadership.

By 1990, AHME was increasingly involved in sponsoring national and international CME efforts in addition to its role as an ACCME-member organization. AHME was represented on the planning committee for the 1992 Congress on CME, which was the first of these congresses. The CME congresses have been held every four years since then and, as a member of the Tri-Group, AHME continues to be involved in their planning.

In 1991, Richards was asked by the board to propose a structure for CME within AHME. Initially, members were surveyed to determine their role and interest in CME. With more than 170 positive responses, an interest group in CME was formed, had its initial meeting in November 1993, and formed a steering committee the next year. Publication of a *JCEHP* article titled "Creating a New Paradigm for CME: Seizing Opportunities within the Health Care Revolution" provided further stimulus for discussion of AHME's CME role.[9]

The new interest group provided leadership in reviewing proposed revisions in the ACCME Essentials and authoring an AHME response. Because of AHME's role as an ACCME member organization, the interest group became a forum for input on ACCME policy matters.

In May 1995, the AHME board authorized formation of a council on CME, and David Marler, PhD, was elected as the first council chair (1995–1997). From the inception of the councils, AHME required each of them to develop specific programs for each of the AHME spring institutes. This process allowed the council to initiate CME oriented sessions each year for the council itself and AHME members. The AHME spring institutes with the council have provided the nuts and bolts of CME accreditation; information sharing between DMEs and other CME educators; ways to organize and manage CME in a community hospital; the use of outcome measures as a means to change physician behavior and improve patient care; and ways to comply with the new ACCME accreditation criteria.

As noted earlier, the AHME role in medical education was not limited to undergraduate, graduate, or continuing medical education; it was an organization that was committed to the continuum of medical education in hospitals. In the early years of AHME, the hospital DME was the focus for the sharing of information relative to medical education. However, with the inception of the Councils in AHME (Council of Administrative Directors of Medical Education; Council on Medical Education Consortia; Council of Transitional Year Program Directors; Council on Continuing Medical Education) the organization increased its membership with other educators as committed members to the association that were not DMEs.

During the past 30 years, there has been an on-going change in medicine not only in modalities of care but also in the organizations that support the changing environment in medicine. AHME member hospitals have developed CME programs that have updated AHME members to the changing environment of CME. The AHME role in CME has been and continues to be a voice of hospital-based medical education.

Canadian Association for Continuing Health Education

The following is a fictitious scene that could have occurred in 1996 at the annual ACME meeting. A special interest group gathers a day prior to the conference for a meeting that has occurred since 1994 and is affectionately called Canada Day. Those in attendance include René Gagnon, MD, associate dean of CME at Laval University; Bernard Marlow, MD, director of continuing health education (CHE) for the University of Toronto; Bob Chester, BSc, CCPE, manager of CHE for a large pharmaceutical company; and Peggy Ahearn, president of a medical communications company. Their conversation may have gone something like this:

Bob: René, I've noticed that a lot of people that come to Canada Day say it is their favourite part of the ACME conference.

Bernard: Well, no surprise to me, Bob. Have you noticed that Canadians are disproportion-

ately represented running workshops, posters, and sessions here?

René: Oui, I feel like we all spend a lot of effort travelling only to talk with and learn from each other.

Peggy: Why don't we just run Canada Day in Canada?

And voila! The seed was planted for the birth of an organization. Or was it? Let us turn the pages back before we look ahead and see how that seed germinated, what it grew into, and the value of that growth. As Malcolm Gladwell discusses in his book *Outliers*, rarely does an idea start where one thinks it does.[10]

Turning the hands of time back to 1991, we find ourselves at a reception party in San Francisco. A group of Canadians gather for discussion and an exchange of ideas. About 50 Canadians involved in CME had for years been attending the annual meeting of ACME in the United States, and they finally set a time to meet with each other while there.

The following year at the ACME meeting in New Orleans, they informally met at the end of the day and declared, "We should meet again next year." In Orlando, the following year, they decided to plan something more formal for years to come. The first planning committee in 1993 consisted of Gagnon; Donna Barber, MEd, University of Saskatchewan; Russell Knaus, MD, Lumsden Medical Clinic; Jane Tipping, MAEd, University of Toronto; and Christopher Dean, BSc, member from a pharmaceutical community.

They, along with people such as Ahearn, Jocelyn Lockyer, Dave Davis, Linda Snell, Vivian Vinet, Céline Monette, Pierre Lavalard, Marcel Doré, Sheila Rivest, Chris West, Annie Barron, and many more, hatched a plan for a half-day meeting during the 1994 ACME annual meeting in San Diego for Canadian CME providers (including individuals from universities, hospitals, associations such as the Royal College, Canadian Medical Association, College of Family Physicians of Canada, and pharmaceutical and communication companies) to share ideas and best practices in CME. They called the day "Ideal Canadian CME: What Is It?" Their goal for the meeting was to create a new paradigm in CME and build collegial networks.

Based on the positive feedback from the 1993 meeting, they decided to expand to a full day the next year and continued this special interest group meeting at ACME for the next six years. Affectionately known as *Canada Day*, it was developed by and for Canadian CHE professionals who appreciated the opportunity to learn and grow from their colleagues working in a similar environment. The meeting, which began as a reporting day, developed into a great educational experience that became so popular that the regular members of the Canadian contingent began to talk about moving Canada Day to Canadian soil. Around the same time that this idea was ruminating, Canadians became acutely aware of the fact that the presenters at the main ACME sessions were disproportionately represented by Canadians. The vision of a Canadian CHE organization was explored, and plans were started for an annual meeting in Canada the following year.

The year 2000 marked the last Canada Day in the United States. In 2001, an annual meeting focused on Canadian CHE issues and bearing the name Canadian Association of Continuing Health Education (CACHE) was officially launched in Ottawa, Canada. Attendees of the 2001 CACHE meeting voted by an 85 percent margin that they "wanted the association to be more than a meeting." Another 83 percent "felt that allied health professionals should join" CACHE.[11] This feedback led to the formation of a strategic planning/special interest group (SIG) in 2002 to begin the process under the leadership of Marlow; Gary Sibbald, MD; and Alex Szucs of building a plan that would see CACHE become a full-service CHE association. If Canada Day was the seed, then the SIG workshops (2002–2004) acted as the germination of the seed. In subsequent years, CACHE held several successful meetings in conjunction with the annual meeting of the Royal College of Physicians and Surgeons of Canada.

To further guide the growth of this new organization, SIG conducted a value audit of the attendees. Using written surveys and telephone interviews, about 40 participants of the SIG vetted the data on the important issues facing the association and presented their findings to the 2002 CACHE General Assembly. In 2004, the 13 participants at a CACHE retreat reviewed and updated the values. While the core values remained the same, members at the retreat introduced new values to reflect current trends. The value words describing CACHE included:

- Uniquely Canadian
- Representative of stakeholders, with balance
- Meeting place, exchange, relationships, networking, forum, home
- Fostering, collaborative
- Interdisciplinary
- Expansion, growth
- Original research, national research, research for all
- Financially sound
- Innovations in education
- Healthcare system, planning, implementing
- Linked to outcomes: patient, research systems, patient care outcomes
- Policy
- Standards, accreditation

As defined by the steering committee in 2002, many individuals and groups have a vested interest in and derive value from CACHE. The annual meeting offers professional development while attendees learn about innovations in CHE and continuing professional development (CPD). Attendees can showcase their work by sharing their research projects and CHE programs. Networking and idea exchanges are common at the annual meeting as are mentorship opportunities. Attendees can also participate in a forum that increases positive working relationships among Canadian CHE/CPD stakeholders. The CHE literature database allows members to receive key publications and the opportunity to publish. CACHE also allows individuals to gain access to fellowships, CHE/CPD experts, and key online CHE/CPD resources.

The first official meeting of the CACHE board of directors was held on September 8, 2006, in St. John's, Newfoundland. The board met prior to the start of the scientific sessions to build a foundation for the CACHE constitution and by-laws and to develop a strategic plan for the newly formed association. They addressed questions such as, why have CACHE? and how does it contribute to CHE? The mission of CACHE became one in which the CACHE organization provides CHE professionals with leadership excellence in CPD and Education Research.

What is the true value of CACHE? Some CHE players were asked this question in 2009 and their responses follow.

Fran Kirby, MEd, director of professional development and conferencing services for the Faculty of Medicine at Memorial University, responded:

CACHE has played a pivotal role in the evolution of CHE. It is the only organization of its kind in Canada to bring together public (government, academia), private (pharmaceutical and medical communication companies) and not-for-profit groups (health care associations) to share best practices in CHE. The CACHE annual meeting has been well recognized as one of the best educational and networking opportunities to connect with colleagues in the field. While the political environment changes around us, CACHE responds to this by fostering collaboration and providing timely education to support CHE professionals.[12]

Denis Drouin, MD, clinical professor of family medicine and associate director of the Continuing Professional Development Centre, Laval University, responded:

I have always been impressed by the quality of Canadian research in the field of medical education. At CACHE, people share experience and expertise on

how to better educate, how to better learn. Over time, we have discovered that professional education was a component of a successful knowledge translation/implementation program. We have discovered that professional education should include other healthcare professionals and not only physicians, that knowledge was not enough, that to enhance quality of care we had to work as well in changing systems, implement a continuous quality improvement program and provide patient/population education. The medical profession is a lifelong learning experience, yes, but the CACHE forum allowed us, Continuing Professional Development Providers, to discover what was the meaning of what we are all accountable for, "Bridging the gap between science and action."[13]

Bob Chester, CHE manager of a pharmaceutical company, responded:

CACHE had its humble beginnings as a Special Interest Group at ACME. Based on the energies of that small dedicated group, CACHE has grown into an association that represents the vision of those CME professionals who are interested in a truly collaborative approach to CME in Canada. Each year through the annual meeting I have been inspired by what I have learned from others and challenged to be a little bit better than I was last year.[14]

Wendy Musselman, vice president of Nuvis Canada, responded:

In this era of CME reform CACHE has and continues to provide its stakeholders with a forum to facilitate opportunities to share a voice, professional development, and peer-to-peer interaction. It is through this medium that we are able to stay current on national and global CME trends. To this end CACHE is an invaluable partner and advisor for continuing medical education in Canada.[15]

Morris Freedman, MD, FRCPC, president of the Federation of National Specialty Societies of Canada, responded:

Since its inception, CACHE has played an important role in bringing together stakeholders and building a collaborative model in the CME/CPD enterprise in Canada. Through its annual conferences and recent Summit, CACHE creates opportunities for health professionals to come together and exchange points of views on current and future needs for a collaborative, professional health education environment.[16]

Ivan Silver, MD, Med, FRCPC, vice-dean of continuing education and professional development, Faculty of Medicine, University of Toronto, responded:

CACHE was born from "Canada Day" at ACME. It is a meeting place and home for all of the players in contemporary Canadian CHE. Its strength is its potential for collaboration, mutual understanding, and trust among all of its partners. I am looking forward to its future![17]

Christie Sterns, MHSc, CTDP, president of Training Makes Cents Inc., responded:

CACHE offers members a great way to stay connected and current on what is happening in the CHE Community both through its Web site and via the national annual meeting.[18]

In summary, just as it takes a community to raise a child, it also takes a community to build an organization. CACHE was built in a professional, iterative, consultative, and collaborative process. After many years of preparation, CACHE has proven its value in just a few short years and should be proud of what has been accomplished. CACHE is now a fully registered association with operational by-laws, strategic documents, insurance, committees, working groups, and membership. An election process for board members and executive has been determined. CACHE hosts an annual meeting as well as a Web site and newsletter. Member benefits such as a subscription to *JCEHP* and fall and spring summits have been added. Moving forward, CACHE intends to focus on the annual meeting, add member benefits, and address the need to have CME provider education and certification.

Finally, it is not known how this young seedling called CACHE will fare, but it currently stands as a shining example of transparency and collaboration that works for a win-win-win outcome in this era of regulation. We all share a desire for optimal patient outcomes. By focusing on this common denominator, it is truly the patient that wins. Will CACHE wither or will it take root and become strong? In the end, the seedling's growth depends on all of us and how we care for it.

Notes

1. "Fact Sheet: Alliance for CME at a Glance," Alliance for Continuing Medical Education Web site, http://www.acme-assn.org/about/media_kit/fact%20sheet.pdf (accessed July 19, 2010).

2. "Alliance 35th Annual Conference," Alliance for Continuing Medical Education Web site http://www.acme-assn.org/about/press_release35ConferencePR.pdf (accessed July 19, 2010).

3. W. C. Felch, *The Alliance for Continuing Medical Education: The First Twenty Years* (Dubuque: Kendall/Hunt, 1996).

4. J. S. Green and others, eds., *Continuing Education for the Health Professions: Developing, Managing, and Evaluating Programs for Maximum Impact on Patient Care* (San Francisco: Jossey-Bass, 1984).

5. Richard V. King and Sterling A. North, "Alliance for Continuing Medical Education Competency Areas for CME Professionals: Competencies Analysis Report," submitted 2008, http://www.acme-assn.org/home/compreport/CompRprt_1.pdf (accessed June 20, 2010).

6. B. J. Bellande, "The State of the Alliance," *Alliance Almanac* 28 (2006): 1–7.

7. Tri-Group Task Force for a New Accreditation System, "A Proposal for a New Accreditation System for Continuing Medical Education," *SMCDCME Intercom* 10 (1996): 1–13.

8. D. E. Moore, Jr., and others, "Creating a New Paradigm for CME: Seizing Opportunities within the Health Care Revolution," *Journal of Continuing Education in the Health Professions* 14 (1994): 4–31.

9. Ibid.

10. Malcolm Gladwell, *Outliers: The Story of Success* (New York: Little, Brown and Company, 2008).

11. Alex Szucs, Minutes of the SIG meeting, 2001.

12. Fran Kirby, e-mail and telephone communication with Jill Donahue, 2009.

13. Denis Drouin, e-mail and telephone communication with Jill Donahue, 2009.

14. Bob Chester, e-mail and telephone communication with Jill Donahue, 2009.

15. Wendy Musselman, e-mail and telephone communication with Jill Donahue, 2009.

16. Morris Freedman, e-mail and telephone communication with Jill Donahue, 2009.

17. Ivan Silver, e-mail and telephone communication with Jill Donahue, 2009.

18. Christie Sterns, e-mail and telephone communication with Jill Donahue, 2009.

National Task Force content authored by
Dennis K. Wentz and Alejandro Aparicio;
NAAMECC content authored by
Karen M. Overstreet

CHAPTER 14

Contemporary Organizations That Influence Continuing Medical Education in the United States: The National Task Force on CME Provider/Industry Collaboration and the North American Association of Medical Education and Communication Companies

As continuing medical education (CME) matured in the 1990s, new entities came into play that affected the field of CME. This chapter describes two of them. The National Task Force on CME Provider/Industry Collaboration (National Task Force) was created in 1990. The National Task Force attempted to improve communication between CME providers and the pharmaceutical and medical device industries as the amount of commercial support and funding for CME was dramatically increasing. Concerns about undue influence on the content and provision of CME due to such commercial support became common, and the National Task Force attempted to bring together all involved parties including the government for informal but intense discussions. The North American Association of Medical Education and Communication Companies, the second entity to be discussed in this chapter, formed to advocate nationally for medical education and communications companies, both for-profit and not-for-profit, who had been approved as accredited providers of CME by the Accreditation Council for CME (ACCME) and experienced rapid growth beginning in the 1990s.

The National Task Force on CME Provider/Industry Collaboration

The mission of the National Task Force is "to provide a leadership forum to impact national policy related to the provision, support, accreditation, and regulation of continuing medical education (CME)."[1]

The National Task Force remains unique and unlike any other forum in CME by virtue of its composition, its structure, and its mission. In our view, the major contribution of the National Task Force has been education and the provision of educational activities and resources. These many-dimensional educational efforts continue to be the dominant theme. Education occurs between and among members of the National Task Force at the three yearly meetings (off-the-record, no holds barred, no minutes, the more debate the better), in frank but engaged discussion. Educational efforts are directed at many groups: to industry regarding CME accreditation and credit, to accrediting organizations about industry policies and constraints, to education of physicians and medical organizations about CME and guidelines from the profession on gifts to physicians from industry, and finally, beginning in 2008, to education of the public, the media, the regulators, and the government. A major new effort has just begun, the issuing of fact sheets developed by the National Task Force to clarify many misperceptions about the organization and delivery of CME.

From its inception, the stated goals of the National Task Force included:

- To bring together individuals from a variety of CME perspectives
- To propose mutually derived ethical solutions to issues in CME
- To disseminate news and information regarding CME
- To safeguard continuing education provider/industry collaboration and support for CME
- To review and recommend guidelines and regulations pertaining to the interface between CME providers and industry
- To provide educational activities that support our mission and goals

How and Why the National Task Force Began

Prior to the National Task Force's initial meeting in 1990, Martin D. Shickman, MD, assistant dean at the University of California–Los Angeles School of Medicine, urged the Society of Medical College Directors of CME (SMCDCME, now the Society for Academic CME [SACME]) to get involved in the issues of industry influence on CME. An ad hoc task force was appointed by SMCDCME leadership; its members met for the first time with representatives of seven pharmaceutical companies in New Orleans in 1986 to discuss issues of mutual concern, including the prevalent industry marketing culture, extremes in company gifts to physicians, and perhaps inappropriate company influence and direction over physician participation in CME. In 1987, the task force became an official committee of the SMCDCME chaired by Shickman, but only three

companies originally present in New Orleans, represented by three individuals, continued to come to the meetings: Robert Orsetti of Ciba Geigy, David Lichtenauer of the Upjohn Company, and Lee Yerkes of Marion Merrell Dow. The discussions were frank, broad reaching, and mutually informative, and the need to create a national forum and debate was clear. Thus, in 1989 Shickman's committee recommended to SMCDCME leadership that a national conference be convened. By this time, committee member and 1987 SMCDCME president Dennis Wentz, MD, became director of the American Medical Association (AMA) Division of CME. The intention of the committee and the interest of the AMA in the issues proved to be a good fit. With the AMA serving as the host organization, a planning committee was appointed that included medical schools, the Alliance for CME, medical specialty societies, ACCME, and SMCDCME.

The first conference on CME Provider and Industry Collaboration was organized and held in Chicago in August 1990. It attracted about 240 individuals interested in the subject; significant industry interest had been piqued by the demanding letters sent to all major pharmaceutical companies by Senator Edward M. Kennedy (D-Mass.) in April 1990 requesting specific data on the amounts companies were spending on physicians, on education, and especially on gifts to physicians. Among the speakers were Theodore Cooper, MD, president of the Upjohn Company, and Ken Feather of the Food and Drug Administration (FDA). Feather described the work of the FDA on regulations for industry support of CME, a project that had extended more than 20 years without reaching a firm conclusion. The attendees agreed on the need for voluntary guidelines applicable to all of the stakeholders in CME as a far better mechanism than FDA or congressional regulations.

In summing up this first conference, James Leist, EdD, then president of the SMCDCME, and Fred Lyons, chairman of Marion Merrell Dow, suggested moving with all possible haste in establishing an inter-organizational national task force. At the time, Lyons was also president of the Washington, DC–based Pharmaceutical Manufacturers Association (PMA, later renamed PhRMA). At the organizational meeting following the conference, Lyons encouraged inviting the FDA to become a member of the national task force, an invitation that the FDA eventually accepted. The first meeting of the National Task Force on CME Collaboration was held in Denver, Colorado, on December 12, 1990. Wentz was elected chair and Robert Cullen, PhD, co-chair.

Confusion between Support of Certified CME and Gifts to Physicians

Prior to the first meeting of the new National Task Force, the AMA Council on Ethical and Judicial Affairs (CEJA), and the AMA House of Delegates issued a key Ethical Opinion 8.061 "Gifts to Physicians from Industry" on December 3, 1990. One week later the Ethical Opinion was officially endorsed by the PMA. It was a whirlwind week, as on December 11, 1990, Senator Kennedy held formal hearings of his Senate Committee on Labor and Health to examine the responses of the pharmaceutical industry to his earlier requests for detailed information. While he and several carefully selected speakers denigrated the behavior of both the industry and the profession, the impending road to congressional regulation was muted by testimony from the AMA president and others that voluntary steps were being taken to correct abuses. The AMA Ethical Opinion was one of these steps (though it had been years in the making and was not developed for this reason).

Just one day later, the National Task Force agreed that a set of Uniform Guidelines about Commercial Support for Continuing Medical Education be developed for use by accrediting bodies. The National Task Force co-chairs organized a series of conference calls extending through winter and spring 1991 to develop these guidelines. These calls, often hours in length and usually with about 30 active participants, were mod-

els of informed discussion, debate, cooperation, and compromise, and progress was made quickly (even without the benefit of e-mail). The Uniform Guidelines were adopted in spring 1991 by the National Task Force and subsequently forwarded to the several accrediting bodies, i.e., the ACCME, American Osteopathic Association (AOA), and American Academy of Family Physicians (AAFP). They were accepted virtually unchanged by the AOA and the AAFP. After discussion, the ACCME voted to replace its existing 1984 Guidelines on Industry Support of CME. The ACCME effort was led by Kevin Bunnell, PhD, a council member, together with ACCME associate director Frances Maitland and J. S. Rheinschmitt, MD. They integrated the Uniform Guidelines of the Task Force into the existing ACCME Essentials and Policies and developed a new ACCME policy on Guidelines for Support of CME by Industry. It was adopted in 1992, and the council members voted to label the new policies as standards rather than guidelines to reinforce their importance. The ACCME also instructed its Accreditation Review Committee (ARC) to enforce adherence to the new Standard with the same vigor as they required documentation of the Essentials.

The National Task Force had fulfilled its first external educational mission. While the rules and regulations for operating the National Task Force were still to develop, there was internal agreement that the National Task Force was to remain a one-of-a-kind invited leadership forum made up of *individuals* representing a variety of CME perspectives that would function without designated organizational representation, an informal and perhaps perpetual, ad hoc group.

The Annual Task Force Conferences

The Second National Conference was held in October 1991 in Chicago. As before, the AMA hosted the event, with a planning committee drawn from the National Task Force. It was a stormy meeting, as the FDA, under new commissioner David

Kessler, MD, unveiled its proposed Guidelines on Industry Supported Continuing Medical Education. These were presented by Ann Witt, JD, the acting director of the FDA Division of Drug Marketing, Advertising, and Communications. While Witt presented the guidelines in draft form prior to being published in the *Federal Register*, the members of the National Task Force and the audience became alarmed at the implications of the proposed regulations. To National Task Force members, the proposed rules were draconian and, if implemented by the FDA, would lead to the collapse of any further efforts at trying to find mutual areas of understanding or cooperation and collaboration between CME providers and industry.

However, frank discussions continued at the National Task Force meetings among CME providers, members of industry, and the FDA. By the time the FDA released the final guidelines in 1997, they were clear, understandable, and acceptable to all parties. While the guidelines were still stringent, the FDA had incorporated an understanding of the dynamics and functioning of the field of CME and clarified many of the gray zones and issues.

The National Task Force annual conferences continue to be held each fall and have achieved unique significance for the CME community. The purpose of the conference is always education: to bring all stakeholders up to date with what is happening at the cutting edge of collaboration between industry and CME; the topics are usually chosen because of the discussions held privately by the National Task Force as a means to gain wider input. An annual lecture honoring the late Martin Shickman, MD, has proven to be an exceedingly diverse forum, featuring speakers like Kenneth Shine, MD, president of the Institute of Medicine; industry chief executive officers such as Robert Ingram, Fred Lyons, and Fred Hassan; government officials such as FDA commissioner Jane Henney, MD; and CME leaders Wentz, George Mejicano, Marcia Jackson, Robert Fox, Barbara Barnes, and Dave Davis.

Current Organization and Initiatives of the National Task Force

Some organizational decisions were made at the beginning and remain. The AMA would serve as official host to the National Task Force and keep the historical but off-the-record notes from meetings. There would be a limitation on membership, no term limits would be imposed, there would be a continuous and deliberate process to broaden the membership so that most stakeholders would be represented, yet only individuals could be nominated and elected to the National Task Force. Once elected, members had to agree to cover their own travel and lodging expenses for attendance to at least two to four annual National Task Force meetings with no substitutions permitted. As at the beginning, there still are no formal bylaws, thus the National Task Force truly remains an ad hoc organization.

The work of the National Task Force is widely recognized and respected. The AMA House of Delegates even cited the role of the National Task Force in working with the FDA and others by adopting Resolution 307 in 1992:

Resolved, that the American Medical Association commend the activities of all parties, including the Food And Drug Administration (FDA), who have worked diligently through the Task Force on Continuing Medical Education Provider/Industry Collaboration in CME to develop guidelines and clear concepts of independence for CME activities supported by commercial companies, and that the AMA continue to monitor the implementation of FDA policies in accredited continuing medical education.

In 1992, the National Task Force reexamined but confirmed the membership policies and procedures that still guide it today. The National Task Force is limited to 45 individual members. Preference and priority in filling vacancies is accorded to individuals employed by umbrella organizations importantly involved in CME. The only standing committee of the National Task Force remains the Committee on Membership, initially chaired by Judith Ribble, PhD, then by Peter Rheinstein, MD, followed by John Burke, PhD, and now Pamela Mason. In 2004, Alejandro Aparicio, MD, director of the AMA Division of Continuing Physician Professional Development, was elected co-chairman of the National Task Force after the retirement of Cullen from the National Task Force. In 2006, Wentz was elected unanimously as chairman emeritus.

Questions raised within the National Task Force about whether it was still useful and needed as a national forum were discussed at a strategic retreat held by the group in May 2006. While it may have been a self-fulfilling prophecy, the need was reaffirmed. One important change in direction was the setting of four-year term limits for members and new appointees; these could be extended only by mutual agreement of the member and the National Task Force. The group carefully considered its membership and decided to do everything possible to keep the National Task Force representational of all of the players and forces in CME today, but it remains an organization of individuals.

Another Educational Project:
Gifts to Physicians from Industry

The second major effort of the National Task Force involved a national campaign to educate (perhaps a better term was *re-educate*) the nation's physicians, physician organizations, and CME providers about the AMA 1990 ethical policies on gifts to physicians from industry (CEJA Ethical Opinion 8.061). After the AMA Council on Ethical and Judicial Affairs (CEJA) guidelines were issued, they received major publicity and many challenges. They were made prominent and given great credence, but this faded over time. The National Task Force remained in the thick of the debate as the media continued to blur the issues of CME and gifts to physicians, and endless discussions consumed National Task Force meetings. Finally, at a fall meeting, frustrated member Linda Raichle gave the group a

challenge—fund a national educational effort—and pledged $100,000 on behalf of her employer (Merck & Company). A consensus quickly developed that the National Task Force was ideally positioned to lead such a concerted national educational effort. At the next meeting, the National Task Force launched a major national effort to better communicate the ideas and principles of the CEJA opinion to the nation's physicians and the public and to find the resources to do so. Significant financial grants came from nine organizations (and not from industry only), the AMA committed staff and major in-kind logistical support, and other organizations contributed in a multitude of ways. In retrospect, the budget for the campaign reached more than $1,000,000, of which $720,000 came from unrestricted financial grants and the remainder was largely in-kind support from the AMA.

A new Working Group on Communication of Ethical Guidelines for Physicians was established in August 2000 and broadly structured to include key individuals from all stakeholders with interest in this issue, obviously many from outside the National Task Force. The group was fully independent from the National Task Force, and Alan R. Nelson, MD, former AMA president, served as its chairman; Beverley Rowley, PhD, served as the project manager. Eventually 42 members made up the Working Group, representing major medical societies, accreditation councils, the public, pharmaceutical and medical device companies and their umbrella groups, the government, and physicians-in-training. A core message was created by the Group:

Physicians have a unique professional relationship with patients and have an ethical responsibility to place the health and welfare of the patient ahead of economic self-interest. Physicians should be mindful that accepting gifts or other remuneration that does not comply with ethical guidelines may give the appearance of undue influence and jeopardize the physician-patient relationship.

Industry and physicians should recognize that gifts

that do not comply with professional guidelines may compromise ethical principles. Industry should share the responsibility to promote the health and welfare of patients by complying with appropriate guidelines.

Guidance for physicians and industry can be found in the current Code of Medical Ethics published by the Council on Ethical and Judicial Affairs of the American Medical Association and the ethics statements of medical specialty societies. In addition, codes of conduct associated with government, industry, or other institutional employment may apply.[2]

The Working Group divided its efforts into two phases: Phase 1 of the initiative was an intensive effort to raise awareness of the CEJA guidelines through a dedicated Web site, direct mailings, journal articles and publications, advertorials in print and in the media, a massive distribution of pocket cards highlighting synopsis of the CEJA Guidelines, and exhibits and special presentations at medical and industry meetings. Phase 2, led by a subcommittee of educators, oversaw the development of educational resources, with four educational activities offered via the Internet. Each educational activity was developed in two formats: (1) self-study activities for individuals, certified for AMA PRA category 1 credit when appropriately used, and (2) curriculum materials including slides and text for teachers and others who would present the material in a variety of settings.

Initially, the results seemed encouraging. More than 465,000 pocket cards were distributed at no cost to physicians via local and national medical and specialty society meetings, and also on request. The Web site was accessed 194,000 times in the first two years, with pages opened or accessed averaging 1,500 a week. Following a public relations release, 5,928 pages were accessed during the week of May 19, 2003. The educational materials appeared on a dedicated Web site that was accessed 152,313 times through May 2003 when tabulation stopped.[3]

Again the results were not long lived. While awareness was created and consciousness raised

about the important ethical implications of industry gifts to physicians, once again little changed in the real world. Speculation as to why usually depends on the perspective and viewpoint of the commentator. But there were many new fiscal and practice pressures on practicing physicians at the time, there was resentment by some physicians at losing some of the freebies once provided, and it seemed to at least several of us that the profession had been slowly moved to behaving more as a trade than as a learned profession. The consequences: consider the new regulations on gifts to physicians from industry that are now being discussed and enacted, from several state governments to the US Congress.

The misconceptions and misunderstandings about CME, CME terms, certified educational activities versus promotional educational activities, off label usage, and others, seemed to increase significantly in 2005 and 2006. Often found in prominent articles in the national media, hearings by lawmakers and even in professional publications, the incorrect information, especially when repeated and quoted, would often be accepted by others, including some in positions of influence or authority who would then seek to make changes to CME based on false premises. The National Task Force, which had reaffirmed its educational mission in its Strategic Retreat described earlier, decided that the Annual Conference was not enough by itself to address this growing problem. At the January 2007 National Task Force meeting, the culmination of the internal discussions on this issue was to create an Ad Hoc group to investigate the feasibility of forming a new committee that "could try to educate specific groups, and the public in general, about issues related to CME and Industry." The Ad Hoc group included 10 members of the National Task Force, including the chairman and the chairman emeritus. The group reported back at the next meeting of the National Task Force in May 2007 and proposed a plan for a standing committee that was to be named the Public Affairs Committee. The committee would develop educational materials about important issues and a distribution plan. The National Task Force agreed to move forward with this latest educational initiative.

Maureen Doyle-Scharff was appointed chair of the Public Affairs Committee in recognition of her earlier work on the Ad Hoc group. The educational strategy evolved by the committee and approved by the National Task Force was the development of a series of fact sheets. They would be exactly that, carefully researched documents, explaining areas, terms, or issues in CME in a factual way. They would not be position papers or opinion pieces but instead would be referenced factual information that anyone could use to inform discussions about CME. The committee worked diligently on the fact sheets through the exchange of e-mails and conference calls every two weeks; these continue as of the writing of this chapter. The work has been significant and emphasizes a very careful review of sources and references to ensure that no personal bias is introduced in the information provided.

The unveiling of the initiative came at the National Task Force annual conference in October 2008. The initiative was very well received within the CME community. Multiple groups have cited the the fact sheets and even provide links to them from their Web sites. The fact sheets that have been issued are titled Continuing Medical Education: Providing Valid and Independent Evidence for Clinical Decisions; Continuing Medical Education: Addressing Conflict of Interest; Pharmaceutical, Biotechnology and Medical Device Company Support of Continuing Medical Education; and On- and Off-Label Usage of Prescription Medicines and Devices, and the Relationship to CME.[4]

As of this writing, the medical profession, industry, and other groups continue to debate the role, if any, of industry in CME. Although the issue of commercial support is often confused with the issues of conflict of interest and gifts to physicians, judgments often end up being made on the basis of perceptions, or misperceptions, instead of on the basis of facts. After 20 years, the National Task Force continues to fill an important role in the CME community providing educational activities and a CME forum for productive, open debate. National Task Force members remain dedicated to the principle that CME improves the knowledge, skills, attitudes, or behaviors used by physicians to serve patients, the public, or the profession.

North American Association of Medical Education and Communication Companies

The North American Association of Medical Education and Communication Companies (NAAMECC) was founded as a nonprofit organization in 2001 by four individuals experienced in CME—Karen Overstreet, EdD, RPh; Jacqueline Parochka, EdD; Mark Schaffer, EdM; and Richard Tischler, Jr., PhD—to promote best practices in CME and to advocate nationally for medical education and communications companies (MECCs). A MECC is an entity (either for-profit or not-for-profit) whose primary business is the dissemination of current information about disease states, therapies, medical products and devices, and other pertinent medical practice topics to physicians and other health-care professionals.[5]

Tischler, the founding treasurer, explained the rationale for forming NAAMECC:

Despite their presence in CME, not just in volume of activities but also the innovation they brought to the industry, MECCs had no voice. Prevented from advocating on their own behalf as a provider group of the Alliance for CME, MECCs were virtually powerless to address misconceptions about their virtue or to tout their significant contributions to quality CME. This need was filled by NAAMECC. The voice became stronger as the organization grew from 4 companies to 100. Those organizations who wanted to work with MECCs to advance CME now had a credible ally. Those organizations that would have preferred to ignore MECCs now had no choice but to address their concerns. The prejudice against MECCs has not disappeared, but the critics have less influence.[6]

Parochka, the founding president of NAAMECC, clarified the need for a new association:

The academics had the Society for Academic CME, the hospital/medical centers had the Association for Hospital Medical Education, but MECCs only had representation in the MECCA section of the Alliance for CME, and, as such, they did not have the ability to create policy or direction for the MECCs. Since MECCs were growing in number and did not have a mechanism to voice concerns and opinions regarding articles in the popular press, four friends and colleagues created NAAMECC. The creation of this organization from scratch will always be one of my fondest memories.[7]

NAAMECC was incorporated in June 2001 in Maryland and held its inaugural meeting at the Baltimore Marriott Waterfront Hotel in October 2001. Current membership includes more than 100 organizations. The mission of NAAMECC is to represent, advocate for, and educate its members. It meets twice yearly, in the fall in conjunction with the Annual Conference of the National Task Force on CME Provider/Industry Collaboration and again in January during the Alliance for CME Annual Conference. The organization has completed several important activities to support its members' efforts to provide high quality, effective CME that is independent of marketing influences and avoids commercial bias, including a code of ethics,[8] a code of conduct for commercially supported CME,[9] the monograph *Industry Funding of CME Under Attack: Enhancing Compliance and Mitigating Risk*[10] based on a roundtable discussion of legal and regulatory experts, and a process for accredited providers to vet unaccredited educational partners (developed with the SACME).

All of the members of NAAMECC are medical education and communication companies. There are several hundred MECCs in the United States; approximately 150 are accredited by the Accreditation Council for CME (ACCME). Accredited MECCs adhere to the same ACCME elements, standards, and policies as do other providers; unaccredited MECCs must also comply with all relevant guidelines. Three profiles of MECCs have been published in the peer-reviewed literature.[11] The most recent describes a largely privately held provider sector that includes a large contingent of physicians and other health-care professionals among its personnel and leadership.

Humble Beginnings but Rapid Growth

Michael Caso, now at Nexus Communications, explained the early role of MECCs:

While at Marion Laboratories (which became Marion Merrill Dow, then Hoechst Marion Roussel, and finally Novartis) in the [1980s], my colleagues managed educational programs divided by disease state. These individuals worked closely with medical schools in the development of educational activities and managed communications agencies to help implement these programs and to develop effective enduring materials.

Before the need for separation of education from marketing, pharma marketing teams worked routinely with agencies, as they had a high level of scientific knowledge about the disease state or therapeutic area. This period of the 1980s demonstrated a rapid upsurge of agencies offering skills in creating and executing educational activities. The need to utilize greater support from MECCs came in the late 1980s when the volume of educational grants at my company alone increased from $15 million to almost $75 million annually.[12]

As it was now obvious that the provision of CME could be a money-making enterprise, the numbers of entrepreneurial providers grew rapidly during the 1980s and 1990s.[13] As Robert Orsetti, MA, editor of *CE Measure,* described:

When pharmaceutical companies (pharma) realized that it was in their best interest to distance themselves from direct involvement, a business opportunity was created and MECCs began to appear. In those days, some pharma companies employed the services of communication companies to prepare publications based on clinical trial results. Some of those later added CME units or evolved into MECCs. Also, some advertising agencies created CME units to extend their operations.[14]

The first MECC was accredited by the ACCME in 1991. This was Professional Postgraduate Services, a division of Physicians World (now KnowledgePoint 360). Since then, the number of MECCs has increased, and the resources and services provided by them have evolved with the continually changing regulatory environment (see Box 14-1).

Mark Schaffer, EdM, founding NAAMECC secretary, explained how MECCs first became organized in the mid-1990s by forming MECCA, a provider section of the Alliance for CME:

In the early 1990s, MECCs were very much on the outside looking in. I was struck by the lack of understanding that, as a group, we had a lot in common and, in order to become accepted, we had to have an organized voice. Several attempts were made to get MECCs to meet as a group, but they were unsuccessful in part because everyone was concerned about sharing "proprietary" information. It wasn't until the Task Force meeting in [1995] that I finally managed to get some individuals together who realized the importance of developing some sort of organization and that not everything we did should be considered proprietary to our own individual organizations. I was later encouraged to apply to the Alliance to become a member section and MECCA was born.[15]

Clearly, MECCs play a crucial role in providing quality continuing education to physicians each year, ultimately affecting millions of patients. Accredited MECCs provide a sizeable percentage (22 percent) of all CME activities, serving about 27 percent of all physician participants.[16] If one were to include activities developed collaboratively with joint sponsors there would be an even larger contribution of MECCs to certified CME.

Where Do MECCs Fit In?
Perception versus Reality

The debate over where CME belongs started in the 1950s, with medical societies and organized medicine claiming authority and other provider groups (e.g., state medical societies, community hospitals) taking a strong stance as well. The de-

---

Box 14-1
Growth and Maturation of MECCs

1970s and 1980s
∓ Establishment of a handful of companies, which then grew rapidly and created the MECC sector. Many developed both promotional and certified education.

1990s
∓ Pharmaceutical industry recognizes the benefits of medical education and has big budgets to spend. Large-scale proliferation of MECCs.
∓ First MECC accredited in 1991.

2000s
∓ NAAMECC created in 2001.
∓ As pharmaceutical pipelines weaken, budgets placed under greater control by procurement teams. Smaller, less efficient MECCs under increasing pressure.
∓ Based on changes in the economy as well as evolving accreditation requirements, several MECCs go out of business or change to promotional education (2008 to 2009).

bate continues to the present day with louder and more frequent calls for MECC's to get out of CME.

Recent proposals calling for elimination of MECCs from CME (e.g., the Macy report[17]) may be based on misperceptions of the role and value of MECCs in CME. Readers of these reports may draw erroneous conclusions; in contrast, the evidence shows that six percent of MECCs are not-for-profit, 80 percent are privately held (20 percent are part of public corporations), 86 percent are not involved in promotional education, seven percent receive no commercial support, 10 percent receive less than 50 percent of their funding from commercial interests, and four percent receive 50 percent to 75 percent of their funding from commercial sources.[18]

MECCs and other stakeholders have continued to adapt as rules and regulations, new accreditation criteria, and new policy have evolved. To enhance their ability to demonstrate exemplary compliance, many MECCs have adopted formal compliance programs similar to those recommended by the OIG for industry. These include staff training, confidential reporting systems, and appointment of a compliance officer.

Future Directions

Most MECC leaders remain committed to collaboration and believe that a variety of providers is required to address the myriad unmet clinical and educational needs within the healthcare system. They also believe that fair competition and plurality in CME lead to innovation. But Orsetti predicts that:

MECCs are likely to remain ripe targets for media criticism and should continue to find ways to reinforce their positive contributions to medical education. MECCs would be well advised to form alliances with academic institutions and to devote more resources to outcomes and performance improvement to demonstrate not only behavior change but also direct patient improvement. A few MECCs are well on their way to transforming for the new realities of

CME. Should direct funding of activities produced by MECCs be disallowed, many companies will have difficulty remaining in business unless they can change their business models to, for example, create partnerships with academic institutions, as a means of being more closely aligned with new pharmaceutical support policies.[19]

The CME enterprise is obviously very different than it was only a few years ago. Heightened sensitivity to regulatory and public scrutiny and evolving guidelines—as well as a deep and genuine desire to create effective practice-based learning and improvement—are allowing both providers and supporters to have a role in the creation of education that makes a difference for practicing clinicians and their patients. NAAMECC leadership and most MECC personnel remain confident that the CME enterprise is moving in the right direction, and are optimistic that their organizations will continue to be vital contributors to the evolution of independent, certified medical education.

Michael Lemon, MBA, former president of NAAMECC, said:

The future role of MECCs will be rooted in collaboration, and the MECC community must forge relationships with hospitals and healthcare providers (e.g., physician private practices, urgent care networks, cancer centers, etc.), as well as other players in the healthcare industry, such as academic medical centers and insurance companies. These collaborative relationships will provide multiple new opportunities for MECCs, including access to patient-level data for performance improvement CME.[20]

Notes

1. National Task Force on CME Provider/Industry Collaboration, unpublished internal documents.

2. Beverly Rowley, telephone conversation with the authors, 2009.

3. Beverley Rowley, e-mail message to the authors, March 29, 2009.

4. "Get the Facts! Campaign," American Medical Association Web site, http://www.ama-assn.org/ama/pub/

education-careers/continuing-medical-education/events/national-task-force-cme-provider-industry/get-the-facts-campaign.shtml (accessed July 15, 2010).

5. "Industry Funding of CME Under Attack: Enhancing Compliance and Mitigating Risk," North American Association of Medical Education and Communication Companies, Inc., Web site, http://www.naamecc.org/downloads/monographweb1.pdf (accessed March 30, 2009).

6. Richard Tischler, conversation with the authors, 2009.

7. Jacqueline Parochka, conversation with the authors, 2009.

8. "Code of Ethics," North American Association of Medical Education and Communication Companies, Inc., Web site, http://www.naamecc.org/About/Ethics/tabid/62/Default.aspx (accessed March 30, 2009).

9. "Code of Conduct for Commercially Supported CME," North American Association of Medical Education and Communication Companies, Inc., Web site, http://www.naamecc.org/About/CodeofConduct/tabid/97/Default.aspx (accessed March 30, 2009).

10. "Industry Funding of CME Under Attack."

11. E. D. Peterson and others, "Medical Education and Communication Companies Involved in CME: An Updated Profile," *Journal of Continuing Education in the Health Professions* 28 (2008): 205–219; J. N. Parochka and J. Cole, "Profile of Medical Education and Communication Company Alliance Members," *Journal of Continuing Education in the Health Professions* 18 (1998): 29–38;

G. A. Golden and others, "Medical Education and Communication Companies: An Updated In-Depth Profile," *Journal of Continuing Education in the Health Professions* 22 (2002): 55–62.

12. Michael Caso, conversation with the authors, 2009.

13. A. B. Rosoff and W. C. Felch, eds., *Continuing Medical Education: A Primer,* 2nd ed. (New York: Praeger, 1992).

14. Robert Orsetti, telephone conversation with the authors, 2009.

15. Mark Schaffer, conversation with the authors, 2009.

16. Accreditation Council for Continuing Medical Education, "Annual Report Data 2006," ACCME Web site, http://www.accme.org/dir_docs/doc_upload/c91205e9 1-7c95-415c-89b3-0a9ff88de363_uploaddocument.pdf (accessed July 13, 2008).

17. S. W. Fletcher, Chairman's Summary of the Conference "Continuing Education in the Health Professions: Improving Healthcare through Lifelong Learning," (New York: Josiah Macy, Jr. Foundation, 2008), http://www.josiahmacyfoundation.org/documents/Macy_ContEd_1_7_08.pdf.

18. E. D. Peterson and others, "Medical Education and Communication Companies Involved in CME: An Updated Profile," *Journal of Continuing Education in the Health Professions* 28 (2008): 205-219.

19. Orsetti, telephone conversation.

20. Michael Lemon, telephone conversation with the authors, 2009.

PART IV

Physician Learning: Research in Continuing Medical Education and Continuing Professional Development

Donald E. Moore, Jr., Nancy Bennett, and
Karen V. Mann

CHAPTER 15

Research in Continuing Medical Education

Research in continuing medical education (CME) has made important contributions to our understanding of how physicians learn and how CME activities support the translation of learning into practice and will lead to improved patient care. Even as CME has developed and become integrated into the missions of medical schools, professional societies, and regulatory bodies, questions about enhancing its effectiveness resonate: Does CME work? CME research can be a critical contributor to a response to this question.

Helping physicians to improve the care they provide to their patients has been one of the strongest motivating factors in the development of CME research. The results of CME research have portrayed how physician learning and practice change are related. At the same time, however, there have been questions about how findings from CME research impact the work of those designing and delivering CME. It is not clear that CME research findings have become part of the day-to-day practice of CME or have been applied to the work of researchers in related fields. This chapter examines the growth of research in CME over the past century, celebrates some of its accomplishments, and suggests strategies that might enhance opportunities for impact.

Early Research in CME

Medicine has always recognized that physicians have an obligation to ensure that the expertise they bring to the clinical encounter is up to date. Throughout the history of medicine, physicians have been mostly left to their own resources to maintain and expand their expertise. Informal gatherings for learning became more formalized courses during the late 18th century into the early 20th century. Early efforts to formalize learning beyond initial training seem to have been based on the thoughts of selected observers of medical education rather than on efforts to systematically assess learning.

Even though the nature of the relationship between participation in an educational activity and the impact of that participation on patient care was not well known, concerns about the quality of patient care around the turn of the 20th century were attributed to deficiencies in education. The Flexner Report, commissioned to address those concerns at the pre-licensure level, focused on structural improvements: a scientific foundation for medical education and practice, teaching by qualified faculty in a university setting, and supervised clinical experience in a hospital.[1] At that time, the prevailing assumption among those educating physicians was that the knowledge, skills, and attitudes students acquired prior to entering practice would last throughout their professional lives. It was assumed that making improvements in initial education would impact the entire continuum. This widely held belief influenced the lack of attention given to graduate and continuing education, and as a result, to the development of research in those areas.

As Abraham Flexner was making recommendations about how the expertise of medical practitioners should be developed, there was increasing recognition that physicians in practice needed to engage in lifelong learning to maintain and expand their expertise. World War II was a significant turning point for CME. Until then CME activities were offered by county medical societies, medical schools, polyclinic hospitals, and proprietary graduate-postgraduate schools (which Flexner called "undergraduate repair shops"). After World War II, a combination of the rapid expansion of biomedical information and the return of health professionals from military service produced a demand for updating and retraining. As a result, medical schools and the newly emerging specialty societies developed and expanded their CME offerings, most often in a traditional lecture format.

Although more CME activities emerged, there was little formal analysis of their effectiveness, with few CME research studies published. Most writing about CME remained in the form of prescriptions for improvement based on authors' opinions rather than evidence or research results. The early research studies more often focused on structural issues and administrative arrangements of CME programs. The first national survey of CME was published by the American Medical Association (AMA) Council on Medical Education in 1938, indicating that state medical societies had assumed leadership responsibilities in CME. It reported, however, that a dual CME system was developing: local CME activities were being coordinated by medical societies; formal postgraduate programs were being coordinated by medical schools. But no indication of quality or effectiveness was included.

Three studies[2] that were conducted in the 1950s focused on the structural characteristics of CME programs in medical schools. They reported that medical schools and free-standing postgraduate institutes were the primary sponsors of CME, with medical schools providing almost all the teaching faculty for all types of activities. Each medical school had a designated person responsible for CME, with limited administrative support. Activities were mostly lectures and were offered as refresher or board preparation courses. As today, criticism based on opinion appeared about inconsistent quality, lack of organization and direction, and low attendance. The tradition and goals of these studies to understand the structure and administration of CME by systematically comparing data have been continued in the biennial Society of Academic CME (SACME) survey, now called the Society-AAMC-Harrison survey.

In a move away from a focus on structural issues, three early studies included an examination of the impact of CME participation on the performance of attendees. John B. Youmans, MD, described a fellowship program offered by Vanderbilt University School of Medicine for local general practitioners.[3] Each course lasted four months, accepted no more than 10 fellows, and included the work-up of patients, rounds in the hospital, conferences, and lectures. A follow-up study was conducted on 75 percent of the fellows through on-site observation in their practices. In addition to structural elements (quality of space, laboratory, office and equipment), measures included practice behaviors such as diagnosis, treatment, public health measures, and quality of patient records. There was also a measure of the quality of the doctor's library and how much he read. Data collected during the observation of the practices were compared to a precourse questionnaire, demonstrating improvements in practice behavior in the 30 offices visited that ranged from 6 percent to 176 percent. Youmans concluded that his findings demonstrated the superiority of practical teaching over didactic instruction. This early report demonstrated some characteristics of relevant, valid research; the intervention was targeted to actual practice, and the measures of change included direct observation of the participants in their practices.

In another early study, Osler L. Peterson, MD, reported that physicians who averaged 50 hours of postgraduate activities provided a somewhat better quality of care.[4] However, while some of the highest rated physicians had attended few CME activities, some of the poorest rated physicians were frequent participants. From these apparently contradictory findings, Peterson concluded that CME had a nebulous effect on the quality of physician performance and suggested a reappraisal of CME methods. Kenneth F. Clute, MD, in his study of physicians in Canada, found no correlation between the quality of the work of general practitioners and the amount of time devoted to postgraduate education.[5] His findings supported Peterson's findings somewhat, but did not agree with Youman's work, which demonstrated improved performance after CME. These studies lacked the sophistication of later CME research, but they identified one of the major questions that continues to characterize efforts in CME research: Does CME work?

Research on CME Focuses on Educational Issues

The 1960s brought significant growth and expansion in the number of CME activities and CME providers. Medical schools were joined by professional societies and hospitals in providing more CME opportunities. At the same time, a new group of CME professionals emerged. Graduate programs in North America provided training in learning, change, and evaluation, developing educators and psychologists who offered those in CME new ideas to expand thinking, and create a new kind of collaboration that introduced educational principles into CME. Leaders in adult education encouraged implementation of ideas about how professionals learn and how to systematically study the questions raised. Their students brought new skills to address questions in CME. Research began to change during this period; the balance shifted from studies of administrative arrangements relying mainly on surveys, to studies examining issues surrounding how to use educational principles to support effective learning and positive behavior change through CME.

Blending the ideas of educators and physicians produced a synergy that resulted in new approaches to CME. In one influential article, George E. Miller, MD, criticized contemporary approaches to CME as ineffective because they were too didactic and not relevant to practice.[6] He recommended that his physician colleagues in CME incorporate the principles of adult education by basing CME activities on the learning needs of the physicians and making learning activities more interactive and relevant.

Following Miller's recommendation, a number of projects sought new ways to make CME activities more relevant by integrating patient care evaluation and quality assessment with CME planning. A planning model emerged from two notable research projects conducted in Utah and Rockford, Illinois. The basic model encouraged a systematic plan to identify problems that face the potential learner, prioritize the problems according to the frequency and intensity of disease, write educational objectives to specify the direction of learning, develop an inventory of available resources that can address the objectives, use interactive techniques, and evaluate the results. The evaluation results would then cycle back to the beginning of the model to provide another source of needs assessment data that identified problems not addressed or incompletely resolved.[7]

Miller further asserted that the purpose of CME was to improve patient care and that systematic planning was central to achieving that purpose. The model reached its fullest form in the "bi-cycle" approach of Clement R. Brown, Jr., MD, which combined a cycle of quality assessment with a cycle of educational planning.[8] The model showed considerable promise for linking CME with quality assurance and improving patient care; however there was little evidence of use of the model or substantial change in physician behavior.[9]

At the same time, educational researchers were increasingly concerned about the lack of evidence demonstrating the effectiveness of CME. Studies found that there was little comprehensive needs assessment, systematic development of objectives rarely occurred, there was continued reliance on didactic techniques, and there was minimal evaluation effort.[10] The findings suggested little progress in use of systematic planning models designed to identify practice-based educational needs and design interactive learning experiences.

In an important precursor to the later emphasis on outcomes, John S. Lloyd, PhD, and Stephen Abrahamson, PhD, identified six levels of CME outcomes: attendance, satisfaction, knowledge, competence, performance, and patient outcomes. At this point, most studies focused on the first two levels (attendance and satisfaction), a modest number focused on knowledge, and few focused on competence, performance, and patient outcomes. What had started to change in this era, however, was the focus of educational researchers in CME. They were beginning to ask specific questions about how CME was being planned and if current approaches were leading to effective learning. The field of CME was poised for major changes in research in its next developmental stage.

Research and the Era of Professionalization (1980–1995)

Professionalization of the field of CME moved research forward. The development of a research community that was specifically concerned with issues related to CME was supported in part by the emergence of the SACME (originally known as the Society of Medical College Directors of Continuing Medical Education) and a journal focused on CME.

While studies of CME to determine "if it worked" were being conducted by those in CME and in the broader field of medical education, the research relied largely on the motivation and resources of individuals and the resulting literature was fragmented and dispersed. To develop the kind of infrastructure that could draw together the CME community, SACME was formed in 1976, to address issues in academic CME in medical schools in North America.

SACME fostered discussion among colleagues, the development of collaborative projects, and new ties among colleagues interested in CME research. Communication was enhanced through a newsletter and informal discussion, but very importantly, meetings focused on CME that included research in the field. For the first time, those in CME had a dedicated professional forum in which to present and critique projects that would add to the literature base and suggest effective translations for CME practitioners to support physician learning. SACME also provided a new kind of meeting place for two critical partners in developing research that focused on physician learning: physicians who were familiar with patient care concerns and the questions raised in clinical practice, and professional educators who were trained in a range of research methods that could assist in answering those relevant questions.

In 1981, the University of California Press published the inaugural issue of *Mobius*, a journal for continuing education professionals in the health sciences. Leadership of the initiative came largely from faculty at the University of California, San Francisco. The editorial board included expertise not only in medicine, nursing, and allied health but also in adult education and extension services. In 1984, the Alliance for Continuing Medical Education (ACME) and SACME adopted the journal as their own; in 1996, the Council on CME of the Association for Hospital Medical Education joined the ACME and SACME in ownership. The mission of the journal has been to promote dissemination of research about the theory and practice of continuing education in the health sciences.

Lucy Ann Geiselman, PhD, was the founding editor and served from 1981 to 1986. Malcolm S. M. Watts, MD, associate dean for CME at the University of California, San Francisco, served as editor from 1986 through 1991. In 1988, *Mobius* became the *Journal of Continuing Education in the Health Professions* (*JCEHP*). Starting in 1992, William Felch, MD, helped the journal expand toward an international presence with commentaries and essays that shed light on contemporary issues, especially those involving accreditation, credit, and newer instructional technologies. In 1995, Robert D. Fox, EdD, accepted the position of editor. Strengthening the theoretical foundation of the field, he introduced a steady stream of highly acclaimed writers in adult and continuing education and enabled stability and growth of the journal into a respected source of scientific information. Paul E. Mazmanian, PhD, became editor of *JCEHP* in 2000 and, in that same year, 20 years of peer-review and on-time publishing were recognized by the National Library of Medicine (NLM). *JCEHP* was listed and indexed in MEDLINE, the NLM on-line literature search service. Key themes of the journal began to shift toward a worldwide audience of health professionals, with increased attention to continuous quality improvement, health policy, performance, competency assessment, knowledge translation, and team learning.

The development of a journal was a signal contribution to the growth of CME research. In presenting a forum in which to disseminate both theoretical and practice-based expertise and to promote each informing the other, the editors provided a rich environment for research to enter a new stage of development.

As *JCEHP* was matured and provided a new way to disseminate information, literature from other sources also affected the field. A major turning point for SACME and its members was triggered in 1982 with publication of a study by John C. Sibley, MD, and his colleagues suggesting that CME "did not work."[11] This study catalyzed research in CME for two reasons. First, it was published in the *New England Journal of Medicine* (*NEJM*). While there were reports of the inadequacies of CME in less well-known educational journals, publication in the highly respected *NEJM* was a very visible public forum. Second, some in CME had concerns about how the study was conducted, believing that a medical research model (randomized controlled trial) might not have been sensitive enough or the appropriate design to detect the complexities of learning. At the same time, Leonard S. Stein, PhD, concluded that CME made a difference under certain conditions, and Lloyd and Abrahamson said its effect was inconsistent. The confusion in the literature and importance of the issues pushed a group of SACME members led by Fox to suggest a major study to develop a more complex understanding of the role of learning and change in medical practice. Under SACME's auspices, a multi-site study was directed by Fox, Mazmanian, and R. Wayne Putnam, MD, to carefully examine the issue of whether CME led to changes in physicians' behavior. Rather than looking at CME as a cause for behavior change, the study explored how and when the complex phenomenon of change occurred and what role CME might have played. The protocol for data collection involved 26 SACME member researchers trained to collect 340 interviews outlining 775 changes that physicians reported. The questions the researchers posed were directed to understanding what changes physicians had made in their care of patients or life during the previous year, what they did to accomplish those changes, and what role learning played in the process. Published in 1989, the Change Study, as it came to be known, was based on a rigorous qualitative design that was unfamiliar to many in the medical field who had more experience with the positivist research paradigm.[12] Based on the findings, the authors proposed a model of learning and change that framed a new understanding of how physicians made changes in their work to stay up to date. The model proposed in the Change Study generated a wide range of questions about how and why continuing education was or was not effective in changing physician behavior, contributing to CME research questions since its publication in 1989.

During the same period, the research committee of SACME recognized the importance of creating an infrastructure to support the research of its members, both in terms of finances and the opportunity to engage in scholarly discussion. One result began in 1984 with the first Research in Continuing Medical Education (RICME) meeting. The quadrennial Congress on CME followed in 1988, broadening the scope of effort to include participation from those involved in CME beyond the university based enterprises of SACME. These meetings continue as an important forum for research.

At the same time another significant activity was under development. A critical part of the research infrastructure for any professional group is access to the publications of others who are researching similar areas. In 1984, the Research and Development Resource Base (RDRB) in CME was created under the leadership of David A. Davis, MD, with partial funding from SACME. Because CME researchers often found that the information they needed was not readily available in existing indexing services, the RDRB was created by continuing education staff at McMaster University and further developed by continuing education staff at the University of Toronto. As a bibliographic database, it collects references to the literature of continuing health professional education. It began as a review of about 200 papers in CME titled "The Impact of CME: An Annotated Bibliography."[13] The focus was the delivery and evaluation of continuing education in the health professions, incorporating information about practitioner performance in such areas as prescribing behaviors, and health-care outcomes. While initially designed around the specifics of continuing education, the RDRB has grown to include all interventions, encompassing such areas as those structured to change practice behavior, optimize performance, and implement guidelines. The RDRB has further expanded and now houses a collection of literature for three inter-related fields: continuing education and knowledge translation, interprofessional education and practice, and faculty development. Although the field offered options to learn about research findings at conferences such as RICME and CME Congresses, and the literature in the RDRB, it became clear that translation and application of research findings was difficult for CME practitioners.

The need for a compilation of knowledge about the practice of CME was recognized at this time to support the growing number of CME professionals. The Association of American Medical Colleges (AAMC) and Department of Veteran Affairs supported a series of working groups that produced the book *Continuing Education in the Health Professions: Developing, Managing, and Evaluating Programs for Maximum Impact on Patient Care.*[14] In another effort, supported by SACME, AMA, and other organizations, small groups of scholars were invited to come together in three consensus conferences (Banff and Beaver Creek I and II) resulting in two books: *The Physician as Learner* and *The Continuing Professional Development of Physicians: From Research to Practice.*[15] The goal of these initiatives was to translate CME research for CME practitioners, and provide a compilation of research literature.

Two other groups have been among those important to the development of the research agenda. The Alliance for CME (ACME) has been a partner in the research effort. The ACME began in 1974 to open discussions about patient care between those in medicine, government, and pharmaceutical companies. Research presentations have become an important part of its annual meeting. In addition, the ACME has long been one of the sponsors of the major conferences, such as RICME and the Congress in CME, and *JCEHP.*

In 1996, the AAMC Group on Educational Affairs underwent a major restructuring with the aim of providing a distinct educational home, in sections for those in medical schools at each of the undergraduate, graduate, and continuing medical education levels, as well as a section for those interested in research across the continuum. This group has provided an additional forum for scholarly work in CME.

Despite the increase in research activity and availability of new information, there was no simple way to begin looking at what was known to define effective CME, and what questions remained to be explored. Davis and colleagues provided leadership to an effort that contributed to the further development of an infrastructure of analyzed results from previous research to support new work in the field.[16] Relevant literature was retrieved for comparison of results from previous studies with differing methodologies, samples, and outcomes in order to combine and synthesize findings. Meta-analysis permitted Davis and his colleagues to identify elements of effective CME activities, i.e., CME that works. Combining the results of Davis's work with the Change Study, a theory of how physicians change and how to plan educational activities to support effective learning was beginning to form. An era that began with uncertainty about the effectiveness of CME ended with an emerging theory about how physicians learn and what CME professionals could do to be effective in support of that learning.

Expanding Research

The end of the 1980s and the beginning of the 1990s marked the emergence of CME as a distinct area of practice and study. Systems of accreditation for CME providers were developed that began to incorporate some of the basic research findings. Accreditation of medical schools in Canada included a mandate for educational research. The Canadian institutional support as part of accreditation led to the addition of educational researchers to many CME offices in Canada, and provided a stimulus for research and development that contributed a large body of work

to the field. There were four major groups of providers: university-based medical schools, professional societies, workplaces like hospitals and health systems, and independent for-profit providers. Web-based learning and other e-technologies provided new delivery options.

Even with the expansion of providers and more CME activities, CME practitioners were not yet working with a common understanding of how to implement effective CME. As in the broader field of medical education, researchers in CME continued to work to develop a theory base that could both effectively guide new questions and inform their interpretation. The Change Study is a significant example of theory-building within the field.

Ideas from related fields have also contributed, enhancing both questions asked and understanding their results. For example, theories of continuing education have built on psychology (such as participation theory of Alan B. Knox, EdD), and within that on motivation (commitment to change) and readiness to change.[17] Social cognitive theories of learning have also been used to frame CME research, especially the concept of self-efficacy as a factor in successful change.[18] Theories of learning through reflection and reflective practice have also been incorporated into the CME literature by the work of Donald A. Schon, PhD.[19] The expansion to include new ideas brought new thinking and discussion, but did not produce great change in the way CME was offered to physicians.

Other broad philosophical shifts beyond CME have also affected the nature of research undertaken and the methodologies used. The positivist view, commonly referred to as the medical model, has heavily influenced CME and, therefore, the research questions asked; preferred designs have been experimental and the methods almost exclusively quantitative. The goal of these studies, to establish generalizable knowledge that can both predict and explain, and to establish causal relationships, remains an important one to researchers in CME. However, reviews of CME research reveal that well-designed and conducted experimental studies have been difficult to implement, and therefore have limited our ability to create the kind of evidence sought by many in the field. More recently, the larger field of medical education has begun to incorporate a different theoretical position, the constructivist view, seeking to describe and understand phenomena, recognizing the possibility of multiple and interacting explanations. This view has led to the use of more qualitative approaches to inquiry. And, there has been a call for increased use of a mixed methods approach, combining both qualitative and quantitative approaches.[20] These developments have broadened ways of understanding and approaches to explore the complexities of physician learning applied to practice and the multiple variables that influence that practice.

New questions, new ideas, and applications of an emerging model resulted in a new creative tension: the juxtaposition of the new understandings gained from research in CME and the challenges of their translation into CME practice. This significant change for CME research moved from an almost exclusively empirical focus to one that includes not only a research-practice praxis but incorporates relevant theory from other fields as well. As an understanding of how physicians learn has become more sophisticated and as the relevance of work in other fields is more accepted, several theoretical orientations and approaches have been used to frame CME research. The generation of theory, expansion of research projects, and increased number of activities all created an impetus for a new view of CME based on evidence that could integrate so many pieces essential for a sufficiently complex picture of learning and change. Putting together all the pieces of theory, methods, and translation of results encouraged a new view of CME, but it was not a cohesive picture. One of the groups that sought ways to crystallize a new picture was supported by the AAMC. An invited group defined the parameters of the new understanding of CME with a list of expanded sources of new ideas in related literature, values for the field, core competencies including those in research, and action steps.[21]

Research in CME: Where Are We Today?

A review of *JCEHP* articles from 1981 to 2006 found that the CME research published in the journal reflected thinking in the field as evolving from a more narrowly focused approach to traditional CME to take into account the broad range of contextual aspects influencing practice improvement and learning in the clinical setting.[22] The number of articles reporting original research increased, reflecting the increased value placed on evidence for improving the design and delivery of CME.

In another approach to systematic review of research on CME, Spyridon Marinopoulos, MD, and his colleagues found that CME is effective in the areas studied, but the authors felt that they were unable to draw firm conclusions due to the generally low quality of study designs, variable quality of reporting in studies, and lack of valid and reliable CME evaluation tools.[23] The authors collected and synthesized evidence regarding the effectiveness of CME and the comparative effectiveness of differing instructional designs in terms of impact on knowledge, attitudes, skills, practice behavior, and clinical practice outcomes. We examined some of the data that they assembled to see if trends were evident in CME research design or the variables measured.

The project by the Johns Hopkins Evidence-based Practice Center (EPC) started with almost 60,000 titles from 1981 to February 2006, reduced to 136 to meet study criteria, oriented toward the traditional medical model. We analyzed the data on knowledge, attitudes, skills, practice behavior, and clinical practice outcomes from articles, from 1981 to 2005, that were listed in appendix F of the report (pp. F-1 to F-25). Several important overall observations resulted. The number of studies published in peer-reviewed journals increased dramatically from nine in

1981 through 1985 to 61 in 2001 through 2005, an increase of almost 600 percent, with publications after 1996 accounting for more than 70 percent of the total. Most articles were published in clinically oriented journals, rather than in medical education journals (80 percent). During the period 1981 to 2005, data were collected on a total of 295 variables in the 140 studies examined. We combined the variables used in the Hopkins EPC study into four categories: satisfaction with curriculum; knowledge, attitudes, and skills; behavior; and patient/clinical outcomes. Two of the categories—(1) knowledge, attitudes, skills and (2) behavior—account for 76 percent of the variables measured.

Research results from the analysis of this select group of articles may be helpful in comparison to other kinds of studies. First, the number of research studies in CME increased dramatically from 1996 through 2005. Second, the majority of these studies (80 percent) were published in non-educational journals, providing information for clinicians but raising concerns that the theoretical basis for physician learning and change that was emerging might not have been reflected in these studies. Third, randomized controlled trials predominated, but selection criteria in the Hopkins EPC study probably caused that result. A review of the literature showed that studies using qualitative approaches increased dramatically from 1996 to 2005, reflecting the increasing acceptance of more constructivist approaches as appropriate for the questions asked. Fourth, self-report methods have been used slightly more often than objective methods. Finally, more than 75 percent of the variables collected fell into two categories: knowledge/attitudes/skills and behavior, reflecting the difficulty of directly addressing the question of the impact of CME on patient health.

The Future of Research on CME

Meaningful historical study goes beyond the essential facts to analysis of trends that provide guidance and direction for the future. Unquestionably the amount of research in CME has expanded dramatically in the last decade and a half. But the evidence that CME is positively impacting changes in physicians' care of patients is modest, and the impact on the health of patients remains unclear. Several factors may be contributing. First, little of what we know about how physicians learn and change has become part of the day-to-day practice of CME. There are probably many reasons for this, including lack of institutional support for CME and the absence of practical guidelines for individuals charged with planning and conducting CME activities.

Another important factor may be the many variables that contribute to patient outcomes in addition to physician behavior. These include, but are not limited to, the health-care delivery system, the variability of individual patients and families, and the social context within which patients live and providers practice.

A third issue concerns the conduct of CME research. Systematic reviews report generally low quality of study designs, variable quality of reporting in studies, and lack of valid and reliable CME evaluation tools. There remains a lack of agreement of the definition of the variables that are being measured and little theory-testing, particularly of the theory describing physician learning and change that has been emerging in the field of CME. In addition, studies contributing to knowledge in CME appear in clinical journals where the review process and criteria may differ from that in educational journals.

The development of CME research described in this chapter highlights major gains, and many changes. Yet it also includes frustrations. The CME field has actively supported several professional groups and created an influential journal that has been included in indexed periodical listings and attracted the attention of many professionals in related fields such as health policy and quality improvement. Regulatory requirements for maintenance of certification of specialty boards and maintenance of licensure of state licensing boards have heightened the awareness of the medical community about the connection between learning and physician performance. Accreditation requirements include some ideas about learning and that are drawn from the results of research. Furthermore, there is more informal discussion that points to the field having moved beyond the idea of simply transmitting knowledge to more complex ideas about supporting effective learning. However, there remain important fields of study, such as clinical practice guidelines, knowledge translation, quality improvement and patient safety, and clinical translational research, with common interests and goals where connections are not yet well established.

Just as in other areas of health care, substantive change can be slow, cumbersome, and complex. The important work of researchers has provided a clearer picture of the role of learning in changing behaviors to produce continually improving care for patients. But, those ideas about effective learning have not become consistently embedded in the daily work of those developing and delivering CME. Institutional support for change in approaches to CME has been inconsistent and funding presents challenges. While change is slow, research provides results that stimulate and inform the conversation among those in the field and create persuasive arguments for change. The idea that CME equates to delivering large amounts of new knowledge to change practice is no longer part of the discussion. There is support for the need to understand how physicians translate new information into practice and make decisions about changing patient management strategies based on evidence and experience. There is a desire in the CME community to make use of research results to help physicians make those changes.

To move forward, priorities in the CME research agenda must align with the needs of CME practitioners as they attempt to function in a health-care environment characterized by change

brought on by health reform, the explosion of biomedical information, and the expansion of information technology and social connectivity. Developing a focused agenda will allow results to build more effectively. Consistent definitions of variables would allow more comparison among projects. Funding must be available. To carry out a research agenda, the field must nurture and encourage capable and productive researchers who will develop and refine theories that undergird the practical tools used by CME practitioners. And, without strategic leadership skills within the CME community focused on the research agenda, the agenda will not move forward. Leadership at both the North American and institutional level is essential. None of the barriers to moving forward are new, but as the health-care field faces new demands, CME research must be part of the effort to support physician learning and change. A better understanding of how to support physicians as they seek to improve health care is essential if CME is to fulfill its promise of guiding change and moving our ideas forward.

Notes

1. A. Flexner, *Medical Education in the United States and Canada: A Report to the Carnegie Foundation for the Advance of Teaching* (New York: Carnegie Foundation for the Advancement of Teaching, 1910).

2. W. F. Norwood, "Observations on the Profile of Continuation Medical Education," *Journal of Medical Education* 30, no. 1 (1955): 31–39; J. E. Deitrick and R. C. Berson, *Medical Schools in the United States at Mid-century* (New York: McGraw-Hill, 1953); D. D. Vollan, *Postgraduate Medical Education in the United States* (Chicago: American Medical Association, 1955).

3. J. B. Youmans, "Experience with a Postgraduate Course for Practitioners: Evaluation of Results," *Journal of the Association of American Medical Colleges* 10, no. 3 (1935): 154–173.

4. O. L. Peterson and others, "An Analytic Study of North Carolina General Practice," *Journal of Medical Education* 31, no. 12 (1956): 1–165.

5. K. F. Clute, *The General Practitioner: Study of Medical Education and Practice in Ontario and Nova Scotia* (Toronto: University of Toronto Press, 1963).

6. G. E. Miller, "Medical Care: Its Social and Orga-

nizational Aspects: The Continuing Education of Physicians," *New England Journal of Medicine* 269 (1963): 295–299.

7. P. B. Storey and others, *Continuing Medical Education: A New Emphasis* (Chicago: American Medical Association, 1968); C. H. Castle and P. B. Storey, "Physicians' Needs and Interests in Continuing Medical Education," *Journal of the American Medical Association* 206, no. 3 (1968): 611–614; J. W. Williamson and others, "Priorities in Patient-care Research and Continuing Medical Education," *Journal of the American Medical Association* 204, no. 4 (1968): 303–308; J. W. Williamson and others, "Continuing Education and Patient Care Research," *Journal of the American Medical Association* 201, no. 12 (1967): 938–942.

8. C. R. Brown and H. S. M. Uhl, "Mandatory Continuing Education: Sense or Nonsense?" *Journal of the American Medical Association* 206, no. 3 (1970): 1660–1668.

9. P. J. Sanazaro, "Medical Audit, Continuing Medical Education and Quality Assurance, *Western Journal of Medicine* 125, no. 3 (1976): 241–252; P. J. Sanazaro, "How Medical Audit and CME Affect Physician Performance—Part 2," *Hospital Medical Staff* 6, no. 2 (1977): 17–26; P. J. Sanazaro, "How Medical Audit and CME Affect Physician Performance—Part 1," *Hospital Medical Staff* 6, no. 1 (1977): 1–11.

10. F. C. Pennington and J. S. Green, "Comparative Analysis of Program Development Processes in Six Professions," *Adult Education Quarterly* 27, no. 1 (1976): 13–23; L. S. Stein, "The Effectiveness of Continuing Medical Education: Eight Research Reports," *Journal of Medical Education* 56 (1980): 103–110; J. S. Lloyd and S. Abrahamson, "Effectiveness of Continuing Medical Education: A Review of the Evidence," *Evaluation in the Health Professions* 2, no. 3 (1979): 251–280; D. A. Bertram and P. A. Brooks-Bertram, "The Evaluation of Continuing Medical Education: A Literature Review," *Health Education Monographs* 5, no. 4 (1977): 330–362.

11. J. C. Sibley and others, "A Randomized Controlled Trial of Continuing Medical Education," *New England Journal of Medicine* 306 (1982): 511–515.

12. R. D. Fox and others, *Changing and Learning in the Lives of Physicians* (New York: Praeger, 1989).

13. D. Davis, "The Impact of CME: A Methodological Review of the Continuing Medical Education Literature," *Evaluation in the Health Professions* 7, no. 4 (1984): 251–283.

14. J. S. Green and others, *Continuing Education for the Health Professions: Developing, Managing, and Evaluating Programs for Maximum Impact on Patient Care* (San Francisco: Jossey-Bass, 1984).

15. D. A. Davis and R. D. Fox, *The Physician as Learner: Linking Research to Practice* (Chicago: American Medical Association, 1994); D. A. Davis and others, eds., *The Continuing Professional Development of Physicians: From Research to Practice* (Chicago: AMA Press, 2003).

16. Davis, "Impact of CME," 251–283; D. A. Davis and others, "Evidence for the Effectiveness of CME. A Review of 50 Randomized Controlled Trials," *Journal of the American Medical Association* 268 (1992):1111–1117; D. A. Davis and others, "Changing Physician Performance. A Systematic Review of the Effect of Continuing Medical Education Strategies," *Journal of the American Medical Association* 274, no. 9 (1995): 700–705.

17. A. B. Knox, "Proficiency Theory of Adult Learning," *Contemporary Educational Psychology* 5 (1980): 378–404; P. E. Mazmanian and others, "Commitment to Change: Ideational Roots, Empirical Evidence, and Ethical Implications," *Journal of Continuing Education in the Health Professions* 17 (1997): 133–144; J. O. Prochaska and W. F. Velicer, "The Transtheoretical Model of Health Behavior Change," *American Journal of Health Promotion* 12 (1997): 38–48.

18. A. Bandura, *Social Foundations of Thought and Action* (Englewood Cliffs: Prentice-Hall, 1986); A. Bandura, "Self-efficacy: Toward a Unifying Theory of Behavioral Change," *Psychological Review* 84, no. 2 (1977): 191–215.

19. D. Schon, *The Reflective Practitioner: How Professionals Think in Action* (New York: Basic Books, 1983), 21–73; D. A. Schon, *Educating the Reflective Practitioner* (San Francisco: Jossey-Bass, 1987).

20. J. W. Creswell and others, "Designing a Mixed Methods Study in Primary Care," *Annals of Family Medicine* 2, no. 1 (2004): 7–12.

21. R. D. Fox, "Using Theory and Research to Shape the Practice of Continuing Professional Development," *Journal of Continuing Education in the Health Professions* 20, no. 4 (2000): 238–246; N. L. Bennett and others, "Continuing Medical Education: A New Vision of the Professional Development of Physicians," *Academic Medicine* 75, no. 12 (2000): 1167–1172.

22. A. MacIntosh-Murray and others, "Research to Practice in *The Journal of Continuing Education in the Health Professions*: A Thematic Analysis of Volumes 1 through 24," *Journal of Continuing Education in the Health Professions* 26, no. 3 (2006): 230–243.

23. S. S. Marinopoulos and others, *Effectiveness of Continuing Medical Education* (Rockville, Md.: Agency for Healthcare Research and Quality, 2007).

CHAPTER 16

The History of Evidence-Based Continuing Medical Education in the United States

The American Academy of General Practice (AAGP), now the American Academy of Family Physicians (AAFP), was the first medical specialty society to require ongoing continuing medical education (CME) for continued membership. In response to its bylaws of incorporation in 1948, the AAGP created a system for reviewing and approving CME activities. AAFP-prescribed credit remains the CME currency for family physicians today and is accepted by all state licensing boards as equivalent to American Medical Association (AMA) Physician's Recognition Award (PRA) Category 1 credit.

The Genesis of Evidence-Based CME

In the late 1990s, the AAFP struggled with how to handle the ever-increasing number of complementary and alternative medicine (CAM) topics being submitted for CME credit approval. Some AAFP members supported these controversial topics while others condemned them. Some felt CAM should be considered within the scope of family medicine, some felt family physicians should be aware of these modalities so they could appropriately counsel their patients, and others felt CAM should not be practiced.

In early 1999, the AAFP Commission on Continuing Medical Education (COCME) led by Washington physician Larry Johnson, MD, made CAM a central focus of its agenda; a decision needed to be made regarding the management of CAM in CME. According to Johnson, the COCME wished to ensure all activities were evaluated consistently.

At its January 1999 meeting, the COCME invited Murray Kopelow, MD, CEO, of the Accreditation Council for Continuing Medical Education (ACCME) as a guest. Dr. Kopelow suggested that if all CME were evidence based, then all CME could be judged by the same consistent standards. There would be no need to single out CAM topics.

As a result of these early discussions, the AAFP formed a Subcommittee on Clinical Content in June 1999 that included members of the AAFP commissions on CME, education, clinical policies and research, health care services, quality, and scope of practice. The subcommittee identified three family physician evidence-based medicine experts to advise the group on an evidence-based approach to CME. Montana State University's Robert Flaherty, MD, had served on the COCME and was named to the subcommittee along with Mark Ebell, MD, of the Medical College of Georgia, and Lee Green, MD, of the University of Michigan. The subcommittee's charge was to design a process for an equitable, evidence-based approach to evaluate CME content and a corresponding process for CME providers to develop evidence-based CME content. The subcommittee accepted evidence-based medicine expert David Sackett's definition of *evidence-based medicine:* "the integration of current best research evidence with clinical expertise and patient values."[1]

In January 2000, the subcommittee invited representatives of external stakeholders in the CME environment to join the group. They included Kopelow of the ACCME; Dennis K. Wentz, MD, AMA Continuing Physician Professional Development (new AMA PRA director Charles Willis, MBA, joined in 2002); Robert Avant, MD, American Board of Family Medicine (ABFM); Delores Rodgers, American Osteopathic Association (AOA); Dale Austin, Federation of State Medical Boards (FSMB); and Bernard Marlow, MD, College of Family Physicians of Canada (CFPC). The addition of these representatives ensured harmonization across the three US and one Canadian CME credit systems and regulators (i.e., AMA, AAFP, ACCME, AOA, and CFPC) and support from the major consumers of CME credit (i.e., the state medical licensing boards—FSMB—and the certifying board in family medicine—ABFM). These stakeholders supported the concept of evidence-based CME (EBCME) content. Willis had a special interest from the perspective of the AMA PRA credit system: "This was useful to the AMA. We did not approve individual activities but were being challenged by 'dangerous' topics, such as anti-aging remedies, that we couldn't counter without some definition of evidence-based CME."[2]

The result of this work was the first iteration of EBCME, which was piloted in 2000–2001. Among the criteria were choices of 10 approved evidence-based medicine sources (see Box 16-1) and six approved evidence-based rating scales (see Box 16-2) that allowed physicians to choose a source and rating scale with which they were familiar. Eventually, this scheme was modified into the Strength of Recommendation Taxonomy (SORT) system that is used to evaluate evidence in medical literature (see Box 16-3). The AAFP

Box 16-1
Original List of AAFP-Approved Evidence-Based Medicine Sources

Agency for Healthcare Research and Quality (AHRQ)
Bandolier
Canadian Task Force on Preventive Health Care
Clinical Evidence
Cochrane Database of Systematic Reviews
Database of Abstracts of Reviews of Effects (DARE)
EBM Online
Effective Health Care
National Guidelines Clearinghouse
US Preventative Services Task Force (USPSTF)

Box 16-2
Original List of AAFP-Approved Grading Scales

AAFP-Recommended Basic Model
American College of Physicians–American Society of Internal Medicine (ACP–ASIM) Model
American Medical Association Model
US Preventive Service Task Force / Canadian Task Force on Preventive Health Care Model
Joint National Committee on Prevention, Detection, Evaluation, and Treatment of High Blood Pressure (JNC VII) Model
Center for Evidence-Based Medicine Model (Sackett et al.)

Box 16-3
AAFP-Recommended Basic Model

Level A: Evidence from meta-analysis or multiple randomized controlled trials
Level B: Evidence from well-designed prospective clinical trials or clinical cohort studies with consistent finding, without randomization
Level C: Evidence from studies other than clinical trials such as epidemiological and physiological studies
Level D: Expert consensus statements

journal *American Family Physician* adopted SORT in 2004.[3]

For an activity to be approved for EBCME credit, the provider needed to use an approved evidence-based medicine source, make evidence-based practice recommendations explicit to learners, and disclose the level of evidence (by using the approved grading scale) for the recommendations.

By 2002, the COCME eliminated the requirement for specific grading scales but continued to require the use of approved evidence-based medicine sources and some accepted grading of the evidence. The process for developing EBCME (see Box 16-4) was disseminated by the AAFP accreditation department with implementation encouraged in AAFP's own CME program as well as those of AAFP constituent chapters.

EBCME Challenges and Barriers

As in the practice of medicine, challenges have arisen for integrating evidence-based medicine into CME. For many topics little or no reviewed evidence may exist. These topics, while not eligible for EBCME credit, should not be excluded from CME programming. As always, physician learners must use their own critical thinking skills to determine what is in the best interests of their patients. While concerns continue about the quality and availability of evidence, it should be the goal of CME providers and faculty to present the highest level of clinical information possible to allow physicians to make informed decisions about their patients' care. By using an evidence-based medicine approach to CME, gaps in clinical research can be found that will stimulate further research in those areas lacking adequate evidence. The goal of this ongoing process is to improve the quality of CME available to physicians. The ultimate goal of the process is to link quality EBCME to changes in physician behavior in their day-to-day process of providing patient care and to measure patient care improvement as a result of EBCME.

The AAFP Home Study Self-Assessment (HSSA) program was the first user of EBCME credit. Nationally recognized, research-oriented family physicians made up the editorial board, and they applauded the concept but challenged the development process, the evidence-level scales required, and the documentation requirements. According to HSSA manager Penny Dove, "EBCME made a real difference in some clinical areas, for example, the overuse of antibiotics. Having the strength of evidence for recommendations really helped to change practice."[4] The HSSA took the issue so seriously that it published a monograph on CAM therapies that was awarded EBCME credit due to its evidence base.[5] California physician Tom Bent, MD, who served on the HSSA board and as chair of AAFP's Commission on Continuing Professional Development (formerly COCME) while EBCME was evolving, stated that "EBCME took the emotion out of complementary and alternative medicine debates. There is now clear evidence for some of the practices. I now use evidence in my exam room every day."[6]

The documentation of the process provided the biggest challenge for implementing EBCME. The onus fell on faculty to develop their content in the prescribed manner. CME providers often were challenged to make the new requirements clear to faculty. Both staff of CME providers and faculty of CME programs complained about the increased workload. Resistance even took the form of "gaming of the system" through retrofitting pre-existing presentations into the evidence-based format by searching approved sources for evidence that would support the existing content.

In 2004, the nation's CME custodians of the CME credit systems in the United States (i.e., AAFP, AMA, and AOA) and the accrediting organizations (i.e., AAFP, AOA, and ACCME) ceased measuring CME in hours and moved to measuring CME in credits. This national decision recognized the evolving value of CME and the growing mismatch between that value and the amount of time required to complete a CME program. The AAFP Commission on Continuing Professional Development followed with a bold and controversial decision to award double credit for CME activities meeting the criteria for EBCME.

This re-inventing of the value of CME credit received criticism and support. The potential for disparity between AAFP EBCME credit and that of AMA, AOA, and CFPC threatened the harmonization of credit across the CME credit systems. Credit for activities designated for both AMA PRA and AAFP could be perceived as unbalanced. Wisely, state licensing boards have taken the position that the credit systems determine what constitutes CME credit, while the licensing boards determine how much credit is required for re-licensure.

The double credit decision awarded extra credit for extra value but not for extra effort on the part of the learner. In fact, the extra burden was on the faculty and, to some degree, the CME provider. A study conducted by the Wisconsin Academy of Family Physicians showed that the biggest barriers to faculty in using the EBCME process was the time required for preparation and documentation and the lack of access to approved EMB sources.[7]

While some expressed concerns that physicians earning double credit would not attend as many activities, other CME providers saw the opportunity to increase their competitive edge with double credit for their EBCME activities. For the AAFP, which tracks CME credit for members, documenting credit for participants of activities that had both double and traditional credit was a challenge. At the same time, AAFP recognized that EBCME was "more justifiable and defensible than previous CME, and physicians valued EBCME more on their transcripts," according to Colleen Lawler, former AAFP director of membership.[8]

Double credit for EBCME served as an incentive to increase the implementation of EBCME. The rationale was that physician learners would value double-credit EBCME and demand more. ACCME promoted the AAFP EBCME criteria as a best practice in validating CME content and mitigating risks of commercial bias.

With just five percent of all AAFP-accredited CME activities designated as EBCME in 2008, the AAFP made the decision in 2009 to sunset double credit and phase it out completely by January 2011.[9] Rationale include the CME environment that expected evidence-base content, a movement toward performance-based CME, and the desire to harmonize CME credit across disciplines.

EBCME and the Future of CME

Ten years after the idea was planted, EBCME has served to facilitate the incorporation of clinical evidence into CME. EBCME was "another strategy to increase the quality and decrease variation in care. Medicine needed to move from 'informed opinion' (white hair + white coat) to evidence," as recalled by Robert Graham, MD, former AAFP executive vice president.[10]

Facilitating the continued integration of evidence into clinical practice is the challenge of all CME. While EBCME was changing the value of CME credit in the early years of the new millennium, the AMA Council on Medical Education convened two task forces to develop two new forms of CME: point-of-care CME and performance-improvement CME. In 2005, the nation's three CME credit systems (i.e., AAFP, AMA, and AOA) adopted standardized criteria for these two revolutionary forms of CME, both of which are based in current best evidence.

CME appears to be evolving from categorizations of *traditional* and *evidence-based* now to *knowledge-based* (e.g., lectures, enduring materials, and journals, any of which can be delivered via the Internet) and *practice-based* (e.g., point-of-care and performance-improvement) CME. It may be that AAFP EBCME will be viewed historically as a catalyst of this process, serving to create a new and improved CME credit from one that served the nation for half a century.

Notes

1. D. L. Sackett and others, *Evidence-Based Medicine: How to Practice and Teach EBM.* 2nd ed. (London: Churchill Livingstone, 2000), 25.

2. Charles Willis, telephone interview with Nancy Davis, March 2, 2009.

3. M. H. Ebell and others, "Strength of Recommendation Taxonomy (SORT): A Patient-Centered Approach to Grading Evidence in the Medical Literature," *American Family Physician* 69, no. 3 (2004): 548–556.

4. Penny Dove, telephone interview with Nancy Davis, February 27, 2009.

5. R. Zoorob and others. Complementary and Alternative Medicine. Family Practice Essentials, Edition No. 293, AAFP Home Study. (Leawood, Kans.: American Academy of Family Physicians, 2003).

6. Tom Bent, telephone interview with Nancy Davis, March 3, 2009.

7. S. L. Lawrence and others, "The Influence of Double-Credit Evidence-Based Continuing Medical Education on Presenters and Learners," *Wisconsin Medical Journal* 107, no. 4 (2008): 181–186.

8. Colleen Lawler, telephone interview with Nancy Davis, March 2, 2009.

9. American Academy of Family Physicians. Board of Directors meeting minutes. April 20–24, 2009.

10. Robert Graham, telephone interview with Nancy Davis, February 26, 2009.

CHAPTER 17

Four Pillars in the Evolution of Continuing Medical Education

In any essay on history, the dates and events need to be correct but the analysis fails if no themes emerge that help readers to understand and explain the present based on the past. Currently, in continuing professional development (CPD),[1] I have seen and heard evidence of many problems, often accompanied by complaints, worries, and very little optimism for a brighter future. What I hear from my colleagues is that the science that underlies the practice of CPD is irrelevant to the everyday problems that those who offer education to physicians face. I also hear that, though there are new standards for quality for CPD activities, those who provide continuing medical education (CME) and those who teach in programs often complain that meeting these standards is too hard if not impossible. It is also common to overhear discussions among my colleagues and to read on a regular basis the belief that any involvement in the enterprise by the pharmaceutical industry is guaranteed to introduce bias, taint the educational effort, and undermine quality. I believe that most see industry as devious and destructive. Finally, when I talk to clinicians and policy makers, they often complain that CME professionals cannot demonstrate that their efforts to facilitate learning are effective or that they are even prepared properly to take on this responsibility.

It is not only what I hear that disturbs me, it is also what I see. The social systems in organizations and the individual actors concerned with improving medical performance and outcomes do not collaborate well or often. In fact, pluralism rules the day as each stakeholder involved in the CME enterprise promotes his or her or its special interests, often in competition with the others in the system. Even specialization within CME, which normally improves practice, in this case has resulted in a disintegration of the CME process into pieces and parts. This is in contrast to the evidence that suggests that learning and change for physicians is holistic, a natural part of the overall process of providing quality care.

I have also observed that the practices most used to develop education for clinicians are primarily a function of mimicry rather than investigation and systematic learning. In fact, rather than sound scientific evidence and reasoning, change is driven by novelty and a "flavor of the month" mentality. In many cases, isolated findings from small, poor studies become justification for the adoption of "innovative" educational methods and techniques that provide a market edge or a public relations advantage. Large literature reviews are often labeled as metanalysis when they do not use common variables, measures, or reanalysis of primary data.

These are the problems I hear about and read about. These are the problems I have seen develop during the 30 years I have studied, written about, and participated in the CME enterprise. This analysis of how we find ourselves plagued by the problems described above is formed around four themes or, if you will, four pillars that form the foundations for CME today and CPD tomorrow. The purpose of this essay is to describe how these themes have emerged from developments in four of the critical systems connected to attempts to offer effective learning and practice improvement in order to explain how we arrived at our present position.

In order to do this I wish to offer a few words about my methodology. Historiography is the research method of historians. Among the many ways it puts structure and process on the study of history, it controls quality by rating the quality of data according to systematic criteria. Secondary data sources, for example, are secondhand accounts written by those who interview or study primary data sources such as eyewitness and written documents of the time. However, one eyewitness is seldom enough. As one eyewitness, I did not feel that I could provide an accurate picture of the history of CME. Since most of this essay is taken from the Shickman lecture delivered at the 2007 American Medical Association Conference on CME Provider/Industry Collaboration, I submitted it in outline form to a panel of nine colleagues, each of whom had experienced the history either fully or in part but from different vantage points than my own. I asked these colleagues to examine my record for accuracy and freedom from bias. What follows, therefore, is an eyewitness account checked for accuracy of events and chronology based on the perspectives and experiences of a panel of colleagues from different facets of CME.

How Did We Get Here?

This may only be considered a brief history since it is a complex field developing within a rapidly changing environment. Nevertheless, like any historical account, certain aspects of that environment have to be examined to understand their role in creating the present. For this essay I will look at four systems: (1) the scientific foundations

of CME as embodied in its research studies and theories that explain how and why physicians learn and change, (2) the systems by which society assigns quality and gives credit to those who provide CME, the accreditation system, (3) the pharmaceutical and medical equipment industry who have provided financial and other support of the enterprise, and (4) the providers of CME, those who work to provide learning opportunities to medical professionals. It is the events and the interactions among these four that offer the best explanation of the present situation.

The Scientific Foundation

Although I was not involved, except as a graduate student, in the literature of CME before the 1980s, I had to study that literature in graduate school and when I began my research career in a medical school in 1979. I observed that there were few studies, and most articles were primarily driven by opinion and oriented towards practice "tips." The few studies that existed were published in literature specific to specialties. Although such works as Brown's bicycle approach to explaining the role of CME were abstract and ultimately very useful, there was little integration of thought or data around very important questions.[2]

In the early 1980s the situation began to change. The Society of Medical College Directors of Continuing Medical Education (now the Society for Academic Continuing Medical Education [SACME]) was populated by a large number of physicians and a few educators who began to push for educating on the basis of scientific knowledge as to how physicians learn and how education should be practiced. Over this decade, *Mobius* was initiated and evolved into the *Journal of Continuing Education in the Health Professions* (*JCEHP*). Standards for articles included in *JCEHP* rose steadily in quantity and quality during the 1990s to the point where in 2001, *JCEHP* was accepted as a MEDLINE publication because it met the highest standards for medical literature.

From 1980 to the early 2000s, leadership in the field moved from the intellectual domination of physicians who developed programs and CME departments to a system driven by those trained formally at the doctoral level in university colleges of education. Educators and physician leaders alike agreed that a scientific foundation in adult learning and development, adult psychology, and systems theory were essential to producing a body of science worth basing practice on.

By 1995, the question of whether CME works had become subsumed into the broader questions of how and why do physicians learn and change. This transformation was a function in part of the change study. This project took five years and involved more than 400 interviews with practicing physicians in the United States and Canada regardless of specialty. Forty CME senior officers from medical schools conducted the interviews. They were conducted in the practice setting and reported in narrative and numerical data. Approximately 20 of these professionals contributed chapters to a book that changed the agenda and the questions that mattered. *Changing and Learning in the Lives of Physicians* demonstrated that doctors learn, that the learning is directed toward changing practices, and finally, that that process could be used to form a fundamental theory for CME.

It is not that today the literature of CPD is complete or that the scientific foundation strong and unshakable. There is much to be done and the field is plagued by the influences of standards of quality for research appropriate to clinical science but not necessarily to the social and behavioral sciences. However, now the field of CPD has books, respected articles in major medical journals, and international journals with special issues on education and CME. *JCEHP*, our professional journal, is indexed in MEDLINE and Science Citations and is a journal that pro-

duces more than 200 pages of research and theory every year along with supplements on important topics. We also have research conferences like Research in CME, now held as a regular part of the SACME meetings and sessions at the Alliance for Continuing Medical Education (ACME), among others, devoted to translating literature into practice. It would appear that we have made important advances but we have not yet succeeded in building a full and complete scientific foundation as envisioned by the early leaders of SACME.

Although we have a complex body of literature, it isn't read very often by very many. When one speaker at a recent conference asked an audience of about 100 how many had read the last issue of *JCEHP*, fewer than half raised their hands. Within the CME community, we have seen a declining interest and weaker support for research in CPD. In the last five years, research training sessions have been poorly attended or canceled for lack of enrollment. There have been no follow-up, large-scale studies like the *change* study, and the notion of consensus conferences targeted to practice principles for quality education has only recently received any traction.

For the scientific foundation to grow it must be built systematically, on three legs. There must be a *theoretical base* that explains physician behavioral change in terms of the relationship among their competencies, their performance, and the outcomes for their patients. There must be a body of *studies that support or challenge the theoretical foundation* of CPD as well as its common practices. The body of literature finally must *connect theory to investigation to practice.*

In order to fulfill the need for quality programs and educational solutions to health-care challenges, the scientific foundation must recognize that collaboration and transparency among a body of scholars is essential if knowledge is to advance. Scholarly practitioners must use the literature we have. They must read it, interact around it, and search for ways to improve it.

CME also must integrate knowledge and practice around the most well supported and useful theories of change and learning, integrating theory and practice perspectives from many sources.

The Growth of Accreditation

Accreditation systems almost always developed out of a desire of a group of organizations to regulate the quality of their work and products. CPD is no different. Current accreditation of CME is based on the belief that with a systematic process in place, standards of practice and self regulation will not only police but also improve the CPD system. The present system of accreditation has experienced notable changes and considerable evolution to become what it is today.

In the early days, the days when the accreditation system took on its basic shape (i.e., the mid-1970s), the system was based on models of education developed in the 1950s by Ralph Tyler intended to heavily influence the form and function of public school education up through universities. This model focused on writing behavioral objectives that were built to integrate educational activities around types and levels of change in human behavior.[3] The Tyler model basically focused on three stages: the development of written behavioral objectives, the design of education appropriate to the type and level of objective, and the evaluation of knowledge gain based on the type of objective.

The "Essentials" of CME were the first standards set by the accreditation organization. The essentials emphasized the same three phases and focused on the organizational characteristics of those who provided CME. As time passed, emphasis on the potential for industrial bias in programs became a larger concern to the medical community and the Accreditation Council for Continuing Medical Education (ACCME). The ways that the ACCME coped with the growing perception of the potential for bias in industry-supported CME was met with an increasingly rigorous set of rules for forcing disclosures of rela-tionships with industry. The underlying principle was to tell the learners about all sources of bias and let the buyer beware.

In 2006, the accumulation of research and sophistication in the underlying literature, along with extensive efforts by the CME professional associations to educate their members to the research base, led to a complete revision of the system for accreditation. The new system focused on standards of quality derived from studies of adult learning and physician education. The standards focused on change and learning theory, the assessment of needs as a necessary step in the planning process, the development of outcomes measures to answer questions of effectiveness, recognition of the self directed nature of much of medical learning, and the important role of quality improvement as an integrated partner in the process. In addition the new criteria reflected a growing body of literature on the role of barriers to learning and the contributions of health-care systems to both problems and solutions.

In terms of issues of bias, however, accreditation continued with the same for controlling commercial bias by not only asking for complete disclosures but also by insisting on the development of strategies to manage bias and conflict in the planning process. For example, if a speaker was conflicted in a way that made bias likely in the presentation, an alternate speaker should be found. Although this evolution helped with the problem, it did not satisfy critics of the system of CME who continued to insist that any industry money represented bias. The advances in the accreditation process were recognition that the system of CME it supported was changing as its scientific foundation evolved. Its relationship with industry changed and the providers, themselves changed.

To date, we have a system of accreditation that applies legitimate criteria for quality to the enterprise based in a robust body of literature on how and why physicians learn and change. The system is developmentally oriented, in that it seeks to provide feedback to providers for improvements but also to regulate behavior that is contrary to standards. It also rewards progress with special designations of excellence and is capable, although reluctant, to withdraw accreditation outright. However, providers criticize the accreditation system and stakeholders have asserted that the accreditation process does not respond effectively in consideration of practical concerns or limitations endemic to the complexities of the health-care environment. It is also charged with being intolerant of industry funding and of unjustly trying industry involvement in a court of assumptions rather than on the basis of the evidence. Finally, the entire feedback and regulatory functions of the accreditation system are built on how capable and insightful site surveyors are. In other words, since the vast majority of site surveyors come from similar situations and backgrounds as those they survey, it is unclear that they bring any extra insight or other perspective to the issues of quality. Any accreditation system dependent upon self-regulation is always problematic if the regulators do not know more about the work than the providers. In the case of the ACCME, observers must ask how improvement can come from a system where the regulators are the other providers sharing the same perspectives about how hard it is to be excellent in this environment. Academicians, research scientists, or expert clinicians are not part of the process.

If the future is to look better than the past, accreditation must be based on common goals, values and beliefs held by highly trained and experienced site surveyors who focus on the direct application of the body of knowledge underlying the practice of CME. The system must effectively train and certify site surveyors and conduct random audits of providers on a frequent basis. The system must demand transparency and must be transparent to the public as to its activities and findings. Finally, the system must report and reward excellence in public forums. It must operate in a goldfish bowl, constantly explaining its actions and positions to a health-care community and public that wants to understand how and why health-care practitioners do what they do.

The Pharmaceutical and Equipment Industry

For the most part, before 2000, industry focused on funding marketing and sales messages about their products. Even though some companies recognized the dangers and pitfalls of outright attempts to buy presentations only if the message they wished to promote was present, they would request opportunities to edit speeches by experts, to produce slides that communicated marketing themes, and to engage their sales force in direct ways in the educational activity. Inside many companies, marketing and sales units controlled all CME funds, speakers were offered through speakers bureaus with company-prepared slides, and disclosures of conflict of interest were made only when required by providers. In this period accreditation was limited to nonprofits, e.g., medical societies, medical schools, and hospitals. It is noteworthy, however, that a few companies worked diligently towards a higher standard of collaboration and actively contributed to the development of the science of CME through support of research; but most saw CME as a tool for marketing drugs.

This era of excess and the desire by pharmaceutical companies to support large-scale programs with national target audiences made it difficult for hospitals and medical schools to compete with newly emerging medical education communication companies (MECCs). Unlike the United States, Canada elected to continue to restrict accreditation to those that provided health care or represented directly and democratically a group of health-care providers. In the United States, the ACCME elected to give accreditation to the organizations that worked for profit, either independently or as an element at arm's length of an advertising agency. The accredited MECCs, for-profit enterprises whose primary business was education rather than patient care, closely aligned with the sources of their funds, pharmaceutical companies. As MECCs' influence grew along with their ability to deliver national audiences of physicians and surgeons, many pharmaceutical companies provided most of their funding to these organizations. Although there were honorable exceptions, the model encouraged the wrong kind of relationships with industry and discouraged locally founded education that was primarily directed towards local problems and communities of practicing health-care providers.

In this situation, growing government concern and involvement was inevitable. By the first decade of 2000, massive fines from increased scrutiny by the Food and Drug Administration and the Office of the Inspector General and headlines in national newspapers reflected growing distrust of the role of industry in CME.

Now, out of these concerns, for almost all companies, marketing and sales can no longer control messages. Company staff, who have had to learn more than most in order to survive, are often more knowledgeable than a large portion of the providers who request funds. Unrestricted grants are the primary mechanism by which CME is supported. Company legal departments restrict and regulate the engagement of those in the pharmaceutical industry with education providers and speakers. Disclosures are more complete and more transparent.

However, now lawyers rule the interaction among providers and representatives of industry, limiting the feedback that one may give to the other related to improving programs and learning or providing support for innovation. The quarter-to-quarter line of sight of industry has made it difficult to create a business case for supporting CME and has led to steadily declining budgets that may be applied to grants in support of programs. The climate also makes collaboration an unacceptable practice. Finally, because the majority of expendable funds lie in marketing and sales, those working in industry in CME must still find ways to please these divisions of a company in order to garner funds necessary to support CME.

For the future, the key is developing honorable means for successful collaboration without intro-duction of bias into efforts to help physicians learn and change. This kind of collaboration depends on transparency among professionals on both sides of the planning table who are highly trained and insightful about the quality of education, especially in terms of its ethics. Support for CME must be aligned with standards of quality. All involved in the educational process, including industry, must be capable of performance at the highest level based on sound knowledge of the field. Once again, the knowledge base of the field predicts its ability to grow and prosper.

Competent Providers

The fourth system, whose changing nature has contributed to the present and future of CME, is the system of providers that delivers CME to practicing physicians and surgeons. This system, like the others mentioned above, has had a tumultuous four decades. In the early days of CME (pre-1976), no formal organization served as a forum and advocate for CME. It was not until 1976 that SACME was formed and in its early days it was almost entirely made up of a group of physicians and surgeons who were chief officers for CME (assistant or associate deans).[4] SACME was formed because, like many groups of professionals working in a new endeavor, these physicians felt they could grow and learn to do their work better through dialogue with their colleagues. Not long after its formation a common theme for meetings was presentations and discussions about how to provide a scientific base for the educational practices used in CME. It was not long before these physicians discovered the rich literature of adult learning and adult education. Given that these medical practitioners were scientifically trained, it became essential immediately that these leaders of the CME enterprise find and apply a scientific base for their actions. This drive was compounded by such events as a *New England Journal of Medicine* article that challenged the effectiveness of CME in changing physician performance.[5] This article, using data to criticize, spurred them to find ways to use data to defend their programs and services.

In the early days of the ACME, under the leadership of William Felch, the association took a more practical rather than theoretical perspective on the field. It also assumed a primary responsibility for educating the others in CME, i.e., those who were directly involved in the day-to-day delivery of CME. This frank educational mission directed towards providers in CME continued to the present but with focus on the increasing diversity of services and products and an ever-widening door open to other stakeholders in the process. And though ACME would offer occasional sessions strongly tied to the research agenda, they were less oriented towards reporting results and more towards teaching practitioners about the results and getting the logistics including budgets in order.

The leaders of SACME felt that the society's responsibilities included engaging in a process of transmitting research findings to the healthcare community. Because more of the literature related to CME was then and continues to be to this day, fugitive, it was essential that a journal be developed that would devote its mission to publishing research and theory related to CME. Fugitive literature refers to the lack of coordination over research that was published in the variety of specialty and other journals of medicine and health care.

Mobius, the first effort at a scientific forum for the field, dedicated a portion of its pages to publication of research and essays related to the CME enterprise. The remainder of the journal was, initially, devoted to policy studies in health care. As time passed, the content devoted to CME grew and eventually included all pages of the journal. ACME joined SACME as copublisher along with the Association for Hospital Medical Education (AHME), and by the late 1980s CME had a research journal, produced quarterly, by ACME, SACME, and AHME that focused on the development of theory and the publication of research. By the 1990s, providers of CME had as-

sociations and publications devoted to reviewing and publishing material to increase their competence and the quality of the learning experiences these providers of CME offered to physicians and surgeons.

It was during this period that the leadership of CME began to shift from physicians to educationalists. Increasingly the literature, the agendas of national programs of SACME and ACME, and the organizational charts of medical schools, associations, and hospitals began to reflect educators as senior actors who were formally trained in adult education or educational psychology. Increasingly physicians who had the title of associate dean or president for CME had many duties in addition to that CME rather than a single focus of the CME of physicians. Increasingly the full-time leaders of the organizations included more PhDs and EdDs rather than MDs. This change indicated a growing professionalization of the field as higher educational standards for employment meant more formal training in education. It also meant the introduction of fierce advocates for research and development enterprises in both SACME and ACME. As noted in other chapters, this group made of partnerships between highly trained PhDs and MDs was responsible for the majority of the literature in the field. They served as teachers of CME on the agendas at national associations and they led efforts to revamp all aspects to better principles of adult learning and adult education. Educationalists trained at the doctoral level joined with a core of physicians in leadership positions who studied education on the job, to work towards new definitions of quality in the field based on a score of the scientific literature of CME.

By the mid-1990s, the literature was rich and complex, but it was also changing. Providers of CME were well informed and they began to articulate a new agenda for CME. The PhDs and MDs along with a limited number of others in the field who had health-care backgrounds began to promote a sense that CME was not just education. Providers began to recognize that the field of

CME was really about changing medical practices and improving patient care rather than teaching physicians things they could remember. This new imperative enhanced efforts to develop funds for research in CME through the professional associations and the publication of serious books devoted to reporting research results (*Changing and Learning in the Lives of Physicians*) and synthesizing and applying studies to practice (*The Physician as Learner* and *The Continuing Professional Development of Physicians*).[6] However, as it was in the beginning, the major question to plague the field was whether CME made a difference in patient care.

During this period of time, a movement was underway to provide CME on a national level by organizations connected strongly to industry, the MECCs. The pharmaceutical and medical manufacturing companies needed to support national programs consistent with their national agenda for sales and marketing. Although specialty societies were well equipped to operate at a national level, medical schools, hospitals, and state medical organizations were not. The CME for-profit industry was born. It was populated with profit driven companies dependent on industry funds and a subset of companies who sold services to these companies.

The imperative for financial success, however, was not limited to those companies who were frankly for profit. Increasing economic pressures, and budget shortfalls changed CME in not-for-profit organizations from a losing enterprise offered for the good of the physician-learner to a potential profit center. Deans and chief executive officers of industry shared a need to associate the education of physicians with the generation of significant discretionary funds for important non CME related activities. Financial success became the measure of worth for almost all who were involved in the CME enterprise, and business models guided practice in some rather than educational models that had characterized the first two decades of the field. Financial success took two forms. It involved either increasing cost and

volume of participants or decreasing the cost and volume of staff. Internal research support dwindled by the late 1990s; the level of education and type of staff who worked as providers in the field showed a decline of MDs and PhDs and a rise in trained professionals holding masters of science and masters of business administration degrees. With this, practices common to business became more common in CME and competition among providers on a program to program basis became commonplace.

Presently, CME has the largest workforce in its history. It offers more lower-cost programs that ever. Providers have endorsed rules that placed limits on their behavior and have insisted on self and peer regulation of the CME product. There is an increasing attendance at national and regional conferences that offer education to CME providers. There are research conferences of activities built into national associations that offer research reports, grants, and awards. The CME provider community (in my experience) exhibits a high motivation to learn more about how to do its work well.

However, proportionately, there are fewer CME professionals with terminal degrees in either medicine or education and more with bachelor's or master's degrees in business or other related fields. This does not mean they cannot learn on the job; it means they have more to learn. More troublesome are the defensive rationales of some that professional training in education or medicine is not essential to the field. Such denial, coupled with standards of practice required today by the ACCME and other agencies, predicts that those who do not know enough will fail. There are few systematic efforts to prepare the workforce in a curriculum based on the science and practice of CME. Charlatans abound, offering quick-fix consultations and workshops designed to shortcut an extensive training process.

To have a competent workforce in CME, it must rest on three legs: (1) a professional staff that can translate scholarship into practice, (2) an organizational culture that accepts CPD and change and learning for health professionals as its primary endpoint, and (3) a collaborating community of actors concerned with changing physicians performance in a way that directly enhances patients' health.

In the future, we must build into the CME enterprise a sense that collaborative learning among equals is essential to achieving common goals. Professional associations in CME must align themselves around the needs of the profession as opposed to the special interest groups and the financial opportunities present in the environment. Practices must become transparent and must be the property of a community of professionals rather than the property of profit centered organizations who set education below financial success. We must train providers to the research base within the context of CPD as participants in the development of solutions to health-care problems. We must continue to focus on incorporating multidisciplinary perspectives that illuminate our understanding of how change occurs and how health-care professionals learn. These are the paths forward.

Conclusion

This essay has focused on the development of four pillars of CME, systems that are independent but interact throughout the history of CME to shape its form and function.

- A body of science that explains and predicts how to intervene in ways that improve the quality of health-care delivery and recognizes that change is a function of education policies and systems designs.
- A set of criteria for excellence that translates the literature and science into standards for practice that the CPD community can adopt.
- The development of a system of support that puts resources to use for the betterment of patient care without bias and in a fair and balanced fashion.
- A competent CPD organization whose

providers can use all of the elements above to offer change strategies that drive towards improvements in the health of the public.

In order to achieve our potential, we must recognize that our failures to achieve fully our ambitions in regard to improving patient health are in part due to the lack of appropriate interaction, collaboration, and professional development of these pillars. We have not been transparent and we have not shared our solutions or our problems. The future depends on an integrated enterprise that bases its strengths on collaboration that connects knowledge, standards of practice, financial support, and competent performance by CME providers. Without integration, our failure to achieve will continue. We will disintegrate into historical oddities who failed to assume their place in a new order, one that bases practice on science, that collaborates in local and national agendas for improving the health of the public, and one that sees learning and change as integral and necessary to quality medical care.

Notes

1. The term *continuing medical education* is used in the chapter title rather than the contemporary *continuing professional development of physicians* because of its historical accuracy, not as a preference of the author.

2. C. R. Brown and H. S. M. Uhl, "Mandatory Continuing Education: Sense or Nonsense?" *Journal of the American Medical Association* 213 (1970): 1660–1667.

3. R. F. Mager, *Preparing Instructional Objectives,* 2nd ed. (Belmont, Calif.: Lake Publishing Co., 1984).

4. R. Caplan, "The Society of Medical College Directors of Continuing Medical Education (SMCDCME): Its Origin in 1976 and First Dozen Years," *Journal of Continuing Education in the Health Professions* 16 (1996): 14–24.

5. J. C. Sibley and others, "A Randomized Trial of Continuing Medical Education," *New England Journal of Medicine* 306 (1982): 511–515.

6. R. D. Fox and others, *Changing and Learning in the Lives of Physicians* (New York: Praeger, 1989); D. A. Davis and R. D. Fox, eds., *The Physician as Learner: From Research to Practice* (Chicago: American Medical Association, 1994); D. A. Davis and others, eds., *The Continuing Professional Development of Physicians: From Theory to Practice* (Chicago: American Medical Association, 2003).

PART V

Continuing Medical Education
and Continuing Professional
Development in Canada

CHAPTER 18

The Evolution of Continuing Medical Education in Canada

The story of continuing medical education (CME) in Canada traces the origins of concepts and ideas, the evolution of processes and structures, and the assessment of impacts, all of which influenced and directed the development of CME in Canada. While physicians and healers long preceded the development of Canada as a nation,[1] the identification of critical background influences, both social and educational, define the purpose of the chapter and, thus, direct the writing plan. The story begins in colonial times and sets the stage for the gradual emergence of medical institutions and the improvement of educational processes and practices.

Phase 1: From Colonial Times to Osler

In colonial times, the first physicians came to Canada after being educated in Europe, and later the United States. The early history has been well described by Heargerty in his book *Four Hundred Years of Medicine in Canada*.[2] Formal medical education in Canada began in Montreal where the Montreal Medical Institution was founded in 1823 by physicians from Edinburgh, Scotland, who worked at the recently opened Montreal General Hospital.[3] By 1829, the institution transformed into a faculty at McGill University where, ironically, the new university needed to have an established program to meet the terms of the James McGill will and its offer of his estate (in the countyside near Mount Royal) for a campus.

Thus, the first faculty at McGill was in medicine, and it was the first Faculty of Medicine in Canada. Schools quickly followed in Toronto and at the Université de Montréal (1843), at Laval in Quebec City (1852), in Kingston, Ontario, with Queens (1854), and Halifax (1867).[4] Preceding the development of schools of medicine, often by decades, was the development of hospitals, although the direct link between hospitals and universities as joint teaching sites was yet to be made in many cases. By the turn of the 20th century, with the addition of the schools at London in western Ontario, and in Manitoba, there were eight medical schools of "varying quality" in Canada, as Flexner was to later describe them in his report to the Carnegie Foundation in 1910.[5]

Meanwhile in the United States, emerging from the time of Andrew Jackson's presidency when deregulation had been widely promoted, was the appearance of many proprietary medical schools of questionable quality. It was a phenomenon that, over time, attracted considerable attention. The outcome was the Flexner Report of 1910.[6] Flexner's influence was as important in Canada as in the United States. The key point is that with the coming of improvement of medical schools and hospitals, there existed structures for promoting better quality educational practices. Thus, with the emergence of new philanthropic bodies such as the Carnegie Foundation from the preceding economic boom, came a new concern with the quality of medical education and the physicians so produced. The Flexner Report focused support for the review of educational processes and the possibility of adopting criteria to guide and improve the quality of medical education. But the ferment of that era, as reflected in Flexner's analyses, was not focused strictly on laboratory-based research, as is often erroneously asserted. Also at that time, the first signs of interest in assessing and improving the outcomes of care in surgery were seen in Codman's work from the Massachusetts General Hospital in 1910. They were the first signs of another influence that would slowly emerge over the next decades: the issue of quality of medical care. These events set the stage for the recognition of what was to emerge over the next years: the need for structures to assess quality. Two of the earliest examples were the creation of the Medical Council of Canada in 1912 and the National Board of Medical Examiners in the United States in 1914.[7] They signaled the coming of standards by which medical licensure would be granted and potentially portable in North America.[8] To re-emphasize the theme and assumptions behind this analysis, the message is that the history of CME and its evolution has to be seen in terms of what was going on in society, in medicine, and in academia on both sides of the Canadian-US border. The impacts from ideas flowing back and forth across the US-Canadian border will be repeated throughout the examination of the history of CME in Canada.

Around the time of Canada's emergence as a country, a physician's sources of continuing education were his colleagues and library. For instance, in 1864, the Medical Society of Nova Scotia received a bequest from Frederick Cogswell, MD, of his medical library. His books were to be used for the benefit of students at the Halifax Medical College and the practitioners of Nova Scotia.[9] In fact, after the Halifax Medical College became part of Dalhousie, the Canadian Medical Association (CMA) brought a suit regarding ownership of the library because of its perceived academic value. One new structure that emerged with Canada's confederation was the

CMA in 1867. Its initial role was primarily educational. It led to many changes, including the origin of the concept of the Medical Council of Canada.

William Osler, as he was leaving North America for Oxford in 1905, spoke frequently about the physician's library and, as always with Osler, learning from the study of one's patients.[10] Osler's description of learned practitioner John Bell illustrates his viewpoint: "Reading in his carriage and by lamplight at Lucinda's bedside, he was able to keep well informed; but he had an insatiable desire to know the true inwardness of a disease, and in this way, I came into contact with him."[11]

In this manner, Osler and Bell learned together and unraveled the mysteries of illness, like pernicious anemia. Clearly, the world of continuing education for physicians was not formally organized, and probably the Canadian approach at the turn of the 20th century was Oslerian: study the patient, talk to respected colleagues, and maintain a good library.

Phase 2: Coming of Accreditation, Processes, and Structures in Medical Education

With the development of institutional structures and interest in educational processes in the early 1920s, the changes in Canada and the United States between 1920 and 1950 were very much in the mindset of developing standards to be applied through these new structures and processes. The attempt to apply the concept of *outcomes* failed after its initial trials in Boston, so the realization of outcome-defined results would have to wait for some time. It would come back into focus with the work of Donabedian in the 1960s when he created the quality of care framework of structures, processes, and outcomes.[12]

Following the First World War, the first attempts at organized CME began to emerge. In Canada, that began in Halifax at Dalhousie with the Annual Refresher Course in 1922.[13] Physicians paid for the course, which consisted of lectures and included a four course dinner for $1.25 at a well known hotel. Sixty-seven physicians attended in 1924 and, by 1953, the Annual Dalhousie Refresher Course attendance had grown to 387. During the 1930s, many other institutions began to offer refresher courses, often through hospitals, particularly in the larger cities.

This time period also marked the development of other medical structures and institutions that were to provide the basis for much of the formal support and promotion of CME or continuing professional development (CPD) in the later part of the 20th century. For example, one critical development was the beginning of both the specialty boards and the professional colleges. This began in the United States, as recounted by Rosemary Stevens in *Medicine and the Public Interest* in 1970.[14] Although specialty boards clearly began on the US side of the border, it was not without significant Canadian participation. Consider that Charles Martin, chair of medicine at McGill, was one of the founders of the American Board of Internal Medicine. In Canada, the founding of the Royal College of Physicians and Surgeons of Canada (RCPSC) was certainly promoted in 1924 at the Conference on Medical Services and, ultimately, it came to pass in 1929 under the leadership of Jonathan Meakins, also from McGill. It signified the emergence of a national dual specialty college in Canada, which offered an educational venue to its small community of specialists similar in principle to the professional colleges in the United States. However, it was only in 1937 that its second role as a certifying body, akin to the board structures in the United States, became established.[15] By that time, the accreditation of medical schools through the Liaison Committee on Medical Education (LCME) was underway sponsored by the American Medical Association (AMA) and the Association of American Medical Colleges (AAMC) in the United States. The same processes were underway in Canada via the CMA and the faculties.[16]

National conferences were held at that time around issues of educational standards and other quality issues. For example, at the previously mentioned 1924 Conference on Medical Services in Canada, George Young, MD, of Toronto highlighted the existence of intramural (within teaching centers) and extramural programs or so-called extension lectures and clinics.[17] Many were intended to provide specialized training in all manner of developing areas, like public health and laboratory medicine. But he also alluded to the development of short intermediate courses for graduates, in addition to training for specialists. He noted that two schools offered opportunities for the practicing physician to partake of the undergraduate programs, but he focused on the fact that several schools of medicine had short postgraduate courses open to all graduates in medicine. He quoted from one of the school's announcements:

The object is in nowise to train specialists in any branch of medicine or surgery, but to afford an annual opportunity to the general practitioner to witness with a minimum expenditure of time and energy the practical and clinical application of those methods of diagnosis and treatment which have come into use since his graduation, or on account of local conditions he may hesitate to adopt in his own practice.[18]

During the same session, it was noted that many local medical societies presented sessions on the latest advances in medicine, hopefully bringing a sense of interest and enthusiasm to the rural physicians, as would be the case in the teaching centers. Suffice to say, that by 1924–1925, the appearance of updates and refresher courses were well established. Yet the tone of the discussion also identified the unmet needs of many communities due to lack of appropriate training or the availability of specialized physicians or surgeons to assist the local doctor. It seemed that the preparation of physicians for the realities of their practice was of great concern. This was an early discussion of what later was to become known as *needs assessment*.

In the meantime, increased interest in CME was underway. In a 1929 issue of the *Canadian*

Medical Association Journal, CMA General Secretary T. C. Routley made reference to the needs of the practitioner for "progressive education,"[19] noting that "the doctor who allows his medical equipment to stand still, stagnates." Each decade, he continued, sees so many contributions to medical learning and achievement that it behooves the doctor in practice to be constantly alert for new ideas, improved methods, and approved help. He stressed the attempts of the CMA to assist organized medicine in furthering postgraduate study, and he noted that support for these programs was coming from the Sun Life Assurance Company. Routley bragged that the picture of growing support for teachers of medicine being sent out to meet the practitioners was "unequalled in any English speaking country in the world." The size of this program rose each year from 169 in 1926 to 329 in 1928, supported to the tune of $30,000 per year by Sun Life. It was also interesting that the members of the CMA also received the *British Medical Journal* at a special rate at that time. Thus, the recognition of the need for continuing education was clearly on the rise, with support coming from the universities, the CMA, and from the life insurance industry.

Subsequently, in the evolution of the specialty boards in the United States, new ideas appeared in terms of the continuing education of specialists. While the first certifying board was the American Board of Ophthalmology, the first certifying board in North America to require CME credits to maintain certification was the American Board of Urology in 1934.[20] The specialty association movement began in Canada with the RCPSC, as noted, but it was only in 1937 that the RCPSC also became the body for issuing certificates of specialization, by examination, and not by election.[21] This development became a key building block for CME and CPD developments in Canada in the 1990s.

Also during this era, support grew for educational infrastructure in Canada from charitable foundations in the United States. This support initially focused on the building of learning and teaching resources. While CME was not the priority of the time, these developments were of interest because they foretold the notion of philanthropic bodies investing in infrastructure for medical education in an era before governments had begun a major increase in funding physician education.[22] Such philanthropic investors included the Carnegie, Kellogg, and Macy foundations.

World War II caused the re-evaluation of educational processes to stall out for a decade, but afterwards, a new period of increased interest emerged for what was often called *postgraduate education.* Such education was to retrain and upgrade physicians returning from military duty or those physicians who in Canada had been trained in special three-year courses often without traditional internships.[23] Above and beyond that, one saw the coming of renewed interest in medical education, in particular, with new focus on the curriculum for medical students. A typical example was the coming of systems learning at Case-Western Reserve in Cleveland, a change that was watched widely across North America. That change was followed by an interest in the quality of practice. Two studies, one in the United States and one in Canada, brought significant focus on general practice and its practitioners' educational needs. They were the Osler-Peterson study in North Carolina and the Clute study on general practice in Ontario and Nova Scotia.[24] From this point onward, a major change occurred in the evolution of CME in Canada and the United States. While collaboration and cross-border fertilization would continue, the balance of influence on CME in Canada would move to the universities, which became increasingly pro-active.

Phase 3: Period of Educational Reorientation to the Student and Learner

In the early 1950s, medical education took on a new focus. That focus shifted from the teacher as the center of the educational endeavor to the student as learner. The greatest interest of this focus was in undergraduate medical education. Yet, concern over the opportunities in continuing education of the practicing physician began to increase. Residencies and research fellowship training opportunities grew, but in contrast to the medical curriculum, improvement in the educational capabilities of postgraduate clinical education had remained relatively stagnant following its expansion in the larger centers like Montreal, Edmonton, Winnipeg, and Toronto. With recovery from World War II underway and with improved economic times, the next two decades of greatly increased public support for medical education and research were beginning. One saw the expansion of University of British Columbia (UBC) to include clinical training and the creation of the medical faculties at Ottawa and Saskatchewan. By 1960, Canada boasted 12 medical schools. The Medical Research Council of Canada (MRC) began offering expanded salary support for researchers, and indirectly (via Medicare and the MRC), the notion of full-time faculty began expanding.[25] These funding changes continued to affect the medical community for the next two decades, during which time Canada also prepared for the coming of universal hospital and then universal medical insurance (Medicare). With that longer term goal, education expanded further in an effort to increase workforce production of all health professionals in the late 1960s.

With rapidly changing health policies, increased funding, and an emphasis on education, the first steps forward in the improvement and expansion of CME were being taken. With the new focus on the learner (and, in the case of CME, the physician as learner), the development of new structures, better processes, and new educational expertise received significantly greater attention. Events in the United States had a significantly positive influence on both medical education and CME in Canada. These events included the development of medical education units in Buffalo; Chicago; East Lansing, Michigan; Los Angeles; Boston; and Seattle.[26] By the mid-1960s, the first group of formally sponsored medical educators

from Canada were being trained in the United States, and the consequences for undergraduate medical education and postgraduate medical education would be significant.[27] The first spin-off from a new breed of educational scholar was a focus on the learning processes as well as learning structures. This would begin impacting CME in the 1960s. In 1961, G. R. Shepherd wrote about the history of CME in the United States since 1930.[28] In 1962, the dean at Minnesota, Robert Howard, addressed the Association of American Medical Colleges in Los Angeles about the future role of the medical school in CME.[29] With Howard as chair, a *Report on the Committee on Continuing Medical Education* was presented to the Association of American Medical Colleges in 1963.[30] The term *CME*, which was not yet widely used before the early 1960s, became an accepted term. This recognition also reflected the creation of specific divisions or departments of CME at many medical institutions. In Canada, the increased interest in CME was highlighted in several medical schools and was greatly re-enforced with the founding of the College of General Practice in 1954, later renamed as the College of Family Physicians of Canada in 1967. The college included CME as an essential part of its activities and included CME requirements for remaining a member in good standing. It held a conference of medical education in 1962 at which the following consensus was reached: "Continuing medical education is an essential feature of the practice of modern medicine as it maintains the doctor's ability to provide quality care. This concept of 'lifelong learning' must be actively developed in undergraduate medical student and be sustained in the graduate doctor, both practitioner and teacher."[31]

At the university level, encouraged by the Kellogg Foundation, formal programs, as opposed to annual courses, emerged in the late 1950s at Dalhousie, Laval, Université de Montréal, and UBC. In 1950, Dean Grant at Dalhousie created a postgraduate committee with financial aid from the Kellogg Foundation in Battle Creek, Michigan, and within six years had created a four-pronged program: visiting professorships, short courses, outside speakers, and a news bulletin. In 1955, Lea Steeves, MD, was appointed as the first full-time director.[32] In 1963, Steeves, having established an extramural program at Dalhousie, wrote about extramural CME.[33] Subsequently in 1965, he argued passionately about the need for CME.[34] He was not alone. On the recommendation of Dean McCreary, UBC developed a department of CME in 1960 and again the Kellogg Foundation offered assistance.[35] Donald Williams was the first chair and was responsible for its development. The University of Alberta opened a department of CME in 1963, under Sam Kling's leadership.[36] Laval University, under Pierre Jobin, had also developed an extramural CME program in 18 regions of Quebec that included presentation and discussion of cases, for which the 1964 program is described in some detail.[37] In Montreal, Doctor DeGuise Vaillancourt had established the division of postgraduate medicine at the Université de Montréal and was offering outreach programs for physicians in the northwest region of Quebec.[38] In 1962, Dean Douglas Bocking at the University of Western Ontario (UWO) asked a committee to look at selected programs for CME in North America. Their report led Bocking to create a CME program in 1964 to serve the physicians of western Ontario. These events dovetailed with the 1964 Association of Canadian Medical Colleges symposium on CME, at which time authors began to differentiate CME as intramural and extramural programs for practicing physicians from the more traditional notions of internships and residencies. However, there was much to do. William Ruhe, from the AMA side of the LCME, reported from a 1960–1961 LCME survey of Canadian and US medical schools that only four of the twelve universities with faculties of medicine in Canada had major responsibilities for CME courses and another six reported subordinate but minor roles in CME. Two did not respond to the survey.[39]

As noted previously, key points of departure that focused attention on CME on both sides of the border were the Clute Report in Canada and the Osler-Peterson report in the United States on the quality of medical practice.[40] Essentially, the two reports documented the gaps between the reality of practice and the state of the knowledge of medical science, clinical laboratory use, and therapy. Both drove major change. Within three or four years, several conferences were held on the future of CME, including the use of new technologies such as television in CME and the use of audio-visual technology in education and CME. The field thrived with ideas about formats and techniques and, most critically, with a clear perception of need. The common practice of offering refresher courses in a lecture format at teaching hospitals presented by academics focused on their areas of expertise clearly had not focused on the learners and their practice needs. The issue of how to best proceed and improve the quality of practice and reduce the time from discovery to the bedside of local doctor's office was still to be the subject of many years of research and study. To that end, at the start of the 1970s, the first of many physicians and PhDs with training in medical education in the United States returned to Canada to pursue these key questions. Amongst those were family physicians Paul Cudmore and Marvin Clarke who returned to Dalhousie to direct the CME division. In fact, the next two decades from the late 1960s onward were to become a point of major departure for CME. With it, came innovative approaches and the use of formal study of the effectiveness of CME processes. Among this change and innovation, some of the old approaches began to die, but the process was slow.

As the chair of the Carnegie Foundation Commission on the Future of Higher Education in 1973, John Millis wrote that North America is moving into a learning society and medicine was to be part of that movement.[41] Millis was well known and spoke at medical education conferences and faculty retreats in Canada in the early 1970s. Educators and academic leaders embraced his ideas and, as a result, both clinical graduate medical education and CME were swept up in that movement.

Phase 4: Major Change—Increased Educational Capacity, Quality, and Accountability

Even as the 1970s began, there were two additional harbingers of the dramatic changes to come in the next three decades. Front and center were activities in the United States where interest in CME was revitalized within AMA, within state regulatory bodies, within certifying bodies, and within universities, including research in education at many levels. In particular, John Williamson and Paul Sanazaro wrote about CME in the context of improving quality of care.[42] George Miller similarly addressed the issue of quality in his article "Continuing Education for What?" He stressed the growing threat to the practitioners' competence due to overwhelming number of new facts and poor educational approaches.[43] He concluded that CME should not be continuing instruction.

The need for a more proactive approach to CME was apparent and reflected in two new trends. A significant number of Canadians returned from the United States—including those studying with Miller—after formal preparation for educational careers.[44] This trend was augmented greatly by the development of four new medical schools, in Newfoundland, Alberta, Ontario, and Quebec. Each of those schools placed great emphasis on preparation in medical education and hired faculty and advisors who could perform that task. The world of CME was influenced greatly by that trend and, in particular, those new schools that placed a major effort on CME.

In Newfoundland, Memorial University, under the direction of Max House, MD, and Judith Roberts, developed particular expertise developed in distance education by means of satellite transmission.[45] The university sought to connect to the outports of Newfoundland and later used its expertise to deliver interactive programs to the Caribbean and Africa. In the latter case, Memorial

University worked with Donald Hillman, MD, and Elizabeth Hillman, MD. The school at McMaster focused on southern Ontario and developed innovative programs under Jack Sibley, MD (who conducted outcomes trials on methods of CME), Jacqui Wakefield, and John Premi. Later at McMaster, Dave Davis created the first warehouse of information on CME trials and other studies in CME and wrote with colleagues on the paucity of CME studies of acceptable quality. That database continues to be maintained. The University of Calgary, in Alberta, started slowly but became a powerhouse in CME under Gerry McDougald and later John Parboosingh, both of whom worked closely with Jocelyn Lockyer. In time, both Lockyer and Parboosingh would become major figures in CME in Canada and across North America. They produced innovative approaches to CME and ran an extensive research program. The school in Sherbrooke, Quebec, also established a successful medical education unit reflecting its innovative curriculum under Roger Dufresne.[46] Its subsequent CME development became associated with the beginning of the Quebec-wide and integrated Conseil de l'Education Médicale Continue. In the meantime, the established programs also made major advances and transitioned to needs-based, quality improvement-oriented CME.

Ottawa and Saskatchewan were among the schools established or expanded in the 1940s and 1950s. Ottawa took a particular interest in computer-based educational methods under Jan Bormanis, MD, and later many of its faculty worked closely with Parboosingh and J. J. Demers, who provided the major leadership at the RCPSC as its role in CPD emerged.[47] In the 1970s, Saskatchewan moved to be a major figure in CME, with Olie Laxdall, MD, and Penny Jennett, MD, carrying out what was then considered by many physicians to be the best practitioner-oriented CME programs in Canada. But their contributions were not limited to course development. They carried out significant research, including randomized trials, well into the 1980s when Jennett moved to Calgary to manage and lead its tele-health development and Laxdal retired. Nearby, Manitoba also had greatly upgraded its CME under Dan Snidal, and its impact and direction were greatly influenced by the fact that the College of Physicians and Surgeons of Manitoba became the first medical regulator in Canada to introduce mandatory CME in the late 1970s. This led Murray Kopelow, MD, and associates to develop innovative approaches to assessment in practice, prior to his leaving for the United States to head the Accreditation Council for Continuing Medical Education (ACCME). The University of Alberta, which worked jointly with Laval and established itself as a major leader in educational assessment through the R. S. McLaughlin Examination and Research Centre, also greatly expanded its programs in CME. Under Sam Kling, appointed director of CME in 1963,[48] the university moved from an annual course to short courses and then extramural programs for all of Alberta, until Calgary, as described previously, developed regional programs in southern Alberta in the mid-1970s. UWO became a major center for the study of patient-centered care under the direction of Ian McWhinney, and its development had a worldwide impact in primary care education. Its programs also followed the emerging pattern of linking CME with improved care and quality outcomes. At Queens, after Garfield Kelly began the Office of CME in 1968, anesthetist Stuart Vandewater initiated programs at regional hospitals in eastern Ontario in the early 1970s. Dalhousie with Ian Purkis, Wayne Putnam, and Lynn Curry and many collaborators, such as David Gass and Karen Mann, was recognized internationally for innovatively designed studies leading to frequent publications on learning and program effectiveness and, of course, an extensive selection of regional programs.[49] During the late 1970s, change also came to the two oldest schools: McGill and Toronto. Given their large number of associated teaching hospitals and their strong hospital-based postgraduate courses, the role of the university in pro-

moting learner-based and coordinated programs emerged under Fred Fallis in Toronto and Guy Joron at McGill. There followed a change in CME emphasis at Toronto with the arrival of Davis from McMaster as director in 1994. The nature of evidence, assessment of impact, and issues of adopting change in practice were emphasized. The larger centers could often offer innovative, hands-on, short training courses featuring new content like divorce mediation or managing behavioral change. These topics broached issues that had not been recognized previously as relevant for the practicing physician, or even lawyers. Similarly, the use of their faculty's expertise in simulation and e-learning decision support led to innovative studies for skills improvement, at Toronto especially, and for on-line decision support for drug prescription with family physicians at McGill.[50]

By the mid-1990s, by virtue of its CME research and its program development, Canada was seen as a major leader and contributor to CME progress. This continued to expand well into the next century. For instance, the first combined meeting of the Society of Medical College Directors of Continuing Medical Education (later to become the Society for Academic Continuing Medical Education or SACME) and the group on Research in CME (RICME) took place in Montreal in 1986. The move to link CME innovation and development with the annual meeting of the directors of university-based CME was refreshing. Furthermore, the RICME conference became a true congress with more international participation at each subsequent meeting. The combined US-Canadian Change Study proved to be another seminal event. The study was a multi-centered effort to understand the phases of the physician's career with real data from the profession and, thus, had implications for CME programming.[51] In 1984, Davis and colleagues, working with the clinical epidemiology group at McMaster, did the initial systematic analysis of the literature on the effectiveness of CME.[52] Other analyses followed, but the concept of reviewing the evidence for the effectiveness of CME was established and it, in turn, led Davis to establish the database known as the *Research and Development Resource Base in CME*. This regularly updated[53] database was made freely available to CMR researchers and was relocated to the University of Toronto in 1995. These events were symbols of the expansion of formal analysis of CME effectiveness and the emergence of research as a regular tool and activity of the CME office at Canadian universities. Questioning, analysis, and empirical studies became established processes in CME across Canada. That work, reflected in the literature of the era, continued to increase into the late 1990s and the new millennium. The list of achievement is too huge to recite herein, but the numbers of CME-related publication from within Canada tell the story. According to a recent SCOPUS search, the number of Canadian publications on CME grew in the following manner: 33 publications from 1960 through 1969, 133 from 1970 through 1979, 134 from 1980 through 1989, 285 from 1990 through 1999, and 749 from 2000 through March 2009.

Thus, this increase of studies in peer-reviewed publications reflected the priority given to developing CME in Canada. In particular, in light of events about to take place, some specific accomplishments linking CME to quality assurance, patient safety, accreditation, and even maintenance of licensure must be recognized. The start of an era of CPD and increased accountability was underway, and such an era would involve many agencies and bodies.

Implications: Widening the Vision, the Scope, and the Partners

The leaders of CME within Canada in the late 1990s realized that their enterprise had evolved from the basic structure of the CME units in the 1970s and 1980s, marketing their various courses, typically based on needs assessment, toward a new vision, new roles, and a new framework for the future. During that time, their vision and scope began to expand. Several trends and new partners had converged on their world. Major background events taking place in the medical-health care world were about to affect greatly CME. They included two Institute of Medicine reports titled "Quality Chasm" and "To Err Is Human."[54] These reports were long overdue in that the concepts and data underlying these reports were well known in the health services research and policy sectors of the health care community. Many of Canada's CME leaders, medical regulatory community, and national medical associations were aware of these developments. Visionaries within Canada's CME community realized the need to form new alliances, many of which were to be outside traditional medical partnerships. As these new relationships developed, these same leaders within Canadian CME sought new partnerships and pushed innovative developments implicating health professions education in expanded roles in quality and systems safety. The early preparatory steps that readied these leaders for this shift can be traced back to the 1980s and 1990s.

First, the offering of regular summer research institutes through SACME had a significant Canadian bent and was often managed and promoted by Lockyer from Calgary and Karen Mann from Dalhousie. It was one of many regular events that gradually introduced new investigators into the CME field in the United States and in many Canadian centers, such as Calgary, Toronto, Hamilton, Montreal, and Halifax. This initiative was greatly augmented by other developments in Canada.

In the mid-1990s, following a written challenge from Malcolm Watts in 1989,[55] an annual meeting was begun around continuing education in the health professions, as more and more interdisciplinary education initiatives emerged. It became an annual event and led to the Canadian Association for Continuing Health Education (CACHE-Canada), which was legally "born" in 2003.[56] It has evolved as a truly interdisciplinary approach, as were a lot of the rapidly changing CME units across Canada. Again McMaster was a leader, but other major developments were soon underway at many settings, such as the University of British Columbia, with Toronto being the site of a particularly large and highly skilled interdisciplinary group. By the early 2000s, foci of interprofessional continuing education research and developmental activities had been established across Canada, from British Columbia to Newfoundland.

Fortunately, these shifts and the resulting impacts were not limited to the universities. By the mid-1990s, an integrated approach to CME gradually expanded the scope to the emerging field of CPD with the significantly expanded interest of well positioned new partners like the certifying bodies and the regulators. This development had origins in the regional programs that were well underway by the 1970s, and it came be argued that the notion of integrated cross-institutional approaches to CME probably first came into existence with the creation of the Council on Continuing Medical Education (Conseil de l'Education Médicale Continue, or Conseil) in Quebec in 1975. It really followed two events: a new professional code placing maintenance of competence with the College of Physicians of Quebec (CMQ) in 1974 and a provocative article by the former dean of medicine at the Université de Montréal, then with the CMQ, Eugene Robillard, on the need for permanent educational partnership between many parties implicated in CME.[57] After its formation, the Conseil was formed, it evolved in the 1980s into a province-wide, integrated, collaborating body, with a secretariat at the College of Physicians of Quebec, under François Laramee. The collaborative was made up of 10 partners: four universities (Laval, Sherbrooke, McGill, and Montreal), the College of Physicians of Quebec (regulatory body), the three professional associations, the two professional syndicates (bargaining units), and the certifying bodies.[58] It took on a completely province-wide approach to program planning and coordinating roles, in-

cluding common ethical principles, conflict of interest principles, and accreditation criteria. This key leverage step to wider intraprofessional integration was highlighted by the developing programs of the regulatory body—the CMQ—from 1974 onward, in continuous quality assurance and maintenance of performance in practice. Given its wider legal mandate in 1974, giving it a greater role in monitoring performance, the college's continuous quality improvement (CQI) roles evolved over the next decade. Planned CME programs were designed to address documented needs through the Conseil, but the CMQ, through its CQI responsibilities, established remedial programs (e.g., for poor prescribing) and performance criteria for other disciplines and conditions.[59]

Similarly, working with their regulator, the College of Physicians and Surgeons of Ontario (CPSO), McMaster faculty members Davis, Norman, Turnbull, Cunnington, et al., formally studied the challenged physicians from the CPSO peer office visit program and offered insights into their cause and management.[60] These innovators and others from across Canada met regularly and exchanged ideas and plans with colleagues engaged in similar work. They also included international colleagues working on similar problems in Australasia and Europe. Gordon Page and several members of the group summarized its evolution in an initial article in 1995 and, in the following year, the group followed with a major article in the *International Journal of Safety and Risk in Medicine*, an interesting commentary on the influence of the Institute of Medicine (IOM) reports.[61] These types of information sharing and collaboration continued in British Columbia, Manitoba, Quebec, and Ontario. At the same time, however, other provinces and university CME units were collaborating on additionally innovative programs around the issues of performance assessment and educational interventions.

Another shift was also underway. This was the introduction of peer assessment of work (practice) performance. Such assessment would, in turn, provide feedback to the individual physician planning his or her individual needs based on his or her own performance. These provincial regulators moved ahead with multi-source assessment, and these major developments, often in tandem with existing educational units in the universities, were well underway by the turn of the millennium. Two excellent examples were the performance activity review (PAR) program in Alberta by (1) the College of Physicians and Surgeons and Jocelyn Lockyer at the University of Calgary group and (2) the College of Physicians and Surgeons in Nova Scotia with Joan Sargeant in CME at Dalhousie University.[62] The era of direct measurement of performance linked with the planning of educational need is well underway.

These performance-based initiatives, in turn, were helped greatly by the increasing interest in the maintenance of competence (MOC) by the major Canadian certifying bodies RCPSC and CFPC. Specifically, with the requirement for MOC by both bodies, most family physicians and specialists were accountable for an annual recording of a variety of documented maintenance activities, including reflecting on what changes they would need to make in their practice profiles. Again, CME and CPD units at the universities were the beneficiaries of more interventional programs. More importantly, the notions of quality improvement and safety were gaining even greater prominence in educational planning.

As a result of these integrated and collaborative developments, the leadership role of the CME community in Canada and on the North American and international scenes has been pushed evermore to the forefront. CME has embraced CPD, MOC, and performance assessment but now even includes interprofessional components to its assessments and in its planning and orientation activities. Combined with the coming of simulation as a feedback tool and as the basis for deliberative and repeated practice, the playing field is now larger and the integrated sources of information and analyses are guiding much of today's CME planning, research, and action steps.

Closing Comments: A Happy Collaboration Continues

It used to be said that if you have seen one CME unit, you have seen one CME unit. While the variety of activities and increasingly direct approaches to quality and safety have been added to the CME mix, as Davis pointed out recently in a national health policy issue, the field has not stood still on its structures, processes, and programs.[63] These Canadian groups have worked to link their CME structures and processes to the third component of Donabedian's quality of care framework: outcomes. The field has now moved to the basic issues of knowledge translation (KT) and skill transfer in the form of trials and demonstration projects. National demonstration projects, pilots, and trials for many KT clinical activities are underway in Canada.[64]

In conclusion, the fields of CME and CPD are now broader based and no longer entirely instructive in their orientation. They are learner friendly, interdisciplinary, and integrated across institutions, professions, and agencies. Leaders in this evolving set of activities are now studying and proposing models that meet the data gathered rather than trying to fit the data into some preconceived concepts. The field of continuing educational development is focused on the real world and working aggressively toward quality improvement based on outcome-based results and on empirical demonstration. What became known as CME in the 1960s has changed. Today, the physician's education is recognized as a life-long process with practice-based programs that provide feedback and direction, focusing on physician needs and performance gaps. The newer programs can measure if the educational intervention has worked. If it is not successful, the plan is revised based on the data and feedback and implemented anew. And the outcomes will be assessed again. After all, it is about the patients and their outcomes. Osler would be pleased.

Notes

1. J. J. Heagerty, *Four Centuries of Medical History in Canada* (New York: Macmillan, 1928), 65, 144, 148.

2. Ibid.

3. R. L. Cruess, "Brief History of Medicine at McGill," McGill University Web site, http://www.mcgill.ca/medicine/about/history (accessed January 19, 2009).

4. N. T. McPhedran, *Canadian Medical Schools: Two Centuries of Medical History* (Montreal: Harvest House, 1993), 1–37, 38–53.

5. Ibid.

6. A. Flexner, *Medical Education in the United States and Canada,* bulletin 4 (New York: Carnegie Foundation for Higher Education, 1910).

7. C. Vodden, "State of the Union," chapter 1 in *Licentiate to Heal: A History of the Medical Council of Canada* (Ottawa: Medical Council of Canada, 2008), 1–6.

8. W. Dale Dauphinee, "Licensure and Certification," in *International Handbook of Research in Medical Education,* edited by G. Norman and others (Dordrecht: D. Kluwer Academic Publishers, 2002), 835–882.

9. W. K. Kellogg Health Sciences Library, *The Kellogg Library's Role in Continuing Medical Education* (Power-Point slides available from Kellogg.library@dal.ca).

10. W. Osler, "The Student Life," in *Sir William Osler, 1849–1919: A Selection for Medical Students,* edited by Charles G. Roland (Toronto: The Hannah Institute for the History of Medicine, 1982), 44.

11. Ibid.

12. A. Donabedian, "Evaluating the Quality of Medical Care," in *Health Services Research,* edited by D. Mainland (New York: Milbank Fund, 1967), 166–201.

13. J. Gray and L. C. Steeves, "Continuing Medical Education: A Pioneering Educational Innovation at Dalhousie University," Dalhousie University Web site, http://cme.medicine.dal.ca/Cmehis.htm (accessed January 14, 2009).

14. R. Stevens, *American Medicine and the Public Interest* (New Haven, Conn.: Yale University Press, 1971), 198–243.

15. C. Vodden, "Changing of the Guard," chapter 6 in *Licentiate to Heal: A History of the Medical Council of Canada* (Ottawa: Medical Council of Canada, 2008), 33–38.

16. American Medical Association, "Dates in the History of the AMA Council on Medical Education," American Medical Association Web site, http://www.ama-assn,org/pub/category/print/3609.html (accessed January 14, 2009).

17. G. S. Young, "Post-Graduate Medical Education in Canada," *Canadian Medical Association Journal* 15 (1925): 312–315.

18. Ibid.

19. T. C. Routley, "Some Facts about the Canadian Medical Association," *Canadian Medical Association Journal* 20 (1929): 173–177.

20. Stevens, *American Medicine,* 198–243.

21. Vodden, "Changing of the Guard," 33–38.

22. McPhedran, *Canadian Medical Schools,* 1–37, 38–53.

23. Ibid.

24. O. L. Peterson, "An Analytic Study of North Carolina General Practice," *Journal of Medical Education* 31 (1956): 1, 74, 165; K. F. Clute and others, *The General Practitioner: A Study of Medical Education and Practice in Ontario and Nova Scotia,* (Toronto: University of Toronto Press, 1956).

25. McPhedran, *Canadian Medical Schools,* 1–37, 38–53.

26. W. Dale Dauphinee, "Canadian Medical Education: 50 Years of Innovation and Leadership," *Canadian Medical Association Journal* 148 (1993): 1582–1588.

27. W. Dale Dauphinee, "Evaluation and the Royal College of Physicians and Surgeons of Canada: A 35-Year Story of Initiatives and Influence," in *The Evolution of Specialty Medicine: 1979–2004* (Ottawa: The Royal College of Physicians and Surgeons of Canada, 2004), 109–124.

28. G. R. Shepherd, "History of Continuing Medical Education in the United States since 1930," *Journal of Medical Education* 35 (1960): 740–758.

29. R. B. Howard, "The Future of the Medical School in Continuing Medical Education," *Journal of Medical Education* 38 (1963): 28–33.

30. R. B. Howard, "Association of American Medical Colleges: Report of the Committee on Continuing Medical Education," *Journal of Medical Education* 38 (1964): 430.

31. L. C. Steeves, "Extramural Continuing Medical Education," *Canadian Medical Association Journal* 88 (1963): 732–735.

32. Gray and Steeves, "Continuing Medical Education."

33. Steeves, "Extramural Continuing Medical Education," 732–735.

34. L. C. Steeves, "The Need for Continuing Medical Education," *Canadian Medical Association Journal* 92 (1965): 758–761.

35. D. H. Williams, "The New Department of Continuing Medical Education, University of British Columbia: Its Comprehensive Co-Operative Purpose," *Canadian Medical Association Journal* 84 (1961): 694–695.

36. E. A. Corbet, "Frontiers of Medicine: A History of Medical Education and Research at the University of Alberta," chapter 6 in *Medical Education* (Edmonton: University of Alberta Press, 1990), 164–167.

37. P. Jobin, "Enseignement médical permanent à Laval: Programme extra-muros (automne 1964)," *Canadian Medical Association Journal* 92 (1965): 762–764.

38. D. Vaillancourt and M. Gill, "Continuing Medical Education by Television: A Canadian Experience," *Canadian Medical Association Journal* 98 (1968): 1136–1139.

39. C. H. W. Ruhe, "A Survey of the Activities of Medical Schools in the Field of Continuing Medical Education," *Journal of Medical Education* 38 (1963): 820–828.

40. Peterson, "North Carolina General Practice," 1, 74, 165; Clute and others, *General Practitioner*.

41. J. S. Millis, *Carnegie Commission on Higher Education, Towards a Learning Society: Alternative Channels to Life, Work, and Serve* (New York: McGraw Hill, 1973); J. S. Millis, "Issues in Graduate Medical Education," *Journal of the American Medical Association* 197 (1966): 159–161.

42. P. J. Sanazaro, "An Agenda for Research in Medical Education," *Journal of the American Medical Association* 197 (1966): 149–154; J. W. Williamson, "Assessing Clinical Competence," *Journal of Medical Education* 40 (1965): 180–187.

43. G. E. Miller, "Continuing Education for What?" *Journal of Medical Education* 42 (1967): 320–326.

44. Dauphinee, "Canadian Medical Education," 1582–1588.

45. A significant portion of the material presented in this and the next two paragraphs represents an informal, composite recollection of the author and various colleagues who had long associations with the centers described, much of which, unfortunately, has not been documented publicly. Time and resources did not permit the on-site searching of archived files and reports for each of the CME offices for further verification or gap analysis.

46. R. R. Dufresne, "Continuing Education in Medicine," *Union Médicale du Canada* 105 (1972): 1705–1708.

47. I. J. Parboosingh and J. J. Demers, "Continuing Professional Development and Maintenance of Certification," in *The Evolution of Specialty Medicine: 1979–2004* (Ottawa: The Royal College of Physicians and Surgeons of Canada, 2004), 51–67.

48. Corbet, "Frontiers of Medicine," 164–167.

49. Gray and Steeves, "Continuing Medical Education."

50. R. K. Reznick and H. MacRae, "Teaching Surgical Skills—Change in the Wind," *New England Journal of Medicine* 355 (2006): 2664–2669; R. Tamblyn and others, "The Medical Office of the 21st Century (MOXXI): Effectiveness of Computerized Decision-Making Support in Reducing Inappropriate Prescribing in Primary Care," *Canadian Medical Association Journal* 169 (2003): 549–556.

51. R. D. Fox and others, eds., *Changing and Learning in the Lives of Physicians* (New York: Praeger, 1989).

52. D. Davis and others, "The Impact of CME: A Methodological Review of the Continuing Medical Literature," *Evaluation and the Health Professions* 7 (1984): 251–283.

53. D. Davis and others, "The Case for Knowledge Translation: Shortening the Journal from Evidence to Effect," *British Medical Journal* 327 (2003): 33–35.

54. Institute of Medicine, *Crossing the Quality Chasm: The IOM Health Care Initiative* (Washington: National Academy of Sciences, 1996); Institute of Medicine, *To Err Is Human: Building a Safer System* (Washington: National Academy of Sciences, 1999).

55. M. S. M. Watt, "CEPH—A New Discipline Rooted in the Practice?" *Journal of Continuing Education in the Health Professions* 9 (1989): 61–65.

56. CACHE Canada, "Who We Are," CACHE Canada Web site, http://cachecanada.org (accessed March 11, 2009).

57. E. Robillard, "Role of Paragovernmental and Governmental Action in Permanent Medical Education," *La vie médicale au Canada français* 1, no. 1 (1972): 12–15.

58. Fédération des Médicins Spécialists du Québec, "Notes on CPD," Fédération des Médicins Spécialists du Québec Web site, http://www.fmsq.org/e/medicins/dpc/dpcenbref.html (accessed January 27, 2009).

59. F. Goulet and others, "An Innovative Approach to Remedial Continuing Medical Education, 1992–2002," *Academic Medicine* 80, no. 6 (2005): 533–540; F. Goulet and others, "Performance Assessment: Family Physicians in Montreal Meet the Mark!" *Canadian Family Physician* 48 (2002): 1338–1342.

60. G. R. Norman and others, "Competency Assessment of Primary Care Physicians as Part of a Peer Review Program," *Journal of the American Medical Association* 270, no. 9 (1993): 1046–1051; J. Turnbull and others, "Cognitive Difficulty in Physicians," *Academic Medicine* 75, no. 2 (2000): 177–181.

61. G. G. Page and others, "Physician-assessment and Physician-enhancement Programs in Canada," *Canadian Medical Association Journal* 131 (1995): 1723–1728; G. G. Page and others, "Physician-Assessment and Physician-Enhancement Programs in Canada," *International Journal of Risk and Safety in Medicine* 8, no. 3 (1996): 217–224.

62. J. M. Lockyer and others, "What Multi-Source Feedback Factors Influence Physician Self-Assessments? A Five-Year Longitudinal Study," *Academic Medicine* 82 (2007): S77–S80; J. Sargeant and others, "Directed Self-Assessment: Practice and Feedback within a Social Context," *Journal of Continuing Education in the Health Professions* 28, no. 1 (2008): 47–54.

63. D. Davis, "Continuing Education, Guideline Implementation, and the Emerging Transdisciplinary Field of Knowledge Translation," *Journal of Continuing Education in the Health Professions* 26, no. 1 (2006): 5–12.

64. I. D. Graham and others, "Lost in Knowledge Translation: Time for a Map," *Journal of Continuing Education in the Health Professions* 26, no. 1 (2006): 13–24.

CHAPTER 19

A History of the Committee on the Accreditation of Continuing Medical Education—Canada

One reasonable reading of the last one hundred years of medical education in North America would indicate that the medical profession is readily committed to visiting educational rigor and surveillance on those who presume to enter the profession but most reluctant to apply the same standards to itself once basic education is complete. While speaking fulsomely about the continuum of lifelong learning, the profession has applied the most intense scrutiny to the first two stages—undergraduate and postgraduate—while leaving the third and longest phase—continuing medical education (CME) or continuing professional development (CPD)—to fend for itself.

The development of the Committee on the Accreditation of Continuing Medical Education (CACME) represents an instructive chapter in the evolution of the medical profession's seriousness in addressing the quality of education required of and for its members. Long dedicated to the quality and nature of education for those *entering* the profession, organized medicine in Canada (and in the United States) has been much more tentative in giving serious, sustained, and critical attention to those already *practicing* the profession.[1]

Flexner Then and Now

Exactly a century ago, the organized professions in the United States and Canada participated in the development of the Flexner Report. This involved an educational assessment of the many medical schools then extant in North America. Many of these were disturbingly commercialized and unscientific. Abraham Flexner eloquently and bitingly described the situation:

First and last, the United States and Canada have in little more than a century produced four hundred and fifty seven medical schools, many, of course, short-lived and perhaps fifty still-born. One hundred and fifty-five survive today. . . . These enterprises—for the most part they can be called schools or institutions only by courtesy—were frequently preempted. Wherever and whenever a roster of untitled practitioners rose above half a dozen, a medical school was likely at any moment to be precipitated. Nothing was really essential but professors. . . .

The teaching was, except for a little anatomy, wholly didactic. The schools were essentially private ventures, money-making in spirit and object. . . .

Income was simply divided among the lecturer, who reaped a rich harvest, besides, through the consultations which the loyalty of their former students threw into their hands.[2]

Well into the last quarter of the twentieth century, one could substitute *CME* for *medical school*, add in the largess of grateful pharmaceutical companies to fees and grateful students, and have a reasonably representative picture of much of the state of affairs in educational offerings for active practitioners.

Even today, as much as half of all such offerings in the United States derive from industry support.[3] It is unlikely that the situation is dramatically different in Canada. While significant advances have been made in the academic CME/CPD community, this has not been the result of substantial commitment or resource support from the medical schools themselves. Until quite recently, virtually all CME units were expected to be cost neutral or profit centers. The situation is aggravated in many schools where successful CME events developed at significant cost are spun off to hospital-based and other entities where income is not provided for further research and development of new CME innovations. This lack of serious commitment is frequently excused on the basis of inadequate resources on the part of the medical school. This can be usefully compared to the following, somewhat plaintive, observation by Flexner:

> There are in the United States and Canada 56 schools whose total annual available resources are below $10,000 each—so small a sum that the endeavor to do anything substantial with it is of course absurdly futile, a fact that is usually made an excuse for doing nothing at all, not even washing the windows, sweeping the floor, or providing a disinfectant for the dissecting room.[4]

While CME/CPD events now frequently take place in luxurious surroundings, this can often be attributed to the largess (and attendant influence) of industry and not to the seriousness of support from medical schools or even the profession itself.

To a great extent the Canadian Forum on CME was animated to change this situation—to define and develop resources such that academic units for CME/CPD would not remain in this situation but might become centers of excellence helping to build the envisioned *system* dedicated to the best possible professional service to Canadians. This is captured in the vision statement endorsed in 1998:

> That Canadian physicians will embrace their responsibility to provide the highest quality care possible by participating in a life-long, self-directed program of effective and practice integrated CME.[5]

The subsequent development of the CACME was an active expression of this vision. It initially focused on the accreditation of academic units of CME and, while primarily representing the pillars of professional accreditation (self assessment and peer review), it represented a broad spectrum of medical constituencies in its attempt to embrace the academic, advocacy, and regulatory branches of the profession as well as those responsible for the earlier portions of the spectrum of lifelong learning. The focus on university units of CME reflected the belief that such academic institutions had a particular responsibility for the disinterested development of effective methods of assessing and responding to the educational needs that underscored ongoing improvement in health-care delivery. This undertaking was grounded in a significant and measurable shift in how those responsible for the CME portion of the medical school curriculum viewed their priorities. This shift took place quite rapidly in the 1980s and was documented in surveys conducted in 1983 and 1988. Given the high response rates of the study, the results are rather robust:

> The CME issues identified in the two surveys had changed considerably, with entirely new issues being identified in 1988 and the emphasis placed on issues having changed. The identification of factors that promote or inhibit application of new knowledge by practicing physicians was of lowest importance in 1983 and of primary importance in 1988, and comparison of the cost-effectiveness of CME methods was an important issue in 1983 and among the least important in 1988. The noted changes mirror developments in Canada's health care milieu.[6]

Two observations are relevant in a historic context. First, by this time, the idea had developed that there was such a thing as a CME portion of the medical school curriculum for which medical schools might be seen as responsible. In the earlier part of the century, this was not evident. Second, changes mirrored developments in Canada's health care milieu. This data underscores the historical emergence of the profession assuming greater responsibility for the ongoing *social responsiveness* of their practitioners and of their practitioners' systems of educational support. However belatedly, the Flexnerian impetus for collective responsibility for educational preparation was extending to a collective responsibility for ongoing education for practice.

Based on a wide but occasionally cursory review of existing schools (one day spent in Halifax looking at Dalhousie medical school), the Flexner Report led fairly directly to the closure of many commercial schools, the curriculum transformation of others, and the eventual development of professional bodies dedicated to medical education and systems of accreditation towards ongoing quality assurance. It is useful to think of this as a time when the profession assumed a collective responsibility towards the education of its neophyte members. Over the ensuing half century, a proliferation of medical organizations (specialty colleges, regulatory colleges, medical councils, faculty organizations, etc.) developed as the profession moved to regularize the standards for both undergraduate and graduate/postgraduate medical education and to assume more defined responsibility for the preparation of both generalists and specialists to be licensed as physicians for independent practice.

The Flexner Report still serves as both a touchstone and a guide and presents opportunities for both those who feel its influence was unbalanced[7] and those wistful that its scientific call to arms has been inadequately followed.[8] Now a century after its initial presentation, it is still called upon as a paradigm of serious intent and is still invoked as a model that should apply to CME/CPD.[9]

It is worth noting that the same alacrity that the profession displayed towards the education of those on the way to the profession was singularly lacking when approaching those already in practice. In short, the same care was not taken in the longest portion of the continuum of lifelong learning as the century came to a close.

A Patchwork Quilt

While many factors led to this unseemly delay, it is only fair to say that there were foci of action where serious attempts were made to advance an agenda for both the encouragement of physician participation in learning and the enhancement of the quality of CME/CPD activities. Many remarkable researchers and leaders emerged to provide ideas, innovations, and insights that paved the way for more organized development. Indeed, with regard to the development of academic CME, Canada became a leader in research and development as well as in the assessment of competence and the design of remedial education.

Significant advances also occurred in other medical educational organizations as they took up aspects of the profession's responsibility for the ongoing quality improvement of medical practice. Beginning shortly after mid-century, the College of Family Physicians of Canada (CFPC) began its educational focus at the CME level, only later becoming involved in postgraduate and then undergraduate education. While this patchwork of initiatives and leaders provided an increasingly rich array of examples of conceptual frameworks, scientific understanding, and deployment of effective CME, an integrated system of education, assessment, and practice change akin to that seen in pre-licensure training remained elusive.

As early as 1978, the Canadian Medical Association (CMA) Council on Medical Education was working to bring these many threads together in order to ensure some minimal quality and resources among CME providers, that individual programs meet some standard of educational excellence, and that the educational experiences result in improvement of physicians' knowledge and performance.[10] In retrospect, this seems a rather modest aspiration, using such words as *minimal* and *some* and not attempting to link physician performance to health outcomes. This is perhaps a reflection of both the scientific and political understandings at the time. However, it did set in motion an increasingly effective working relationship between the major national professional bodies that, over time, resulted in the creation of CACME and the development of an accreditation system more akin to that present for undergraduate and postgraduate medical education.

National Development

Under the Canadian Constitution (repatriated in 1982), health and education are primarily subjects of provincial rather than federal jurisdiction. However, for a number of historical, financial, and practical reasons, a greater degree of consultation, coordination, and even collaboration evolved between provinces and the federal government. The nature of these interactions, together with the major national debates on the meaning of *federalism*, is well beyond the scope of this chapter. However, they do form an important background for understanding the impetus for the many "solitudes" of medical politics to begin the bridge-building necessary to create systems of both health care and medical education. As the main national professional organizations saw increasing need to coordinate their activities in the national policy arena in the 1980s, they formed a Canadian Medical Forum wherein their respective presidents and chief executive officers met on a regular basis to explore common issues and reach consensus on joint action. After tentative progress at first, the last three decades have seen a greater capacity for the many branches of the profession to work together for the benefit of Canadian health care. The Canadian Medical Forum represented a serious and ongoing commitment of the various branches of the profession that had developed over the preceding decades to participate together in the national issues of the day. One such issue was the state of CME/CPD in Canada.

As the CMA, through its Council on Medical Education, reviewed the rich array of initiatives and actors in CME, it sought to provide support for coordination of a joint commitment to this third phase of lifelong learning. With the Association of Canadian Medical Colleges (ACMC), CFPC, Royal College of Physicians and Surgeons of Canada (RCPSC), Medical Council of Canada (MCC), Federation of Medical Licensing Authorities (FMLAC), Canadian Federation of Medical Students (CFMS/FMSQ), Canadian Association for Medical Education (CAME), Pharmaceutical Manufacturers Association of Canada (PMAC), Canadian Association of Interns and Residents (CAIR), and Conseil de l'éducation médicale continue du Québec (CMQ), they began the Canadian Forum on CME in the mid-1990s. The Forum met regularly and, by 1998, developed a consensus statement that represented a vision of CME as a system of responsive education capable of assessing the need for new knowledge through understanding the needs of patients, and ensuring the timely deployment of that knowledge through educational processes that reliably lead to changes in practice that were, in turn, assessed regularly for their impact on health outcomes among patients.

Again, this is captured in the vision statement endorsed in 1998:

> That Canadian physicians will embrace their responsibility to provide the highest quality care possible by participating in a life-long, self-directed program of effective and practice integrated CME.[11]

There was no naivete about the challenge in building such a complex adaptive system, but a clear and mutual desire to see it be achieved emerged: "The unwavering focus of professional continuing education should be to improve clinical performance and patients' health."[12] All of the

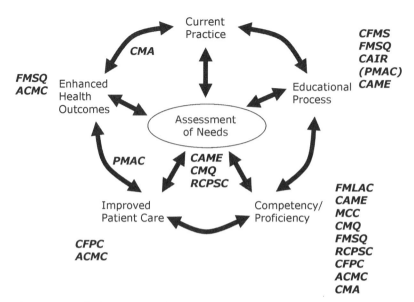

Figure 19-1 Linked Learning Cycle Featuring Associations. *Source: R. F. Woollard and others, "Proceedings of the National Forum on Continuing Medical Education" (CMA House, Ottawa, January 22, 1997).*

organizations signed on to move this vision forward. A model of a linked learning cycle formed the basis of the relationships within such a system. The consensus statement represented more than rhetoric. The Forum went on to define the roles of its member organizations and to situate their various functions within the linked learning cycle (see Figure 19-1).

During the course of these deliberations, the ghost of Flexner was always close at hand. This was not so much because of his focus on scientific education. It was more a hopeful desire to have the profession apply the same level of rigor and commitment to organizing CME as had already gone into undergraduate education. Subsequent to Flexner's articulate and sharp critique of the commercialized and self-serving medical schools that dotted North America in the early 20th century, the bulk of them closed. The passing of these unlamented schools had resulted in a remarkable flowering of medical education and the later development of academic medical centers that became a prime focus for research and medical advances in the 20th century. It also re-

sulted in an extensive bi-national accreditation partnership—Committee on the Accreditation of Canadian Medical Schools (CACMS) and Liaison Committee on Medical Education (LCME)—that serves as a world leader in ongoing quality enhancement of physician preparation. The Canadian Forum on CME looked to the possibility that the highly commercial influences and self-serving features of contemporary CME might similarly become a historical artifact by the turn of the century.

The Forum and the Origins of CACME

Under the initial leadership of Dean Doug Wilson, chair of ACMC, and Bob Woollard, MD, chair of the CMA Council on Medical Education, the Forum worked to establish principles and the basis for a system of CME embracing the regulatory bodies and the other parent organizations of what became CACME. Challenges emerged in building an integrated system of this nature. For one thing, the two national colleges were developing increasingly sophisticated credit recognition systems of their own. In addition, FMLAC (now known as the Federation of Medical Regulatory Authorities of Canada [FMRAC]) was developing an extensive competency assessment process to ensure the ongoing quality of care provided by its licensees. Known as the Monitoring and Enhancement of Physician Performance, this commendably innovative and consultative project sought to use the best available evidence in order to address some of the gaps later identified in the linked learning cycle model. The core role of education in addressing at least some of the needs identified through monitoring made the need for a collaborative profession-wide relationship evident.

Various scandals involving physician and industry relationships brought ethical concerns to the fore. Under the chairmanship of Woollard, the three councils of the CMA held countrywide hearings and developed guidelines for the ethical relationships between physicians and industry. Other bodies adopted the guidelines and influenced the manner in which CME was funded and provided. While industry continued (and still continues[13]) to provide a major source of funds for what is called CME, the increasingly effective academic divisions of CME/CPD in the medical schools began to practice greater control over these relationships.

During the course of their development in the last quarter of the century, the academic divisions formed a Standing Subcommittee on CME (SCCME) within the ACMC (now known as the Association of Faculties of Medicine of Canada [AFMC]). This became a venue for sharing work, experiences, and research. It also provided a basis for developing a system of self-assessment and peer review—the essential features of a professional accreditation system.

While the Forum had provided one helpful model for inter-organizational collaboration, the CACMS in its bi-national relationship with the LCME provided a model for the functioning of an accreditation system. However, while CACMS and LCME constitutes a partnership between the

advocacy (CMA and American Medical Association) and academic (ACMC and Association of American Medical Colleges) branches of the profession, it was apparent that a body seeking to address the quality of educational activities by practicing physicians would require an even broader range of perspectives. As it happened, the physicians of Quebec had been developing a sophisticated collaboration and effective system for integrated assessment, educational organization, and competency surveillance. The lessons learned from that process were freely shared, and the resulting Conseil de l'éducation médicale continue du Québec became one of the founding members of CACME. The other members were (and are) the AFMC, CMA, CFPC, RCPSC, and FMRAC.

CACME Is Born

CACME was established in 1996 as a subcommittee of CACMS, with the CACMS chair also being the CACME chair (a joint chairmanship that continued until 2007). Standards were worked out in conjunction with SCCME and a regular system of accreditation developed. Initially, divisions of CME had been reviewed as part of the CACMS-LCME process, but these were more ancillary to the undergraduate process and lacked fully developed standards. The initial reviews resulted in variable terms of accreditation based on the assessed quality and challenges of the unit in question. This soon gave way to a five-year accreditation cycle modeled on the CACMS-LCME process with potential for interim reports, interim visits, shortened cycles, probation, and removal of accreditation. As CACME gained experience in the process and the units provided feedback, a review and revision of the standards were undertaken and the process became increasingly more marked by the use of more objective standards and compliance measures.

By 1999, CACME was operating as an independent entity and no longer as a CACMS subcommittee; and the joint chairmanship ended in 2007 with the conclusion of Woollard's second term. There had been some hope of closing the circle of lifelong learning by linking the accreditation of undergraduate and CME/CPD components. In practical terms this proved more challenging than helpful. Indeed, in recent years more appropriate effort has been put into linking with the accreditation processes of other professionals in the health-care domain.[14]

As CACME looked to adapt its work to the evolving trends in health services and education, it engaged in the movement towards enhancing the social accountability of medical schools. Focused by a seminal World Health Organization initiative in 1995, this international effort became an increasing focus of work in Canadian medicine.[15] A major effort led by the AFMC formed the basis for reviewing CME/CPD not only in the framework of science and pedagogy but within the values that society might reasonably expect from its doctors.[16] Thus, CACME undertook a complete revision of its standards and procedure in order to put them explicitly within a framework of social accountability.

In 2005, the CACME standards were completely rewritten using social accountability principles.[17] In this formulation the organization of the committee is described thus:

The Committee on Accreditation of Continuing Medical Education (CACME) accredits the Continuing Medical Education/Continuing Professional Development (CME/CPD) offices of all Canadian faculties of medicine.

The current accreditation standards used by CACME were introduced in 2005. There are 15 standards, which cover a wide array of administrative, educational and research issues. They are divided into four categories:

- Responding to societal needs
- Organization and administration
- Provision of educational services
- Research and innovation

Each standard includes evaluation criteria to determine one of four levels of compliance: non-

compliance, partial compliance, compliance, or exemplary compliance.

CACME is an independent committee with representation from and appointed by:

- The Association of Faculties of Medicine of Canada (AFMC)
- The Canadian Medical Association
- The Collège des médecins du Québec
- The Royal College of Physicians and Surgeons of Canada
- The College of Family Physicians of Canada
- The Federation of Medical Regulatory Authorities of Canada

Each university CME/CPD office is subject to a periodic accreditation survey visit by two to three assessors, each of whom is experienced in academic or association CME/CPD. The visits last two days and comprise a series of interviews with key stakeholders in the office, including the dean of the faculty, office administrators, and physicians who have attended the office's education activities.

Based on the survey teams' reports, which include decisions on the level of compliance for each standard, CACME determines the offices' terms of accreditation, which can be for a maximum of five years. Interim progress reports are often requested to address areas deemed to be partially compliant or non-compliant.

Other activities of CACME include contributing to the advancement of CME/CPD standards generally in Canada and liaising with other CME/CPD accreditation bodies, including the Accreditation Council for Continuing Medical Education [ACCME] in the United States.[18]

The accreditation system currently embraces all 17 Canadian medical schools and has established a robust working relationship with the parallel evolution of ACCME. Under the leadership of Canadian Murray Kopelow, MD, the ACCME has moved forward in a complex environment to foster changes in the American CME/CPD environment. As part of this, he initiated the concept of *substantial equivalency* in order to address the challenges of international comparisons as information technology and point-of-service education blur the traditional geographic constituencies in CPD. With CACME, this concept was developed into a practical expression of collaboration across borders. The jointly developed policy paper on Substantial Equivalency has gone on to form the basis of evolving international initiatives as CME/CPD enters the realm of cybernetic globalization. It was taken forward to Europe to work towards an international agreement on standards.

Are We There Yet?

The full achievement of the National Forum on CME vision of a coordinated and adaptive national system for CME/CPD in Canada that embraces the accreditation activities of the CFPC, RCPSC, SCCME, CACME, and the national specialty societies is a focus of ongoing activities. CACME has hosted meetings to gain a new consensus on this next stage of the evolution of Canadian CME/CPD. An initial discussion paper by Richard Handfield-Jones, MD, has formed the basis for fruitful explorations.

However, if we revisit the linked learning cycle and the responsibilities resting with the many constituencies in Canadian medicine, we see that considerable room for action remains. As we become more aware of the conceptual basis for complex adaptive systems and more fully realize the health system and its educational supports are complex rather than complicated,[19] it is apparent that we must create a web of viable feedback loops in order to make the linked learning cycle work. Some of these are in place, but we have yet to achieve the success hoped for in 1997:

If the [National Forum on CME] is to be a success, it must provide value added such that our collective efforts add up to more than the sum of our individual and organizational contributions. This will not be achieved by compromising the autonomy of our various organizations—it will be achieved by forging a shared vision whereby the actions of our individual organizations can be focused on our common purpose of serving the Canadian public.[20]

The history of CACME advises us that this is an ongoing task but a worthy one.

Notes

1. R. Woollard, "Continuing Medical Education in the 21st Century," *British Medical Journal* 337 (2008): a119.

2. A. Flexner, *Medical Education in the United States and Canada: A Report to the Carnegie Foundation for the Advancement of Teaching* (New York: The Foundation, 1910), http://www.carnegiefoundation.org/eLibrary/docs/flexner_report.pdf.

3. Macy Foundation, "Continuing Education in the Health Professions" (conference proceedings, Josiah Macy, Jr. Foundation, Bermuda, November 28–December 1, 2007), http://www.josiahmacyfoundation.org/documents/pub_ContEd_inHealthProf.pdf.

4. Flexner, *Medical Education.*

5. National Forum on CME: Consensus Statement on CME, CMA Council on Medical Education, 1998.

6. L. Curry and K. V. Mann, "Priority Issues in Continuing Medical Education Show Sensitivity to Change in Canadian Health Care," *Canadian Medical Association Journal* 142 (1990): 299–302.

7. "Editorial: Academic Medicine: Resuscitation in Progress," *Canadian Medical Association Journal* 170, no. 3 (2004).

8. Academy of Medical Sciences, *Strengthening Clinical Research* (United Kingdom: Academy of Medical Sciences, 2003), http://www.acmedsci.ac.uk/p_scr.pdf.

9. Macy Foundation, "Continuing Education."

10. "CMA Council on Medical Education Discusses Substandard Medical Schools and Accreditation Problems," *Canadian Medical Association Journal* 118 (1978).

11. National Forum on CME: Consensus Statement.

12. Woollard, "Continuing Medical Education," a119.

13. Ibid.; National Forum on CME: Consensus Statement.

14. "Accreditation of Interprofessional Health Education, AIPHE: Community Home Page," Canadian Interprofessional Health Collaborative Web site, https://www.cihc.ca/library/handle/10296/351 (accessed June 26, 2010).

15. R. F. Woollard, "Caring for a Common Future: Medical Schools' Social Accountability," *Medical Education* 40 (2006): 301–313.

16. "Association of Faculties of Medicine Proceedings" (inaugural meeting, Partners' Forum on Social Ac-

countability of Canadian Medical Schools, Halifax, Nova Scotia, April 27–28, 2004).

17. Woollard, "Caring for a Common Future," 301–313.

18. "Committee on Accreditation of Continuing Medical Education (CACME)," Association of Faculties of Medicine of Canada Web site, http://www.afmc.ca/education-cacme-e.php (accessed June 26, 2010).

19. S. Glouberman and B. Zimmerman, "Compli-

cated and Complex Systems: What Would Successful Reform of Medicare Look Like?" Health and Everything Web site, http://www.healthandeverything.org/files/Glouberman_E.pdf (accessed July 25, 2010).

20. R. F. Woollard and others, "Proceedings of the National Forum on Continuing Medical Education" (CMA House, Ottawa, January 22, 1997).

Craig M. Campbell and I. John Parboosingh

CHAPTER 20

The Evolution of Continuing Professional Development at the Royal College of Physicians and Surgeons of Canada: Setting Standards for Canadian Specialists

The major role envisioned for the Royal College of Physicians and Surgeons of Canada, when it was created by an Act of Parliament on June 14, 1929, was to develop national standards for specialty education and establish the certification process by which specialty designation and qualifications for Canada would be based. However, its role in continuing medical education (CME) was not formally expressed until 1971 when renewal of the Letters Patent of Continuance included a role for the College "to encourage, assist and promote continuing medical education." This chapter describes the changes in CME and the health care environment that influenced the College to assume a leadership role in setting standards for specialty CME in Canada. The Royal College commenced an active program of research into innovative CME/CPD models in 1990, established a new Directorate of Professional Development in 1998, and implemented a mandatory maintenance of certification (MOC) program to sustain membership and fellowship in the Royal College in 2000.

The College's Response to US Programs of Recertification: 1975–1985

As early as 1973, recertification was a subject of intense debate at the American Board of Medical Specialties (ABMS). Several specialty boards had already formulated policies and set dates to initiate time-limited certification. In Canada, a survey of the fellowship on the College's role in CME and recertification was met with little response. However, the apparent lack of interest of fellows was not shared by the Presidential Committee on Horizons. The Committee's report to Council in 1977 recommended that the College take a leadership role, working with the medical schools and the national specialty societies, to ensure that effective CME programs would be available for specialists. It also recommended that Council declare its support for recertification and create a task force to advise the College on how this might be implemented. The Council of the Royal College, reaffirming its position that maintenance of competence is the responsibility of the individual fellow, voted against the implementation of recertification and instead established a Committee on Maintenance of Competence to foster the development of practice specific CME plans for fellows.

Events Leading to the Development of a System of Maintenance of Competence for Fellows: 1986–1993

In 1986 the newly formed Communications Publications and Continuing Medical Education

(CPCME) Committee, chaired by A. R. Cox, recognized the central position of maintenance of competence in the changing environment in which specialists practiced. Increasing subspecialization, rapid expansion of knowledge, and introduction of new technologies created demands for specialists to seek effective methods of keeping up to date. Changes in public attitudes were considered to be of great importance by members of the CPCME Committee: fellows had to recognize that consumers (patients) were not only highly educated and better informed, but also had increasing expectations of specialty care. The concept of the *social contract* between professionals and the public, whereby professionals have rights and responsibilities, was central to the discussion. Other points of view such as increasing medical liability, development of quality assurance and risk management programs in hospitals, new directions of licensing bodies, and pending legislation in some provinces were considered by the committee. Feedback from the regional advisory committees of the College supported the recommendations of the CPCME Committee. Trends in other countries such as the United States and Australia to introduce mandatory CME also influenced the recommendations of the CPCME Committee.

The Royal College Council in 1988, receiving recommendations from the Regional Advisory Committee for region 3 and the CPCME Committee, approved a new mission statement for the College that included the following: "to promote the continuing professional competence of specialist physicians and surgeons . . . and establish efficient and effective strategies for the maintenance of competence of specialists in collaboration with other organizations."[1] The "other organizations" referred to the faculties of medicine and the national specialty societies. Council, influenced by the recommendations made by Cox on behalf of the CPCME Committee and P. P. Demers, MD, Director of Fellowship Affairs, passed a resolution that the College accept the responsibility in principle for the development of a system geared to the maintenance of competence of specialists.

An innovative system that rewarded fellows for practice-based learning, driven by self-assessment of knowledge and peer review of practice performance, was outlined at a workshop sponsored by the CPCME Committee and chaired by C. R. Woolf, MD, in 1988. Council, at its September 1989 meeting, received the report of the workshop and requested the Office of Fellowship Affairs develop a Maintenance of Competence (MOCOMP) pilot project. The 10th Conference on Specialties in 1990, chaired by President D. R. Wilson, was devoted to reaching agreement with representatives from the university faculties of medicine and the national specialty societies on the principles that would govern a voluntary MOCOMP program. The system was to be based on the principle of continuous improvement and enhancement of competence rather than a punitive or coercive approach.[2]

The principles and outline for a MOCOMP pilot were summarized in a College publication entitled RCPSC Maintenance of Competence System that was distributed at the 1990 annual meeting. Alan Hewson, MD, who had spearheaded the maintenance of competence program of the Royal Australasian College of Obstetricians and Gynaecologists, was the guest speaker at a seminar on maintenance of competence. After the meeting, Hewson accepted to participate in a Royal College–sponsored lecture tour that enabled him to meet with fellows in major cities across Canada and discuss issues and strategies to promote and support maintenance of competence.

The goal of the MOCOMP pilot project was a departure from the original project proposed by the CPCME Committee. A planning group consisting of the CME coordinators or chairs from 10 participating national specialty societies was convened under the leadership of I. J. Parboosingh, MD, associate dean of CME at the University of Calgary, who was appointed to the position of associate director of the Office of Fellowship Affairs. This planning group invited R. Fox, professor of adult education at the University of Oklahoma, to serve as an advisor to the development of the pilot project. The planning group met to explore ways to develop an innovative program based on the principles of adult learning. A draft pilot project was outlined that assessed the feasibility and acceptability of developing a pilot project built on the principles of practice-based self-managed continuing education. The initial proposal envisioned inviting participation by fellows of the Royal College who were members of the 10 national specialty societies that volunteered to support the development of the pilot project. However, persistent interest from other national specialty societies to participate in the pilot project led Council to make the MOCOMP program a voluntary activity open to all Royal College members.

The MOCOMP Program: 1993–1999

The MOCOMP program included the approval of accredited traditional CME conferences, self-directed learning activities (termed *personal learning projects*), and provided participants with an annual profile of their CME activities. The MOCOMP program provided all participating specialists with a learning diary to support and structure reflection on practice and to facilitate the recording of self-directed learning projects stimulated by their professional practice. The theoretical principles and educational construct that supported the MOCOMP program were based in part on Donald Schon's theory of reflective practice.[3] The standards for practice-based learning included within the MOCOMP program were developed from the results of a research project, led by C. M. Campbell, Parboosingh, and T. Gondocz and funded by a generous grant from Searle Canada. This research project studied the self-learning experiences of 65 volunteer fellows in internal medicine.

PCDiary, the electronic version of MOCOMP's learning diary, and the Question Library, a search-able database of individual diary items, was generously funded by GlaxoWellcome Canada and offered to physicians in 1996. PCDiary was probably the first generation of e-portfolios and social network software that was made available to practicing physician as tools to support the development and recording of their continuing professional development activities and identified outcomes. In 1996, MOCOMP was awarded the CPE Award of Excellence by the American Association of Adult and Continuing Education. The educational principles behind PCDiary and the results of an evaluation of its impact were published in peer reviewed journals.[4] These publications, spearheaded by Campbell, led to requests from sister colleges abroad to pilot the e-learning tools. Between 1997 and 2000, pilot projects were established in Australia, England, Scotland, and Denmark. In Canada, the Ontario College of Physiotherapists piloted PCDiary. Several other organizations produced their own versions. University of Newcastle, New South Wales, developed an e-learning diary for undergraduate medical students, and the Australasian College of Pathologists established its CPD e-diary from PCDiary. The Scottish Postgraduate Medical and Dental Board developed its own learning diary (CELT). The first Internet version of PCDiary was launched by the Australasian Society of Ultrasound Medicine in 1998. Within a period of five years, the Royal College of Physicians and Surgeons of Canada had established an international reputation for innovations in CME and learning technologies. These tools were developed at a time when medical educators saw the need for the medical profession to adopt the concepts embraced in the term *continuing professional development (CPD)*. CPD included educational activities relevant to a physician's discipline-specific knowledge or skills (the domain of traditional CME) but embraced learning activities linked to a broader set of competencies, enabling the inclusion of educational offerings that addressed doctor-patient communication, interdisciplinary team skills, risk management, medical ethics, health advocacy, use of health technologies (to name a few) as central components of a practice-specific learning strategy. In Canada, the essential competencies for continuing professional development were defined within the Royal College's CanMEDS 2000 project Skills for the New Millennium. The competences defined within these seven essential roles provided the framework for linking engagement in continuing professional development to the quality of specialty care provided to patients.

At the time of the development of a voluntary MOCOMP program there was an assumption that this would attract a modest but enthusiastic group of volunteers. Although the initial hope was to recruit approximately 2,000 volunteers, almost 4,000 initially agreed to participate in the pilot project. However, only a portion of these early adopters participated on an annual basis, and when the pilot project was discontinued in 1999 to make way for the mandatory program of maintenance of certification, only 30 percent of fellows had registered, and 13 percent received an annual profile. Fewer than 10 percent of fellows voluntarily recorded their self-directed learning projects using either the electronic or paper versions of the learning diary.[5] Very few members of Council participated in the pilot project, and several questioned the validity of the learning strategies and requirements to document activities and outcomes. Until the Royal College felt it important enough to mandate participation, many fellows refused to participate in a voluntary program, and participation quickly reached a plateau. Fellows, already overcommitted with busy practice schedules, felt that external pressures or incentives would be required to promote participation in a national CPD program designed to achieve the goal of enhancing standards of practice.

The Case for Mandatory CPD and Maintenance of Certification

The report from the external strategic review of College activities undertaken in 1997 recom-

mended that mandatory maintenance of certification be adopted within five years. The report raised the College's awareness of pressures for specialists to show evidence they were keeping up to date. The provincial licensing authorities, cognizant of pressures from the public, reaffirmed that commitment to continue learning is an integral part of the social contract that underpins the transparency and accountability of a self-regulating profession. These conclusions were shared by other countries throughout the world. For example, several Australasian royal colleges and the American Board of Medical Specialties (ABMS) expressed the view that in the absence of a commitment to maintenance of certification, specialty certificates would likely lose their value by society over several years.

Receiving the report from the External Strategic Review, the Royal College Council recommended establishing a mandatory continuing professional development program to promote continued learning after certification. A task force was struck in summer 1997 and chaired by J. W. D. McDonald, MD, to explore the options for the creation of such a program. Leaders in medical education and assessment from national specialty societies, the university offices of CME, and the Federation of Medical Specialists of Quebec were recruited to participate in the task force.

Recertification by Examination or MOC?

The task force joined the debate on the pros and cons of recertification by examination and the approach to MOC, which was already in progress in several international royal colleges and at the ABMS. Most US specialty boards accepted that time-limited certification was inevitable, although the traditional approach to recertification, consisting of examinations every 10 years, was considered a crude form of assessment of the continuing competence of specialists. Recognizing that Canadian law mandates each provincial medical regulatory authority to establish programs to identify physicians who are not fit to practice or fall below established professional standards, the task force elected not to recommend formal assessments of competence or performance. Instead, the task force recommended that the Royal College follow the Australasian colleges and establish a mandatory program of continuing education for maintenance of certification with the intent to promote a culture of continuous quality improvement and the pursuit of excellence in specialty medicine.

Maintenance of Fellowship or MOC?

The debate on whether the new program should be called maintenance of fellowship or MOC provided the opportunity to review the meaning of the terms *specialty certification* and *fellowship in the College*. The practical implications were debated at meetings of the regional advisory committees, and the fellowship at large was drawn into the discussions. Fellows were assured that the Royal College would not remove specialty certification (a historical event) from individuals who have justly earned that status. However, it was decided that participation in a mandatory program of continuing professional development should be an absolute requirement to maintain fellowship in the Royal College and use of the designation FRCPC and FRCSC. This decision fundamentally changed the meaning of the designation as not only the achievement of initial certification but a commitment to sustain the quality of specialty care through engaging in lifelong learning activities designed to enhance the quality of professional specialty practices.

At a meeting of the presidents of the national specialty societies, registrars of the licensing (now known as medical regulatory) authorities, and the CME deans or directors within the faculties of medicine, held at Royal College headquarters in February 1998, Luc Deschenes, MD, president of the Royal College, presented the case for the implementation of a mandatory program of continuing learning in practice. By the end of this meeting, there was consensus that the Royal College, in collaboration with the national specialty societies and the university CME offices, should initiate a continuing education program that should be called the maintenance of certification program.

Accepting the report of the task force, Council in April 1998 passed a motion in support of the principles for the development of a maintenance of certification program. In September of that year, Council passed the second set of motions relating to maintenance of certification: "that participation in the program be a requirement for admission to Fellowship, effective December 31, 2000" and "that participation in the program be normally required for maintenance of Fellowship, as prescribed by regulations approved by Council."[6]

A Directorate of Professional Development was established in July 1998, and Parboosingh was appointed as its first director. The decision was made to discontinue the MOCOMP program at the end of 1999. Fellows of the Royal College could begin to participate in the new MOC program on a voluntary basis on January 1, 2000. Participation was mandatory by January 1, 2001, for all active, active senior, and emeritus members engaged in full-time or part-time practice or related professional activities such as teaching, research, or administration. Unlike MOCOMP, the new mandatory program was not given a formal acronym but is still referred today as the *MOC program*. A committee was struck with representation from regional advisory committees, national specialty societies, and CME deans to begin planning the educational framework for the new mandatory program.

The new organizational structure for the College recommended by the External Strategic Review Committee was implemented in the fall of 1998. McDonald was appointed vice president of professional development and chair of the professional development committee (PDC), a standing committee of Council. Ten national specialty societies, the Federation of Medical Regulatory Authorities of Canada, the Federation of Medical

Specialists of Quebec, deans or directors of CME in the faculties of medicine, and one representative of the pharmaceutical industry (Rx&D) were represented on the PDC. Three subcommittees reported to the PDC: the standards committee, charged with developing the educational framework for the maintenance of certification program; the information management committee, charged with establishing methods for fellows to document participation in the program; and the accredited providers committee, who were charged with establishing standards for the accreditation of CME providers.

Consultation with Fellows, Stakeholder Organizations, and the Public

Resistance to the establishment of MOC, encountered among some fellows and fueled by the leadership in a few national specialty societies, became more vocal when the starting date of the program was announced. Concern was expressed that specialists working in rural areas had less access to CME programs compared with their colleagues in the larger towns and teaching hospitals and would find it harder to meet the requirements for MOC. Articles eloquently penned in the *Medical Post* accused the Royal College of not consulting its fellows. The accusations could not have been further from the truth. The fellows were surveyed as part of the external review undertaken by the College. Of the 3,655 who responded, 2,569 (or 70.3 percent) agreed that CME should be a regular requirement to maintain their specialty certificate.[7] These findings, and the extensive consultation undertaken by the task force, were published in the *Annals* of the Royal College of Physicians and Surgeons of Canada and on its Web site. In 1999, after a year of public debate, the Medical Post commissioned an external (Gallup) poll of fellows. The results showed that nearly 70 percent of fellows accepted the College's decision to establish MOC.[8] This was reassuring news, especially for senior officers of the College who, remembering the last divisive debate in the College in 1972, expressed concern for the future of the College should a significant number of fellows choose to resign.

The educational framework of the MOC program, drafted in the fall of 1998 by members of three large specialty societies, was continuously revised in response to feedback from the societies and from fellows. Most fellows understood that inclusion of a credit validation process based on a random sample of self-reported entries was required to add credibility to the program. Indeed, 40 of the 43 presidents of national specialty societies who responded to a survey concurred with the need for a credit validation process within MOC program. In addition, 36 presidents thought the minimal standard of 80 credits per year required to comply with the program was "just right," with six indicating that they perceived the standard was "too low."[9]

Research into public opinion, undertaken by a public relations firm on behalf of the College in 2000, indicated that the public's traditional acceptance of specialists had changed in recent years. Two-thirds of respondents indicated that they were interested in the credentials of specialists and would access a public listing to reassure themselves of the qualifications of their specialist. In helping the public to select a specialist, respondents indicated that knowledge of the initial certification and CME profiles of a specialist were more important than a recommendation from a family physician or friend. The results of these studies suggested that the public would likely equate the designation FRCPC and FRCSC not only with quality training and certification, but also with participation in an accredited program of continuing professional development.[10]

The results of the public survey came as a surprise to many fellows, though the changing climate of transparency and accountability had already started to have an impact on their daily activities. For instance, an increasing number of hospitals, regulatory authorities, and the law courts were requiring physicians to document their participation in CPD activities as part of a privileging or renewal of licensure process or to establish the basis for testifying as an expert. Therefore, an important goal of the maintenance of certification program was to provide fellows with a standard method of documentation and to ensure that benchmarks for CPD were fair and consistent across provincial and territorial jurisdictions.

Town hall sessions were held at national specialty society meetings to obtain feedback from fellows as the final design of the program took shape. The experiences of fellows who participated in the voluntary program in 2000 informed the final revisions to the program's framework and credit system before it was formally rolled out as a mandatory program on January 1, 2001. The College had taken every opportunity to ensure that its fellows, the national specialty societies, and the CME deans in the faculties of medicine participated in the design of the program.

The Regulations for MOC

To many fellows, the program became a reality when the Royal College Bylaws were revised and unanimously accepted by fellows attending the Annual Business Meeting held in Edmonton in 2000. A *fellow* was now defined as "a person who was admitted to Fellowship in the Royal College in accordance with Article 5 of Bylaw No. 13 and who is in compliance with the Maintenance of Certification requirements of Article 7 of Bylaw No. 15."[11] There were initial concerns that fellows who obtained fellowship by examination prior to 1972 would be able to retain the designation without participating in the MOC program. This issue was resolved by legal advice, which indicated that the term *fellow* in the bylaws applies to all members of the College regardless of how membership was achieved. Completion of the first five-year cycle (January 1, 2001, to December 31, 2005) by documenting accredited learning activities that achieved a minimum of 400 credits was the basis of continuing fellowship, the use of the designations FRCSC and FRCPC, and listing on the public directory of fellows hosted on the College's Web site. The MOC program selected a 3 percent random sample of fellows who participated in the MOC program in the previous year to participate in a review and validation of the required documentation for each activity that was submitted. Fellows who are fully retired from clinical or laboratory practice were exempted from participating in the MOC program.

A unique component of the program is that fellows who retired from clinical activities but continued to participate in medical administration, research, and education (referred to as *related professional activities*) were required to participate in the MOC program. In addition, the Royal College Council in 2001 accepted recommendations from the professional development committee, led by L. Samson, MD, vice president of professional development, that fellows residing in the United States who are engaged in programs of maintenance of certification or recertification of one of the American specialty boards could maintain their membership and fellowship by participating in these programs without having to participate in the MOC program. Finally, specialists who were not certified by the Royal College but had obtained a license to practice in a province or territory were able to participate in the Royal College CPD program, a mirror image of the MOC program. In this manner all specialists practicing in Canada could use the same framework and tools to support their continuing professional development for the benefit of the Canadian public.

The Education Components of the MOC Program

The presidents of national specialty societies, at their annual meeting with Royal College officials in February 1998, recommended that the program extend beyond traditional CME, which was perceived to focus on updating medical knowledge. They wanted the new program to be more comprehensive and facilitate the CPD of fellows.

TABLE 20-1 *The Framework of CPD Options for MOC*

Section	Examples of CPD activities	Assignment of credits
1. Accredited group learning activities: education sessions produced by accredited providers of CPD activities*	Rounds, journal clubs, workshops, courses, conferences, distance education programs	1 credit per hour, no maximum
2. Other learning activities: learning activities that are not necessarily affiliated with an accredited provider	Nonaccredited rounds and meetings; reading journals and texts; information (MEDLINE®) searches; audiotape, videotape, computer, or Internet CME	1 credit per hour, maximum of 100 credits per 5-year period
3. Accredited self-assessment program: programs designed to assist the specialist to identify his/her educational needs	Self-assessment programs developed or sponsored by NSS, faculties, and colleges; training or virtual reality simulators used for the purpose of self-assessment	2 credits per hour, no maximum
4. Structured learning projects: learning activities are planned and the outcome is recorded and evaluated	Personal learning projects generated from participating in a CPD activity, traineeships, preceptored courses, masters and PhD studies	1 credit per hour, no maximum
5. Practice review and appraisal: activities that assist specialists to review their practice	Practice audits and patient surveys, institution audits, incident reports, utilization studies	2 credits per hour, no maximum
6. Educational development, teaching, and research: activities that involve setting standards for practice	Publications (e.g., manuscript reviews), preparation of presentations, teaching, examinations (question writing), research (e.g., grant proposals and trials), setting standards (CPG development)	1 credit per hour, maximum of 100 credits per 5-year period

*Accredited providers are organizations that are reviewed and approved by the Royal College based on their ability to adhere to a defined set of accreditation standards.

A program founded on the concept of continuing professional development would encourage fellows to link their engagement in learning activities to defined competencies that were relevant to each fellow's professional practice profile. The final education framework, shown in Table 20-1, resulted from two years of intensive consultation with the stakeholder organizations.

MOC program educational framework, designed by the standards committee under the leadership of J. Toews and D. Wooster, is innovative. Traditional group learning activities where participants listen to presentations given by experts, participate in interactive learning workshops or seminars, and engage in informal learning with colleagues constituted only one of six categories or options of educational activities that fellows could use to earn credits. The program provided fellows with the opportunity to plan their own continuing professional development program based on their professional roles and responsibilities, identified needs, and the competencies they required to deliver the highest quality of specialty care. Fellows who use self-administered assessments of their knowledge (accredited self-assessment programs) or engaged in reviews of their performance in practice (practice review and appraisal) earned double credits. These incentives were based in part on the educational value of activities that enabled the identification of unperceived needs but also the time and effort required to complete such activities. Finally, fellows could earn credits for engaging in self-directed, practice-based learning and improvement activities by creating personal learning projects (PLPs), designing traineeships, or developing plans to participate in perceptored courses. The emphasis on reflective learning in practice, recognized internationally as a unique feature of the program, is based on years of experience with portfolio-based learning in the MOCOMP program.[12] It recognizes the need for fellows to be competent in the management of clinical situations of uncertainty, ambiguity, and conflict, as well as in the practice of evidence-based medicine. Knowledge required to maintain skills in these competencies is as much tacit as it is explicit, and is largely acquired by practice reflection, communication with colleagues, and the critical reconstruction of practice. When faced with a learning need, fellows can select CPD activities from one or more sections of the framework, like using tools in a toolbox to complete the learning task. The latter concept was termed "educational re-engineering" by Wooster, chair of the standards committee. It demonstrated that MOC was not just about counting hours or credits but had the potential to teach fellows how to enhance their learning through judicious use of an educational framework.

The Role of Information Technology

While fellows accepted the principles behind MOC, they perceived keeping records of CPD activities to be a time-consuming chore. Members of the information management committee felt the use of technology might make record keeping more user-friendly. As mentioned earlier, the potential of electronic records, explored during the MOCOMP program, initiated the development of a program of research into e-learning tools. Two-thirds of fellows participating in the pilot program in 2000 entered their CPD hours into a database built on the College's Web site. Web Diary, the Web version of PCDiary, and the Question Library, a searchable repository of PLPs built for MOCOMP by ADGA Group Consultants Inc., were maintained outside the Royal College by ADGA on a dedicated server. The need for fellows to submit activities and data on two Web sites created general dissatisfaction with the technical support of the program. This led the College to commission ADGA to build a comprehensive Internet portal (www.Mainport.org) for fellows to track their CPD activities. In Mainport, fellows enter CPD activities through an ATM-like Web tool and see their updated MOC credit summary before leaving the site. Mainport hosted Web Diary and Question Library and provided one-stop shopping for fellows to submit CPD activities. Working with ADGA Group Consultants, Inc., the College had its first experience to partner with an information technology (IT) firm. Mixed feelings were expressed by some members of staff who felt that the IT needs of the College should be met by internal resources. Reliance on external agencies was believed to threaten the security of Royal College data. However, Mainport's technical infrastructure and support enabled it to handle data entries from several thousand fellows simultaneously, particularly in the final hours before the MOC deadline on January 31 each year. Mainport proved to be both reliable and robust.

Mainport has attracted interest from other organizations around the world and was piloted by the Bavarian Chamber of Physicians in Munich. In 2003 the College received a grant from CANARIE Inc. to build and test a browser plug-in, called PLP Enabler, to assist users to capture text from digital sources, create PLPs and, synchronizing with Mainport, automatically make entries into Web Diary.

The program of research into e-learning tools continues to grow. In 2003, under the leadership of Campbell and Gondocz, the Centre for Learning and Practice was established within the Office of Professional Development to focus on education research and development. A revised version of e-tools for MOC was made available to fellows in 2007. As well as a modernised IT platform, the new Mainport included more options for fellows to manage and record practice-based learning for MOC credit.

Participation in the First Cycle of MOC

While only 44 percent of fellows in active practice in Canada voluntarily submitted CPD hours in 2000, an information center had to be established in the Office of Professional Development (OPD) to cope with the increasing number of calls from fellows requesting information on the program. In 2002, 90 percent of fellows in Canada participated in the program, up from 84 percent in 2001, when the first five-year cycle commenced. Participation rates were the same for fellows in academic and community-based practices. Annual participation rates in Canada ranged between 85 to 90 percent. Over the course of the first cycle approximately 50 percent of the recorded credits were for attending accredited group learning activities (section 1 of the education framework). The other credits were for completing self-assessment programs, practice reviews, teaching, research, standard setting, and for completing structured learning projects such as PLPs. While many keep paper records of PLPs, 600 recorded more than 3,000 PLPs in Web Diary in 2002. Throughout the first cycle approximately 40 percent of fellows submitted one or more personal learning projects each year. This indicated the beginning of a culture shift from counting hours of participation in CPD activities to documenting what was learned and how it impacts practice.

At the end of the first cycle on December 31, 2005, 90 percent of fellows had submitted at least 400 credits, one percent had not engaged in the program at any level despite multiple offers of support, and nine percent of fellows participated in the program but had not achieved the required 400 credits to complete the cycle. During the first cycle the OPD transitioned the information center into an education support program to provide support and assistance for fellows who were struggling to understand the program, how it could be embedded within their current practice context, or how to document their learning activities in Mainport. In addition, the education support program continued to be a single point source for fellows to call for educational advice or technical support or to e-mail questions or concerns.

Because the MOC program required all fellows to submit a minimum of 40 credits in each year of a five-year cycle, the education support program was able to track the number of fellows who were struggling to complete their cycle requirements. This enabled the professional development committee under the leadership of V. Bernier, MD, to request the executive committee and council to allow fellows who participated in the program but did not achieve the required credits to be automatically eligible to have up to a two-year extension to complete their cycle requirements. During the extension period fellows were required to achieve 400 credits plus an additional 40 credits for each extension year. All credits were subjected to credit validation. Approximately 1,800 fellows entered this extension period to their first cycle, and by the end of the second year only 220 failed to achieve the credit requirements. Therefore the overall success rate during the first cycle of the MOC program was 98 percent.

Nonparticipants and fellows who failed to achieve the required credit requirements reflected a range of specialties, geographic location of practice, and years spent in practice. Although it is difficult to fully understand the reasons why some fellows chose not to engage, conversations and e-mails from those who choose to communicate reflected three main concerns or objections: the lack of evidence that engaging in the MOC program would make better doctors, the lack of time to document learning activities, and the rejection of MOC as a role for the Royal College. These objections occurred despite the Canadian Medical Association Physician Code of Ethics listing, as a fundamental responsibility, that physicians "engage in lifelong learning to maintain and improve [their] professional knowledge, skills and attitudes" and the importance of ongoing competence and performance of physicians as a pillar of professional self-regulation.

In 2006, the Federation of Medical Regulatory Authorities of Canada developed an internal working group to develop and define a program of Physician Revalidation. By 2007 an external Revalidation Working Group was formed that included representation from the Association of Faculties of Medicine of Canada, the Canadian Medical Association, the College of Family Physicians of Canada, the Medical Council of Canada, and the Royal College of Physicians and Surgeons of Canada.

Physician revalidation was defined as "a quality assurance process in which members of a provincial/territorial medical regulatory authority are required to provide satisfactory evidence of their commitment to continued competence in their practice." The purpose of physician revalidation was "to reaffirm, in a framework of professional accountability, that physicians' competence and performance are maintained in accordance with professional standards."

The resulting position statement of physician revalidation required that "all licensed physicians in Canada must participate in a recognized revalidation process in which they demonstrate their commitment to continued competent performance in a framework that is fair, relevant, inclusive, transferable and formative." Since the Royal College of Physicians and Surgeons of Canada had already recognized lifelong learning as a fundamental component of maintaining certifi-

cation, the principle and goals of the MOC program were deemed to meet the requirements of revalidation, enabling fellows of the Royal College to meet the requirements of revalidation through their participation in the MOC program.

Innovations Introduced in the Second Cycle of MOC: 2005–2009

The implementation of the MOC program was developed to occur over three phases. The first phase was the implementation phase (2001–2005), where the primary goal was to encourage fellows to participate in the program, develop an accreditation system of CPD providers, and create an education support strategy. The second phase on implementation (2006–2009) was an improvement phase to address the issues or concerns identified during the first five years. The key changes to the MOC program during this second phase were to promote the documentation of all learning activities (not just total hours per section) and to move the entire MOC framework to focus more on the documentation of outcomes from engaging in learning activities, not just the documentation of participation. Throughout this second phase the program reviewed and revised the standards for self-assessment programs to promote greater access to such tools across the 63 specialties and subspecialties. In addition, the standards and processes to promote e-group learning, the use of hand-held devices in promoting the documentation of learning activities, and the identification of simulation as an effective formative assessment strategy were important innovations in promoting the link between learning and identified professional needs. Finally, the ability to formally link the MOC program to individual CanMEDS Roles was the focus of three task forces under the leadership of G. Kane, S. Tallett, and E. Keely. Their deliberations and recommendations resulted in CanMEDS Roles being added to documentation templates within Mainport to strengthen the link between learning and all of the CanMEDS Roles and competencies. Revisions to Mainport included a new feature called the Holding Area, where fellows could record an idea, thought, or issue that they deemed important but did not have the time to pursue at that particular time. Items in the Holding Area could be reviewed, revised, deleted, or transferred to an appropriate template for submission for credit. Lastly, in the later part of this phase, strategies to enhance the automatic transfer of participation in learning activities was developed with various rounds chairs and conference planners. These strategies were intended to provide additional support to fellows in documenting their participation in accredited learning activities and lessening the burden of documenting the clerical requirements of the MOC program.

The Future of CME at the College Involves Exploring Models that Promote and Reward Interdisciplinary Collaborative Team Learning and Changing in Practice

Plans for future MOC cycles, influenced by pressure from external organizations such as the Institute of Medicine and Canadian medical regulatory authorities, include shifting learning strategies to focus on the achievement of improvements in performance, practice, and health outcomes through engaging in lifelong learning. Also, the educational delivery model should incorporate techniques that change behaviors in the complex adaptive systems that are typical of the inter-professional health-care workplace. These ambitious goals require transformative change in how CME is delivered, and not surprisingly, change in the CME community in general has been slow, as reported by an expert panel on Continuing Education in the Health Professions published by Josiah Macy, Jr. Foundation in 2008. Towards this end, the College has a series of pilot projects in place that explore the introduction of MOC credits for individual and team-based achievements in complexity-based inter-professional practice improvement programs.

Summary

Since its foundation, the primary function of the Royal College of Physicians and Surgeons of Canada has been the setting of standards for postgraduate education and certifying specialists. Advances in specialty medicine and the changing environment in which specialists practice have created the need for the College to set standards and implement a program of continuing professional development. The Royal College explored a voluntary system in MOCOMP. This program proved to be useful in developing CPD activities that fostered practice-based learning and improvement. Equally important, MOCOMP launched the College as an international leader in research into the use of information and communication technologies in CPD.

In 1998, the Council recommended the establishment of a mandatory program of continuing professional development, the Royal College Maintenance of Certification program. Participation rates in the first cycle and subsequent cycles have been exceptionally high. Credit for making a user-friendly yet credible program must go first to the effective communications between the College and its fellows, and second to collaboration with the national specialty societies, the Federation of Medical Specialists of Quebec, the university offices of CME within the faculties of medicine, and the Federation of Medical Regulatory Authorities of Canada.

The MOC program is the first national program to provide physicians with a template that fosters learning in practice. A thorough evaluation of the program was initiated in October 2008 to seek to understand the perspectives, frustrations, and recommendations on the MOC program, Mainport, and its future directions. The executive summary resulting from the qualitative and quantitative data makes 24 recommendations within five themes. In the coming years, the relevance and effectiveness of the MOC program will be based in part on our ability to embed assessment strategies within specialty practices, enhance the link between the intentional integration of group learning, self-learning, and assessment with defined practice and patient outcomes, the promotion of inter-professional team-based learning strategies, and solving the barriers to the documentation of learning activities and outcomes. It is anticipated that the MOC program will prove to be an effective vehicle to assist the Royal College in achieving its vision of "working together for excellence in specialty medicine for the health of Canadians" and its mission as an organization "dedicated to excellence in specialty medical care, the highest standards in medical education and lifelong learning, and the promotion of sound health policy."[13]

Notes

1. Royal College of Physicians and Surgeons of Canada, minutes of meeting of Council, 1988.

2. D. G. Sinclair, "Continuing Medical Education as a Cardinal Responsibility of Academic Health Centres," *Annals of the Royal College of Physicians and Surgeons of Canada* 28, no. 2 (1995): 73–74.

3. C. Campbell and others, "Study of Physicians' Use of a Software Program to Create a Portfolio of Their Self-directed Learning," *Academic Medicine* 71, no. 10 (1996): S49–S51.

4. C. Campbell and others, "A Study of the Factors Which Influence a Commitment to Change Practice in Physicians Using Learning Diaries," *Academic Medicine* 79, no. 10 (1999): S34–S36; J. Parboosingh, "Tools to Assist Physicians to Manage Their Information Needs," in *Information Literacy: Models for the Future,* ed. Christine Bruce and Phil Candy, 121–136 (Wagga Wagga, Australia: Charles Stuart University Centre for Information Studies, 2000).

5. D. A. Schon, *Educating the Reflective Practitioner* (San Francisco: Jossey Bass, 1987), 22–40.

6. Royal College, minutes of meeting of Council, 1988.

7. Survey of College fellows conducted by Ernst & Young, 1997–1998, Royal College of Physicians and Surgeons of Canada Archives.

8. "Mandatory Maintenance of Certification," *Medical Post* (December 1999).

9. Report on the Conference of Presidents, February 1998, Royal College of Physicians and Surgeons of Canada Archives.

10. Findings collected by Vision Research, a Delta Media Company, 1999, Royal College of Physicians and Surgeons of Canada Archives.

11. "Bylaw No. 15, Amended," Royal College of Physicians and Surgeons of Canada Web site, http://rcpsc.medical.org/publications/Bylaw15-Amended_e.pdf (accessed July 21, 2010).

12. Parboosingh, "Tools to Assist," 121–136.

13. "About the Royal College," Royal College of Physicians and Surgeons of Canada Web site, http://rcpsc.medical.org/about/ (accessed July 21, 2010).

CHAPTER 21

The College of Family Physicians of Canada: Continuing Medical Education and Continuing Professional Development in Canada

Continuing medical education (CME) has been an integral part of the College of Family Physicians of Canada (CFPC) since its beginning in 1954 at the Palomar Supper Club in Vancouver, British Columbia. Even before that first meeting, Victor Johnston, MD, who was to become the first CFPC executive director, mentioned the importance of CME in his rallying cry to form a new college of general practice:

I have intimated that though we all leave college with considerable knowledge, and full of enthusiasm and the wine of life, some of our number as the years go by become less than competent. They neglect to take refresher courses, and refuse to meet frequently with their fellows or pull their full weight in medical organizations. . . . To attempt to correct this is one of the most compelling reasons for the formation of sections of general practice. Some of us believe the time is ripe to make a sturdy effort to improve the calibre of general practice through imposing more discipline and responsibility on ourselves and by ourselves.[1]

Dissatisfaction on the part of some general practitioners of the time with their education and their image was one of the reasons for the formation of the CFPC. Detailed plans to address this dissatisfaction were presented early in the college's life. As recorded in David Woods's history of the CFPC, first CFPC president Murray Stalker said in his inaugural address:

It is too often taken for granted that because of the rapid advances in science the general practitioner has not been able to keep up to date. A very large number of good practitioners across Canada has proven that this is not true. It is our hope that this new College of General Practice will help and stimulate the family doctor to retain his position in this changing world, to the advantage of both the profession and the public. . . . Our program for the continuing education of the general practitioner throughout his career is much more concrete. It will be necessary for a member of the college to partake in a minimum amount of postgraduate activity throughout his life if he is to maintain his membership. It is in this manner that we have faith in the development of unity between scientist, teacher, specialist and practitioner.[2]

The educational requirements of members of the young college are also recorded in Woods's history:

(a) One hundred hours of postgraduate study each two-year period.

(b) A minimum of 25 hours of this must be for attendance at formal medical scientific meetings such as the Canadian Medical Association, L'Association des Médecins de Langue Française du Canada, divisional, district or county meetings.

(c) A minimum of 25 hours of this must be for attendance at planned postgraduate courses.

(d) Credits toward the other 50 hours will be given

for approved hospital rounds, medical papers submitted or published, planned reading courses, book reviews, case-history reports submitted for publication, community health service, etc.[3]

A look at the college's organizational structure, programs, and activities in the years since 1954 confirms the ongoing importance of CME. Today, this is reflected in the first sentence of the CFPC mission statement: "The College of Family Physicians of Canada is a national voluntary organization of family physicians that makes continuing medical education of its members mandatory."[4]

CFPC Organizational Structure

The work of the CFPC is conducted by its officers and staff and by committees of member volunteers. The committee responsible for CME is one of CFPC's longest standing committees. The earliest CME committees were the responsibility of Paul Rainsberry, MD, who was hired in 1976 as coordinator of the CFPC education committees. Rainsberry later became CFPC director of education, and today is associate executive director of academic family medicine. In 1993, the CME portfolio became the responsibility of Richard Handfield-Jones, MD, who joined the CFPC as its first director of CME. Handfield-Jones was succeeded in 2003 by Bernard Marlow, MD, the current director of continuing professional development (CPD).

The terms of the original Committee on Education, established in 1954 and chaired by E. C. McCoy, MD, were as follows:

1. To evaluate the various types of post-graduate training as to their acceptability for fulfilling the requirements for continued membership in the [CFPC] and to assess the credits for membership attendance.

2. To conduct, develop or assist in the programs, lectures, courses, or other means of post-graduate medical education for the benefit of the members and of the profession at large.

3. To encourage and assist medical schools and hospitals in developing and maintaining adequate courses and facilities for the education and training of general practitioners.

4. To encourage medical graduates to enter the field of general practice.[5]

In April 1964, the report of the Coordinating Committee on Education recommended that there be only two standing committees on education within the college, one of which was to be the Committee on Continuing Education for General Practitioners, "to deal with all matters pertaining to the pattern of general practice in Canada and the facilities for education and research in education."[6]

By 1975, the Committee on CME, under the chairmanship of G. Gibson, MD, had developed the following somewhat more specific terms of reference:

1. To further continuing medical education of family physicians in all possible ways.

2. To maintain liaison with other interested national organizations.

3. To encourage the establishment and operation of Provincial Committees on Continuing Education and particularly to encourage liaison between the provincial committees and various provincial university departments of continuing education.

4. To further the utilization of all the various types and techniques of continuing education.

5. To develop methods of evaluation and assessment in the various techniques of continuing education and postgraduate study credits.[7]

Today, the committee is called the National Committee on CPD. The name reflects a shift in emphasis from clinical activities to include all the activities that lead physicians to enhance their knowledge and skills in all of their roles. The current committee has a chair and representative from each of the 10 CFPC provincial chapters, and it reports to the CFPC board of directors.

From 1954 to 2009, many subcommittees, working groups, and task forces of the national continuing education committee have been responsible for specific activities and programs such as Self Evaluation and Mainpro®.

Another department that has provided strong support for CFPC members' CME and CPD activities is the Canadian Library of Family Medicine (CLFM), the CFPC library service, which began in the early 1970s. CLFM supports members by offering a complete range of library services, including in-depth literature searching, quick reference, document delivery, and instruction. This service began in the days of print and books and now flourishes in the digital environment, which offers rapid, efficient, and effective information management. Library staff offer personalized service, customized to specific needs of CFPC members.

Maintenance of Certification and Mainpro

In the history of the CFPC, certification and CME are inseparable. Woods's history records that before CFPC's formation, Wallace Wilson, chair of the Canadian Medical Association (CMA) general practitioners committee, asked CMA members in a letter to consider "certification of a first class or Grade A General Practitioner which would involve among other things attendance at a certain number of refresher courses."[8] This became a reality in 1969, when the CFPC introduced certification to recognize physicians who demonstrated acquisition of knowledge, skills, and attitudes integral to the discipline and practice of family medicine. Today, eligibility for certification in family medicine is granted by the CFPC to those individuals who have either completed approved residency training in family medicine or become eligible for certification through a combination of training and practice experience. Certification in family medicine is a special designation of CFPC membership. Certificants may use the designation CCFP (certificant of the College of Family Physicians).

Those attaining certification have always been expected to maintain it, as opposed to undergoing a recertification process. In 1977, maintenance of

certification (MOC) was formally endorsed by the CFPC. Since then, the granting of certification has been accompanied by the requirement that certificants participate in a MOC program.

In 1995, the CFPC introduced Mainpro, which stands for Maintenance of Proficiency/Maintien de la compétence professionnelle, to "bring structure to a loosely coordinated system of credentials and requirements for members and certificants."[9] With Mainpro, all members, certificants and noncertificants, were required to complete the equivalent of 50 hours of CME each year, at least half of which were to be for accredited activities. Accredited activities were termed *Mainpro-M1* and other activities *Mainpro-M2*. CFPC certificants were also required to accumulate Mainpro-C credits, credits acquired from learning experiences that the MOC program identified as being self directed, based on the individual family physician's practice-related needs, evidence-based, and reflective.

Mainpro-C credits are earned by participating in CFPC accredited programs that focus on performance or quality improvement. Handfield-Jones described the CFPC aim for the activity: "We would like individual family physicians to have control of their learning, and we would like our members to see their professional development as a positive part of their work. We hope to put increasing emphasis on this individual responsibility, encouraging members to be critical and reflective about what they do and how they incorporate new ideas and knowledge into their practices."[10]

There are two categories of Mainpro-C eligible learning activities: CFPC pre-accredited and self-directed. Pre-accredited learning activities include conferences, courses, workshops, advanced life-support programs, independent and practice-based small group learning, and organized clinical traineeships and fellowships. Self-directed activities include Pearls™, practice audits and quality assurance programs, provincial practice review and enhancement programs, university degree and diploma programs relevant to the practice of family medicine, and the Linking Learning to Practice (LLP) program. The latter program awards Mainpro-C credits for a variety of activities, including conducting a research project, developing educational materials and/or clinical practice guidelines, committee work that involves the review of family medicine content, and being an examiner for a family medicine or emergency medicine examination.

In 2000, the CFPC board of directors approved moving to a five-year reporting cycle for its members. A total of 250 credits were required over five years. Half of those could be Mainpro-M2 credits; half were required to be Mainpro-M1 credits. For certificants, 24 of the 125 approved credits were to be from Mainpro-C-accredited activities.[11]

Accreditation

As mandated through federal government charter, the CFPC establishes accreditation standards and accredits CME and CPD programs for family physicians in Canada. Accreditation of the CME and CPD programs occupies a significant amount of time on the part of CFPC staff and provincial chapter accreditation reviewers. In 1985, Rainsberry, then CFPC director of education, outlined the CFPC policy for accrediting programs:

The new policy requires that programs provide an opportunity for audience participation or discussion and have some form of evaluation so that participants may relay their impressions of the meeting not only to the planners but also to the speakers. To assure the relevance of the meeting the program planners are encouraged to write educational objectives and to include members of the College of Family Physicians of Canada on their Planning Committee. The College will not usually approve any program that does not have a College member as part of the Planning Committee.[12]

To promote uniformity of accreditation, the CFPC held the first workshop for CME accredi-

tors from each province in 1996. This workshop provided an opportunity to share ideas on guideline interpretation and to ensure standardization of guideline application across Canada. The CFPC has continued to promote Canada-wide standards.

The CFPC has always been responsive to concerns from both members and program developers. In 1997, the criteria used to accredit freestanding CME courses for Mainpro-C credits were modified so that CME program developers could more easily devise programs to meet accreditation criteria. Until then, the only freestanding program to receive Mainpro credits was the Practice-Based Small Group Learning Program. After that date, activities eligible for Mainpro-C credits were significantly increased.

Mainpro programs increasingly address the broadest spectrum of responsibilities and roles assumed by family physicians in Canada. Marlow outlines the current accreditation criteria as follows:

Every CME and CPD program seeking accreditation from the College must have at least 1 CFPC member on its planning committee right from the initiation of the design of the program. The CFPC member is responsible for ensuring "quality control" of the program and maintaining the standards of the College. National programs must have CFPC representatives from each of our 5 national regions on their planning committees.

All CME and CPD program applications are subjected to a rigorous review by up to three experienced, CFPC-trained reviewers, who check programs specifically for balance, lack of bias, and lack of overt commercial support. There must be objective evidence confirming the need for the educational intervention, and budgets must be submitted for review. Conflicts of interest must be declared. The content of all commercially sponsored programs is submitted for peer review. In some cases, specialist content experts are also consulted.[13]

The CFPC and the American Academy of Family Physicians (AAFP) established a reciprocity agreement for CME credits early in the CFPC history. It was formally confirmed after a 1974 visit of the subcommittee of the AAFP CME commission to the CFPC. The current agreement states that AAFP members attending Mainpro-accredited programs in Canada may claim M1 credits as prescribed credits, and vice versa for CFPC members attending AAFP accredited programs in the United States. The CFPC has no reciprocity agreements with any other organizations.

The CFPC National Annual Meeting

Another important CME activity, dating from the earliest days of the CFPC, is its annual meeting. Wilson, in the previously mentioned letter, also asked CMA members to consider "establishment of a General Practitioners' Section within the CMA which would have its own Scientific Program at CMA annual meetings."[14] The scientific program became a reality in March 1957, when the College of General Practice held its first Annual Scientific Assembly separately from the CMA at the Mount Royal Hotel in Montréal. These annual meetings provide a focal point for CME and CFPC business activities. For the most part, the meetings are co-hosted with the annual meetings of the CFPC provincial chapters/ colleges, but they have sometimes been held as independent national meetings. In 1994, Annual Scientific Assembly Committee chair Brian Morris expressed well the spirit of the meetings when he said, "This is the vision that I have for the national ASA: family physicians being active contributors to CME and being speakers and workshop leaders with the skills and expertise to educate their peers effectively."[15]

Beginning in 2000, the national Annual Scientific Assembly was renamed the Family Medicine Forum and combined with the Section of Teachers' and the Section of Researchers' annual workshops. In 2008, more than 3,200 delegates attended, and the scientific program included 25 Mainpro-C sessions and approximately 225 clinical, teaching, and research sessions. Eight satel-

lite symposia and more than 40 meetings were held in conjunction with the 2008 meeting.

Innovative Programs

The CFPC CME programs have incorporated both pedagogic innovations and innovations in communications technology. One of the earliest programs was Medifacts, the CFPC audiocassette CME program that launched in 1972. Medifacts Ltd., a commercial company, produced the tapes, and the CFPC committee on audiovisual aids acted as an editorial advisory board. Advertising revenue covered the production costs. The company returned a portion of the voluntary handling charge to the CFPC to acknowledge the contribution being made by CFPC members on the editorial advisory board. This successful program lasted well into the 1980s.[16]

Provincial chapters are continually developing relevant and innovative CME programs. In the 1980s, the Ontario Chapter of the CFPC, together with several other organizations, was involved in the Telemedicine for Ontario project. Telemedicine for Ontario offered CME by teleconference to audiences of health professionals at 185 learning sites across Ontario. The live courses lasted 45 to 60 minutes and allowed for questions and discussions. The project was sponsored by five Ontario universities, the Ontario Ministry of Health, and Toronto General Hospital.[17]

Also in the 1980s, in response to the rapidly escalating AIDS crisis, the communications committee of the British Columbia Chapter of the CFPC commissioned Vancouver family physician and AIDS specialist Jay Wortman, MD, to present AIDS-testing information seminars throughout the entire province. The program toured 35 communities across British Columbia. Although the program was designed primarily for family doctors, all health professionals were welcomed to attend. Among the resources distributed by the program was a 15-minute video titled "Counselling the HIV-Positive Patient."[18]

A very successful program, the Problem-

Based Small Group Learning Program (PBSGL) began in 1992 as a collaborative effort between the Ontario College of Family Physicians and McMaster University in Hamilton, Ontario. The program has been described as follows:

The PBSGL uses an interactive educational approach to continuing professional development. In small, self-formed groups within their local communities, family physicians discuss clinical topics using prepared modules that provide sample patient cases and accompanying information that distils the best evidence. Participants are guided by peer facilitators to reflect on the discussion and commit to appropriate practice changes.[19]

When the CFPC introduced Mainpro-C credits, the PBSGL was the first to be awarded these credits. The program continues today under the administration of the nonprofit organization Foundation for Medical Practice Education.

In 2009, a look at the eCME Resource Centre on the CFPC Web site reveals the application of new electronic technologies to CME; dozens of online courses and educational opportunities are offered on diverse topics such as management of chronic noncancer pain, tools and strategies managing for infectious disease outbreaks, and assessing child development. Two well-established CFPC programs that incorporate both pedagogic and technologic innovations are the Self Evaluation program and the Pearls program.

Self Evaluation

The Self Evaluation program, the CFPC premier CME product, began its development under the chairmanship of Walter W. Rosser, MD.[20] The program began originally as a question bank for the CFPC certification examination in family medicine. Its potential as a CME tool was quickly recognized and, in 1972, Self Evaluation questions began to be published in *Canadian Family Physician*, the CFPC journal. The first program, published in the October 1972 issue, is freely available online through the PubMed Central archive.

Although the mode of presentation has changed over the years, the process of producing the questions that make up the program has remained the same. Practicing family physicians who are CFPC members develop all questions. Members of the national Self Evaluation program committee form local subcommittees, whose members read a group of peer-reviewed journals and write questions based on what they have read. The questions are reviewed at subcommittee meetings and at the national committee meeting. Questions judged relevant, valid, and well-constructed make it into the program.

In the early 1990s, the Self Evaluation program became computerized and evolved into the Self Learning Suite. The new software allowed flexible access to the questions and provided faster feedback to participants.[21]

Today, Self Learning/Autoapprentissage® (as it is now called) is available on the Web and in print in English and in French. Each issue contains a blend of multiple-choice questions and short-answer management problems. Educational points provide a concise summary of relevant information and highlight major points. The online version links to PubMed abstracts and to available full-text articles. The program has powerful search capabilities and allows creation of customized question sets. Self Learning is a valuable educational opportunity for family medicine residents, to whom it is available at no charge. In 2009, Self Learning had more than 6,000 subscribers worldwide.

Pearls

In 1998, as the evidence-based medicine movement grew stronger, the CFPC released Pearls, an evidence-based practice reflection exercise. Pearls is a self-directed activity that can be completed by CFPC members on their own time regardless of practice location, language preference, or practice profile. Rather than being a pass/fail activity, it is intended as a self-directed, structured, learning activity designed to enhance the introduction of new knowledge into practice. Participants use the medical literature to answer their own practice questions and later reflect on how well decisions have been integrated into their practice. Based on Donald Schön's reflective learning cycle, a Pearls exercise has five steps: formulating a practice-based question, seeking information from peer-reviewed literature, evaluating and critically appraising the articles, making a practice decision based on what was learned, and indicating the effect of this decision on patient outcome.[22] Pearls exercises are accredited for Mainpro-C credits.

There have been two versions of Pearls: a program customized for residents and a Pearls.ce™ program for candidates following the practice-eligible route to CFPC certification. In 2009, a Web-based desktop version of Pearls was introduced.

Relationships with Pharmaceutical Industry

In the first five years of CFPC history, Wyeth, Ltd., furnished an annual sum of $7,500 for payment and travel expenses of speakers at CFPC meetings and funded the CFPC medical recording service, which evolved into the Medifacts audiotape program. Woods lists other pharmaceutical companies that supported CFPC CME programs in the early years. These companies and others continue to support CFPC CME initiatives.

In 1996, Cal Gutkin, MD, the CFPC executive director, outlined the CFPC position with regard to these relationships:

The CFPC formally supports the [CMA] Policy Summary on Physicians and the Pharmaceutical Industry and the Pharmaceutical Manufacturers Association of Canada's (PMAC) Code of Marketing Practices, both published in 1994. By doing so, the CFPC acknowledges the role of the pharmaceutical industry in organized CME. We support the pharmaceutical companies with respect to their responsibility to edu-

cate physicians in the appropriate use of their products. We applaud those companies that have successfully transferred this educational responsibility out of their departments of marketing and promotion and who have been working cooperatively with CME planners in organized medicine to develop progressive educational activities. The policies of both the CMA and the PMAC stipulate that responsibility for program content and choice of speakers should rest with the physician CME program organizers. This position is also supported in our CFPC-CME accreditation criteria.[23]

Currently, the influence of pharmaceutical companies on CME and CPD is the focus of much discussion. Marlow has described the CFPC accreditation processes that guard against bias:

Upon conclusion of all CME and CPD programs, attendees are asked to complete evaluations. These evaluations must include a question asking attendees whether they perceived any bias in the program. The CFPC is developing processes for auditing these responses. We are also developing a new tool to detect and measure bias that will be used in the accreditation review and program audit.

In addition, the College is in the process of developing a policy of co-sponsorship wherein programs will no longer be submitted by individual companies, but rather by physician organizations. These organizations will be responsible for quality control as well as for payment of all expenses associated with CME and CPD programs. Many other new safeguards are also in development.[24]

The Future

Mandatory CPD is coming to Canada. Gutkin explains how CFPC programs support members and will also support nonmembers:

The CFPC membership fees include access to Mainpro® and all the program supports offered by our College, including maintaining and managing each member's CPD record and verifying or providing reports of credits earned as required by the licensing authorities. Participation in a single program—Mainpro®—will ensure that family physicians can meet the CPD requirements of many different organizations at the same time, including our College, the provincial licensing bodies, regional health authorities, and hospital or other institutional boards.

Because some provincial regulatory authorities have stated that the only CPD programs they will recognize as meeting their requirements are those offered by the CFPC or RCPSC, the Boards of both Colleges have agreed to offer non-members access to our Mainpro® and Maintenance of Certification programs. An annual fee for this service will ensure that non-members can access the Mainpro® credit record system and can have our College maintain their records and provide required reports on their behalf.[25]

Gutkin has emphasized that research in CME and CPD is essential to determine the best learning strategies and their effect on physicians' competence and performance in practice.[26] Research is beginning to show the value of practice-focused, evidence-based, reflective learning, which is the basis of the CFPC Mainpro-C program. Marlow, director of CPD, is involved in several major research projects to study the delivery and effectiveness of CPD. With committed leadership, the CFPC continues to affirm the importance of CME and CPD to its members and the medical community.

Notes

1. W. V. Johnston, "General Practice in the Changing Order," *Canadian Medical Association Journal* 59, no. 2 (1948): 167–170.

2. D. Woods, *Strength in Study: An Informal History of the College of Family Physicians of Canada* (Toronto: The College, 1979).

3. Woods, *Strength in Study*.

4. "Mission and Goals," College of Family Physicians of Canada Web site, http://www.cfpc.ca/English/cfpc/about%20us/mission/default.asp?s=1 (accessed July 18, 2010).

5. E. C. McCoy, *Article 2: Report of the Committee on Education* (Winnipeg: College of General Practice of Canada executive minutes, October 27–28, 1954).

6. B. M. Stephenson, *Report to the Board of Directors, Coordinating Committee on Education* (Toronto, annual meeting of the College of General Practice of Canada, 1964).

7. G. A. Gibson, *Report to the Board of Directors, Committee on Continuing Medical Education, semi-annual meeting* (Vancouver: College of Family Physicians of Canada, August 8–9, 1975).

8. Woods, *Strength in Study*.

9. R. Handfield-Jones, "MAINPRO®. Working toward a More Flexible, Accessible, and Meaningful Program for Members," *Canadian Family Physician* 43, no. 4 (1997): 721–723.

10. Handfield-Jones, "MAINPRO®."

11. C. Gutkin, "MAINPRO® 2000," *Canadian Family Physician* 46 (2000): 1399–1400.

12. P. Rainsberry, "Dr. Rainsberry Replies," *Canadian Family Physician* 31, no. 2 (1985): 232–233.

13. B. Marlow, "Is Continuing Medical Education a Drug-Promotion Tool? No," *Canadian Family Physician* 53, no. 10 (2007): 1650–1652.

14. Woods, *Strength in Study*.

15. B. A. Morris, "The Annual Scientific Assembly Wants You!" *Canadian Family Physician* 40, no. 4 (1994): 644–645, 653–654.

16. "Medifacts Celebrates 10 Years," *Canadian Family Physician* 27, no. 2 (1981): 200.

17. "News," *Canadian Family Physician* 32, no. 9 (1986): 1773.

18. "News," *Canadian Family Physician* 34 (1988): 1273, 1275–1279, 1281–1286.

19. H. Armson and others, "Translating Learning into Practice: Lessons from the Practice-based Small Group Learning Program," *Canadian Family Physician* 53, no. 9 (2007): 1477–1485.

20. "Profiles," *Canadian Family Physician* 19, no. 5 (1973): 31.

21. "Self Learning Suite," *Canadian Family Physician* 45 (1999): 136, 138.

22. T. Elmslie and R. Handfield-Jones, "Pearls™: Using Evidence to Develop Your Own Practice Gems," *Canadian Family Physician* 44 (1998): 1322–1324.

23. C. Gutkin and R. Handfield-Jones, "Response [letter]" *Canadian Family Physician* 42, no. 7 (1996): 1296–1297.

24. Marlow, "Drug-Promotion Tool?" 1650–1652.

25. C. Gutkin, Mandatory Continuing Professional Development: Helping Family Physicians Meet the Requirements," *Canadian Family Physician* 53, no. 8 (2007): 1396.

26. C. Gutkin, "Certification, Fellowship, and Lifelong Learning: Recognizing Achievement in a Special Discipline," *Canadian Family Physician* 51, no. 3 (2005): 464–463.

PART VI

The External Environment of
Continuing Medical Education

Barbara Barnes, Bruce Bellande, and
Lewis A. Miller

CHAPTER 22

Regulation of Continuing Medical Education in the United States: A Historical Perspective and View of the Future

When compared to undergraduate and graduate medical education, continuing medical education (CME) spans the longest portion of a physician's career. However, in the United States, the development of formal structures to standardize requirements evolved rather slowly. Across the world, regulation of CME dates as far back as fourteenth-century Venice, with an ongoing requirement for participation in lifelong learning to gain specialty certification and maintain a basic level of professional competence remaining in place for five hundred years. In the United States, leaders such as William Osler, MD, and William Henry Welch, MD, asserted that medical education be grounded in science and that doctors continue to learn throughout their careers. They thus underscored the commitment of the profession of medicine to CME.[1] In 1900, Osler expressed this well: "More clearly than any other, the physician should illustrate the truth of Plato's saying that education is a life-long process. The training of medical school gives a man his direction, points him the way, and furnishes him a chart, fairly incomplete, for the voyage, but nothing more."[2]

What would Osler say today about the maze of regulations—voluntary and mandatory—surrounding CME and affecting the learner, the educator, and the funder? As the twentieth century evolved, the content and extent of a physician's CME became increasingly regulated by a variety of professional and legislative bodies and executive agencies. As a result, the purpose of CME has been extended from a professional responsibility for lifelong learning to a means of qualification for maintaining a medical license, specialty certification, and hospital privileges. Regulation has limited who can provide CME, how it is funded, and whether the CME courses a physician attends will meet the standards for the qualifications listed.

Regulation is a general term covering those restrictions that are legal and those that are defined in guidelines, codes, rules, and standards. Box 22-1 provides a clear distinction among these.

This chapter describes how and why CME evolved from an activity driven by a practitioner's discretion to one that is more and more closely driven by requirements that are promulgated both within and outside of the profession.

Regulation through Self-Reliance

Until the middle of the twentiethth century, the core principles of professionalism, such as those articulated by Osler and Welch, were the major forces guiding physicians' CME activities. According to this philosophy, professionals are responsible for remaining competent and assumed to be motivated and capable of determining what they need to know, accessing resources to impart

Box 22-1
Defining Regulation

1. Regulation
   a. Legal restrictions defined by a government authority
   b. Supported by the threat of sanction or fine
2. Rule or Standard
   a. A widely accepted statement or definition
   b. Criterion established by an authority
   c. Potential for sanction if violated
3. Guideline
   a. Document that attempts to streamline or standardize a process; a recommendation
   b. Not mandatory
4. Code
   a. Outlines responsibilities or appropriate practice for an individual or organization

Adapted from L. Klein, "Navigating Restricted Waters," *Medical Marketing & Media* (April 2008): 49–54.

that knowledge, and developing strategies to incorporate learning into practice. Professional organizations, such as the American Medical Association (AMA) and specialty societies, emphasized the importance of lifelong learning and encouraged doctors to remain current. In 1938, the AMA began publishing lists of available CME activities to help make doctors aware of courses conducted across the country, though there was no endorsement of particular courses or evaluation of their quality. By 1962, the list included 1,146 activities offered by 208 institutions (mostly medical schools, hospitals, and specialty societies) in 38 states and the District of Columbia.[3] There was no formal mechanism for documenting attendance at these activities and little support provided to assist physicians in determining their specific learning needs.

Prior to the post–World War II era, the responsibility of determining the various aspects of one's lifelong learning plan (i.e., the what, how,

and when) was largely placed on the individual practitioner. This philosophy changed rather rapidly as a result of various environmental forces.

Regulation through Professional Standards

In 1940, the Commission on Graduate Medical Education predicted the evolution of specialization and recommended that hospitals formalize their graduate medical education (GME) and continuing education programs under a position of director of medical education. Major forces driving the growth and structure of CME in the post–World War II era included a significant rise in the numbers of practitioners and specialties within medicine, advances in technology, and expansion of GME programs into community hospitals. In addition, hospitals with increasingly formalized medical staff structures assumed a more central role in the health care delivery system, employer-based health insurance enhanced access to more highly technical services, and expansion of the National Institutes of Health fostered research and development. With the rise in specialization and growth in malpractice claims, hospitals in the 1970s began implementing re-credentialing processes, which required use of metrics, such as participation in CME, to determine maintenance of competence. As far back as 1932, the Association of American Medical Colleges called for mandatory CME, as part of its study of medical education. In 1934, the American Board of Urology required CME for physicians seeking certification as a core organizing principle.[4]

The growth in medical knowledge and technology led the profession to create more-formal standards for CME, which were imposed on physician participants (in terms of the amount and nature of education required), as well as on organizations that delivered programming (in terms of the quality of education offered). The latter was accomplished through accreditation: a mechanism by which professions, through the development of quasi-independent bodies, promulgate standards on which organizations, their programs, and individuals can voluntarily be assessed. These organizations serve the public interest by assuring a certain standard of quality, without direct intervention by government or other regulators.[5] Those who successfully meet these requirements can use the imprimatur of accreditation as a marker of quality and compliance with generally accepted requirements.

Accreditation first became employed in various US professions in the 1880s to validate educational programs, primarily on a regional basis. It gained much more prominence within postsecondary education by the 1950s and 1960s, as a means to develop a non-governmental mechanism for oversight and quality control. In 1947, the American Academy of General Practice (AAGP), now the American Academy of Family Physicians (AAFP), developed the first accreditation system for CME, through the development of guidelines against which individual learning activities could be assessed in order to assure educational quality. In addition to accrediting courses, the AAGP established requirements for the amount of CME to be taken by its members, which involved at least 50 hours of accredited programs and 100 hours of "informal" education every three years. Beginning in 1955, the category of "formal" CME was changed to Categories I and II, which included as Category I formal activities sponsored by the AAGP or medical schools, with all remaining activities classified as Category II. Three years later, mechanisms were established by which organizations outside of AAGP and its affiliates could develop CME activities for credit.[6] In 1966, the Academy changed from Categories I and II to Prescribed and Elective CME. To this day, the AAFP continues to accredit individual CME activities offered by a variety of institutions, so long as an Academy member is part of the planning committee, and allows members to satisfy up to half of the required 150 hours every three years through activities that it does not accredit or otherwise designate for Elective credit.

In 1955, the AMA Council on Medical Education issued a review of postgraduate education in the United States and, in 1957, published a "Guide Regarding Objectives and Basic Principles of Postgraduate Medical Education Programs," urging organizes producing CME to adhere to the "highest possible educational standards." In the early 1960s, the AMA Advisory Committee on CME conducted a pilot project involving surveys of Midwest institutions offering CME. In its 1962 listing of CME courses, the AMA announced that its evaluation and subsequent standards would focus on institutions rather than individual courses, "based on the fact that specific courses are so numerous and varied in nature that a standard approach to appraisal would probably be impossible." In 1962, the House of Delegates approved a national accreditation system. The first set of "CME Essentials" for accreditation of institutions was released in 1970, being designed "to lift from above and to goose from below."[7]

The AMA addressed concerns among physicians that development of an accreditation program would ultimately lead to mandatory requirements for physicians to participate in CME, affirming that "there is no such intent by the Council on Medical Education and Hospitals or by any part of the AMA."[8] Following initial oversight by the Council on Medical Education's Advisory Committee on CME, in 1977 responsibility for CME accreditation was transferred to the newly established Liaison Commission on CME (LCCME), which reviewed both individual institutions and state medical societies on the basis of the 1970 "Essentials" and was financed in large part by the AMA. The LCCME governance included the AMA, Association of American Medical Colleges, American Board of Medical Specialists, Council of Medical Specialty Societies, and the American Hospital Association. In 1982, the Accreditation Council for Continuing Medical Education supplanted the LCCME, adding the Association for Hospital Medical Education, and Federation of State Medical Boards, as well as a public and state member, to the governance of the new organization.

Building on the principles established in 1970, accreditation requirements were redesigned into seven "Essentials" and subsequently updated in 1998 and 2006. In response to mounting concerns about potential influence on CME by the drug and medical device industries and its potential use as a subtle marketing tool, guidelines for commercial support were issued in 1984, forming the basis for the Standards for Commercial Support promulgated in 1992 and refined in 2004. The role of the AMA within the ACCME has steadily decreased over time, with financing of the accreditation system being assumed by provider fees and other revenue sources such as investments and workshop fees, incorporation of the ACCME as a 501(c)(3) organization, and relocation to non-AMA facilities. Although the roles of the member organizations have also waned over time, they retain key governance roles, such as approval of bylaws changes and veto authority over other key organizational decisions.

In contrast to the AAFP system, the ACCME requirements for accreditation and the AMA guidelines for "credits" (indicating the level of participation in CME) are related but yet discrete. In 1969, the AMA's Physician Recognition Award (PRA) criteria were released. The AMA specifies the types of activities—both formal, accredited venues, as well as informal, self-directed undertakings—that qualify as CME. In addition to recognizing activities developed by ACCME providers, the AMA also directly awards credit for certain types of education, such as that associated with specialty board recertification and educational degrees. Credits are used by hospital credentialing committees, insurance networks, and state licensure boards as a metric of CME participation. The AMA's PRA defines the number of credits and types of learning activities, similar to the system of the AAFP, to demonstrate adequate CME participation. The system is largely quantitative (based on the total number of credits and minimum number of formal learning activities) rather than qualitative (the types of activities undertaken and their relationship to the scope of

a physician's professional practice). Several specialty organizations, such as the American College of Obstetrics and Gynecology, American College of Emergency Physicians, and American Academy of Dermatology, have developed specific CME requirements for their members.

The American Osteopathic Association (AOA) established its CME requirements in 1973, combining accreditation of providers with credit requirements. Its Council on CME is responsible for the structure, process, and governance. Accreditation is limited to AOA-accredited medical schools and hospitals as well as AOA-affiliated organizations. Other organizations can submit CME programs for approval. Categories of credit include osteopathic versus non-osteopathic programs as well as formal versus informal activities.

The AAFP, ACCME, AMA, and AOA systems have been developed by professional organizations in an attempt to self-regulate, advance practice standards, and respond to environmental pressures for advancement of health-care quality and insulation of education from commercial influence. Compared to the other portions of the medical education continuum, CME regulation has been relatively recent and has evolved quickly, with standards becoming incrementally more stringent, particularly within the ACCME system. From a quantitative perspective, CME has thrived within this environment. Based on the AMA report of 1962 and the ACCME statistics of 2008, the number of institutions and organizations providing CME has risen from 208 to more than 2,500, with the number of activities rising from 1,146 to 100,898.[9] The increase has been particularly dramatic in the last 10 years, in which just the ACCME-accredited portion of CME (not including the AAFP and AOA) has grown to a $2.3 billion industry. During this period, the number of physician participants has grown by almost 300 percent, with the majority of the increase being derived from self-study activities such as Internet-based enduring materials and journal-based CME.[10]

Although the ACCME and AMA have devised

mechanisms for physicians to gain credit from participating in new formats, such as performance improvement and point of care learning, these activities comprise a small component of the CME enterprise. Concern about the impact of traditional CME formats (such as courses and grand rounds) on change in physician practice was a stimulus for the ACCME's development of the Updated Criteria introduced in 2006, which focus on using CME, in conjunction with other interventions, to effect improvements in physician competence and performance, as well as patient outcomes.[11]

Organizational providers of CME have remained concerned about the costs of compliance with accreditation requirements. In the 1992–1993 Survey of the Society of Medical Directors of CME (now know as the Society for Academic CME [SACME]), 90 percent of respondents found the these expectations created a "fair amount" or "a lot" of additional work, with about one-half of the schools reporting difficulty in funding this extra effort and a similar proportion expressing the opinion that the standards yielded little or no benefit.[12] Two years later, 79 percent said that the "documentation required to show compliance is operationally difficult to achieve" and 51 percent raised concerns about their ability to pay recent fee increases imposed by the ACCME. By 2008, 80 percent of medical schools responding to the SACME survey reported having to make moderate or extensive changes to their operations as a result of new ACCME requirements.[13] The burden of administrative work required to meet accreditation standards has become increasingly problematic as sources of revenue such as commercial support become more limited and organizational sponsors of CME seek cost reduction to meet the challenges of the emerging healthcare environment.

Regulation Relating to CME Funding

The funding of CME was originally borne primarily by institutions (hospitals and medical schools) offering educational opportunities at little or no cost to learners, who were largely internal to these organizations. With the advent of larger venues attracting national and regional audiences, medical associations and societies began to assess fees for annual meetings and courses. Beginning in the early 1980s, pharmaceutical companies became interested in funding CME activities, in order to assist physicians in learning about the use of the burgeoning therapeutic armamentarium. Although this began at a fairly modest level and originally was targeted at local and regional activities such as courses and grand rounds, industry support soon grew in scope and size, creating concerns about the potential influence of pharmaceutical funding on the content of CME. The amount of commercial support and funding of exhibits and advertising quickly grew throughout the 1990s reaching a peak of $1.485 billion in 2008 (58.5 percent of total CME provider income).

The first effort to self-regulate commercial support of CME arose when the AMA Council on Ethical and Judicial Affairs issued its opinion on "Gifts to Physicians from Industry" (Opinion 8.0601) as part of its *Code on Medical Ethics* in 1990, followed by the issuance of the opinion on Continuing Medical Education (Opinion 9.011 in 1991) (see Table 22-1). In the 1980s the ACCME used a set of loosely crafted Guidelines regarding the separation of education from promotional activities in CME that was commercially supported. In 1992, the ACCME issued its Standards for Commercial Support (SCS), which provided guidelines for the conditions under which industry funding could be accepted and also required disclosure of conflict of interest by course faculty. The Standards were updated in 2004 with emphasis on managing conflict of interest and further defining the level of independence required of the CME provider and entities that were deemed to be commercial interests (see Table 22-1). CME providers that do not adhere to ACCME Essentials and SCS can lose their accreditation.

TABLE 22-1 *Examples of Regulatory Requirements*

	Enforcement	Description	Impact on CME
Professional Standards and Guidelines AMA Opinions on Gifts to Physicians, Code of Medical Ethics, 1990 (Opinion 8.061) and AMA Opinion on CME, 1991 (Opinion 9.011)	Mandatory for CME providers; voluntarily for physicians	Espouses ethical conduct for physicians regarding the receipt of gifts of any value and type from pharmaceutical and device manufacturers. Defines appropriate standards of conduct for physicians regarding promotional gifts to physicians from industry.	In order to award AMA PRA Category I credit, CME providers must comply with the AMA opinions.
PhRMA Code on Interactions with Healthcare Professionals, January 2009	Voluntary for manufacturers of drugs	Describes appropriate conduct of pharmaceutical companies and their employees with health-care professionals focusing on interactions with health-care professionals that relate to marketing of pharmaceutical products and the roles and responsibilities of everyone involved.	Most commercial supporters have adopted the PhRMA Code and require compliance by CME providers they support.
AdvaMed Code of Ethics on Interactions with Healthcare Professionals, July 2009	Voluntary for device manufacturers	Describes appropriate conduct of medical technology companies and their employees with health-care professionals focusing on those interactions that relate to marketing of medical technology products and the roles and responsibilities of everyone involved.	Most commercial supporters have adopted the AdvaMed Code and require compliance by CME providers they support.
Industry Funding of Medical Education Report of an AAMC Task Force, June 2008	Voluntary	Urges all academic medical centers to accelerate their adoption of policies that better manage, and when necessary, prohibit, academic-industry interactions that can inherently create conflicts of interest and undermine standards of professionalism.	Academic medical centers and other institutions have and are adopting the recommendations of the report.
Institute of Medicine Conflict of Interest in Medical Research, Education and Practice Report, 2009	Voluntary	Urges medical education institutions and similar membership organizations to continue or initiate survey, monitoring, and other activities to promote the reform of conflict of interest in medical education.	Academic medical centers and medical membership organizations, public policy makers and regulators will heed to IOM recommendations in reforming conflicts of interest.

TABLE 22-1 *Continued*

	Enforcement	Description	Impact on CME
Accreditation Standards ACCME Standards for Commercial Support	Mandatory for accredited providers	Describes compliant practices regarding independence, management of funds, disclosure, resolution of conflicts of interest and other requirements associated with commercial support of CME.	Full compliance with the Standards is required for accreditation.
Guidances OIG Compliance Program Guidance for Pharmaceutical Manufacturers, April 2003	Voluntary	Assists companies that develop, manufacture, market and sell pharmaceutical drugs and biological products in developing and implementing internal controls and procedures that promote adherence to applicable statutes, regulations, and requirements of the federal health-care programs and in evaluating and as necessary, refining existing compliance programs.	Drug manufacturers comply with the guidance and require CME providers they support to do so as well.
FDA Guidance on Industry-Supported Scientific and Educational Activities, 1997	Mandatory	Differentiates company-sponsored marketing and promotional activities from independent certified CME and requires independence and complete separation of CME from promotion. Defines "off label," and prohibits its use, in promotional activities.	Drug manufacturers must comply with the guidance and require CME providers to do so as well. Separation of independent, certified CME from promotional, marketing activities supported by companies. Permits appropriate off label discussions in CME, journals, and textbooks.
Laws Food, Drug, and Cosmetic Act, 1938	Mandatory	Gives authority to the FDA to oversee the safety of food, drugs and cosmetics; the efficacy of drugs; biological and medical devices and the marketing and promotion of drug and devices.	Law that authorizes the FDA to regulate the marketing and promotional practices of drug and device manufacturers.
False Claims Acts of the Deficit Reduction Act and Fraud and Abuse Statute, April 2007	Mandatory	Addresses Medicare and Medicaid programs integrity and targets fraud and abuse. Includes provisions for "whistleblowers" by permitting a person with knowledge of fraud against the US government to file a lawsuit	Prohibits fraudulent practices against the government related to reimbursement or other means of illegal personal gain at the government's expense.

TABLE 22-1 *Continued*

	Enforcement	Description	Impact on CME
		on behalf of the government against the entity allegedly committing the fraud.	
Anti-Kickback Statute	Mandatory	Makes it a criminal offense knowingly and willfully to offer pay, solicit, or receive any remuneration to induce or reward referrals of items or services reimbursable by federal health-care program.	Prohibits kickbacks, rebates, fraud, and other inappropriate reimbursement and remuneration that will benefit individuals outside the approved practices authorized by federal and state laws.
Stark Law: Omnibus Budget Reconciliation Act of 1989, Stark I of 1993, Stark II of 2007, Stark III	Mandatory	Three separate provisions govern self-referral for Medicare and Medicaid patients (i.e., removal of potential conflicts of interest from physician decision making). Relates to, but not the same as, the federal anti-kickback law.	Providing free CME to physicians not employed by or affiliated with hospitals may be in violation of the Stark laws if they exceed the $300 exemption permitted by law.
State laws	Mandatory	Laws enacted by state mandating public disclosure of all payments made to physicians by or on behalf of pharmaceutical and device manufacturers.	Commercial supporters are required to report payments made by them or report the entity that made payments as a part of educational grants.
Physician's Payment Sunshine Act, 2009 (proposed legislation)	Mandatory, if enacted	Federal law that requires full public disclosure of all payments made by or on behalf of pharmaceutical and device manufacturers.	Commercial supporters are required to report all payments made by them or report the entity that made payments.

The AMA Council on Ethical and Judicial Affairs (CEJA) also continues to press the House of Delegates to take a position limiting, if not eliminating, commercial support of CME. Updated positions were presented to the House of Delegates in 2008, 2009, and 2010 but have been referred back to CEJA each time for further refinement. In 2006, the Association of American Medical Colleges convened a task force on industry support of funding of medical education, composed of participants from academic medicine, the drug and medical device industries, and the public. The final report has formed the basis of many academic medical centers' policies, including their positions on commercial support for CME. In addition, the Institute of Medicine (IOM) published a consensus report on conflicts of interest in 2009, which examined the impact of conflicts of interest, proposed principles to address them, and explored mechanisms to disseminate these principles.[14] Recommendations included strategies for educating health-care professionals about the implications for conflicts of interest, challenges for accrediting bodies to develop standards requiring education on these topics, and development of new mechanisms for funding of CME.

Professional Regulations and Standards That Include and Affect CME

Specialty board certification represents another voluntary process within the profession to determine metrics for standards of practice and competency. The idea of a specialty board was first mentioned in 1908 in a meeting of the American Academy of Ophthalmology and Otolaryngology. In 1933, the Advisory Board for Medical Specialties (ABMS) was established as federation of the four existing specialty boards (dermatology, obstetrics/gynecology, ophthalmology, and otolaryngology) for the purpose of overseeing the examination and certification of specialists. In 1970, the organization assumed a more formal role in coordinating the requirements of its member boards and was renamed the American Board of Medical Specialties. Other than in family medicine, board certification was traditionally a one-time process, occurring at the completion of residency or early in practice (sometimes with both an oral and written examination). Certification was therefore an initial demonstration of competency following training, with CME being the mechanism to demonstrate the practitioner's commitment to remaining competent through lifelong education, with absence of any standard assessment tool to assure that competence indeed was maintained. In 2000, 24 member boards of the ABMS endorsed the concept of ongoing maintenance of certification (ABMS MOC®), which involves continuous professional development assessment. By 2006, all of these member boards had their MOC plans approved by ABMS, with each comprising four elements to be assessed on a recurring basis throughout a physician's career: licensure and professional standing (Part I), lifelong learning and self-assessment (Part II), cognitive expertise (Part III), and practice performance assessment (Part IV). CME is therefore incorporated into this new certification process, through both Parts II and IV, with the specific requirements varying by individual specialty board. In addition to the 24 ABMS boards, the 18 boards of the American Osteopathic Association Bureau of Osteopathic Specialties (AOA-BOS) anticipate having MOC programs fully operational by 2012.

Attempts at developing voluntary standards for CME have not been limited to medical professional organizations. In 2002, the Pharmaceutical Research and Manufacturers of America (PhRMA) released its *Code on Interaction with Healthcare Professionals*. Likewise, the trade association representing the medical device manufacturers, the Advanced Medical Technology Association (AdvaMed), issued its *Code of Ethics on Interactions with Health Care Professionals* in 2003. Both codes, revised in 2009, call for restrictions on lavish accommodations and meals in association with CME events but are voluntary for association members (see Table 22-1). The guidelines contained in the 2009 revisions are more stringent than the prior versions but are not entirely consistent with the ACCME Standards for Commercial Support.

While the Joint Commission, which accredits health-care facilities, has never been highly prescriptive about CME requirements for medical staff, the 2009 standards stipulate that CME be closely aligned with privileging and credentialing requirements (moving to a qualitative assessment of the concurrence between scope of practice and CME rather than merely a quantitative measurement of credits earned).

Professional organizations and accrediting bodies have clearly played an increasing role in setting standards for organizations that offer CME and physicians who participate in lifelong learning. However, there are a variety of entities involved in these processes, often with inconsistent expectations. In an era of concern about health-care quality and cost, increasing questions are being raised about the profession's ability and willingness to self-regulate.

Regulation through Government Requirements

In the early part of the twenty-first century, it is difficult to pick up a newspaper without seeing an article about regional variation in physician practice, medical errors, and commercial influence on physician decision-making. As representatives of the public interest as well as major payers for health-care services, it is not surprising that federal and state governments have been increasingly engaged in discussions about how to assure physician competence and evidence-based, cost-effective care.

The earliest involvement of government in medical education was through licensing boards. Although New York City had some local processes for this purpose dating back to the late eighteenth century, boards did not appear on a large scale until the end of the 19th century, initially focusing on assessing the quality of medical schools and specifically their graduates. The Federation of State Medical Boards (FSMB) was formed in 1912 as a means of helping to coordinate the activities of the individual states and subsequently as a central information repository. In contrast to accrediting bodies and professional organizations, the current 70 licensing boards (representing states and territories and covering allopathic and osteopathic physicians) have been established by state legislatures and are bound by the laws and regulations of their respective governments. Boards are commonly composed of both physicians and non-physicians, representing a potential continuum of "friendly" (professionally controlled) and "hostile" (externally controlled) regulation.[15] In addition to assuring the qualification of providers, they can also function as a means for regulating the supply of physicians within a state. State boards have traditionally provided oversight of physician qualifications through three mechanisms: initial applications requiring documentation of training and other credentials, prior disciplinary actions, etc.; periodic license renewal to provide self-attestation of

good professional standing; and review of specific complaints with the potential for disciplinary action. State boards have struggled to develop mechanisms to assure ongoing physician competence. New Mexico was the first state to require CME for licensure in 1971. Currently, 44 states have CME mandates, with variation in the number of credits required during the licensure period and some expectations for CME in specific topic areas (such as patient safety, cultural competence, domestic violence, and so forth). The FSMB is currently assessing additional requirements for maintenance of licensure, particularly in regard to physicians who do not participate in the AMBS MOC process. The development of consistent, national standards for licensure is inherently challenging, given the purview of individual state legislatures in determining these requirements.

The enactment of the Medicare and Medicaid programs in 1965 ushered in major public funding of health care, resulting in a variety of federal and state regulations to fill a void that self-regulation could not address. Precedent in addressing fraud dates back to the False Claims Act, originally passed in 1863 to deal with abuses by defense contractors. A key provision (*qui tam*) provided for payment of a substantial portion of the final settlement (15–30 percent) for "insiders" (e.g., contractors' employees) who offered information critical to the prosecution of the case. These principles were subsequently applied to fraud and abuse associated with medical billing and then to other relationships, such as inurements and kickbacks to health-care professionals by manufacturers of goods and services paid for by Medicare and Medicaid. Until the 1990s, however, the federal government had not been heavily involved in the regulation of CME, from the perspectives of either physician participants or the organizations that offer educational programming. However, there has been growing concern within the legislative, executive, and judicial branches about the impact of conflict of interest between individuals in control of content of CME and commercial support on the over-use and misuse of governmentally unded services.

In 1997 the US Food and Drug Administration (FDA) issued the *Final Guidance on Industry-Supported Scientific and Educational Activities,* which provided guidelines differentiating promotional activities from independently produced CME, particularly for the discussion of unapproved uses of a product.[16] Such discussion is not permissible in "programs subject to substantive influence by companies" marketing the products, the FDA guidance said, adding that the primary responsibility for overseeing independence lies with the scientific community and accrediting organizations. The publication of the *Final Guidance* has led to a series of federal actions designed to force separation of promotion and independent medical education.

In 2003 the Office of the Inspector General's *Compliance Program Guidance for Pharmaceutical Manufacturers* offered additional clarification of the FDA expectations.[17] (See Table 22-1.) Although these documents were directed at the drug and device industries, the FDA and OIG guidances helped to substantiate the role of CME as a vehicle for disseminating balanced information, including off-label uses, and underscored the appropriateness of commercial support for CME under specified conditions. As a result of the OIG guidance, manufacturers began a major internal reorganization of functions, moving responsibility for CME grants funding from marketing to newly created medical education divisions of non-marketing departments such as medical/scientific affairs. Despite this change, most funds still emanated from product marketing budgets, maintaining companies' interest in supporting CME that related to their product line.

The ACCME responded by stronger requirements for provider accreditation, forcing any accredited medical education/communication company (MECC) provider to demonstrate clear separation of most functions from any parent or affiliated companies if the latter were engaged in noncertified CME promotional activities. A major pharmaceutical company, followed by others, said it would no longer fund any accredited MECC directly, though did not bar the MECC from becoming a joint sponsor with an educational institution or society. A committee of the US Senate began hearings on the influence of pharmaceutical company funding on CME presentations and speakers, and on physician prescribing that might result in higher cost to federally funded programs such as Medicare and Medicaid. Simultaneously, the federal government began to prosecute pharmaceutical companies for violation of federal statutes, including the criminal anti-kickback statute, the Food, Drug, and Cosmetic Act, and the False Claims Act.

A highly publicized case involving all three statutes implicated CME as a vehicle for promotion of off-label uses of gabapentin, which resulted in a $430 million settlement.[18] The government also alleged that the company paid kickbacks to doctors in the form of lavish trips to attend CME presentations about such off-label uses. In another case, the government charged the company with hiring "thought leaders" to read CME presentations on off-label uses prepared by marketing staff.[19] There have been numerous subsequent state and federal investigations of both drug and device manufacturers that have led to not only large financial settlements, but also to compliance agreements requiring public disclosure of financial relationships with physicians and restrictions on the ability of individuals who participate in industry speakers bureaus to function as CME faculty.

An era of full public disclosure and transparency regarding payments to physicians is now under way. Sixteen states have enacted laws requiring that payments to physicians by pharmaceutical and device manufacturers be reported publicly. It is highly likely that additional states will enact such legislation. The Physician Payments Sunshine Act has been introduced each year since 2007 to increase the transparency of the financial relationships between physicians and industry, and many of its provisions were incorporated into the health-care reform legislation passed in 2010.[20] It is likely that federal legislation will pre-empt many current state laws.[21] One benefit of this act would be a central, national database of financial relationships that would help CME providers verify disclosure information that is now supplied to CME providers by faculty and planning committee members and through mandated and voluntary Web sites created by some drug and device manufacturers.

Implications for CME Professionals

The current regulatory environment represents a patchwork of voluntary and involuntary requirements promulgated by professional organizations, accrediting bodies, and state and local governments. It is imperative for physician learners and organizations providing CME to understand the expectations of these various bodies, the benefits of meeting requirements, and the consequences of non-compliance.

Table 22-1 illustrates the different categories of requirements and regulations. Professional guidelines, standards, codes, and position statements function as recommendations for appropriate conduct. (See Box 22-1.) They often begin as recommendations that are completely voluntary, but may subsequently be used as criteria for membership in professional societies and as the basis of institutional policy. They also may inform legislators and regulatory bodies in developing laws and regulations. Efforts to clarify appropriate processes for industry funding of education serve as a good example. Following publication of a policy paper developed by key thought leaders in January 2006 that recommended examination of commercial support for CME and management of personal and institutional conflicts of interest, the Association of American Medical Colleges formed a multi-disciplinary task force that

created detailed recommendations for academic medical centers to consider in managing industry relationships, including those related to CME. Following the schema and suggestions offered in these two publications, many academic medical centers have created more-rigorous processes for overseeing industry funding of education (including graduate as well as continuing education) and have restricted the level of participation of physicians in promotional speaking engagements. These initiatives, as well as increasing interest by government in addressing the influence of industry on health care, continue to inform professional standards and guidance, as evidenced by a recent report by the Institute of Medicine and proposals to amend the AMA Council on Ethical and Judicial Affairs opinions.[22]

As previously noted, accreditation involves the development of standards by an independent professional organization, and institutions voluntarily agree to be assessed. Accreditation can be used by government to determine compliance with certain standards, as in the acceptance by the Centers for Medicare and Medicaid Services of Joint Commission accreditation to determine whether an institution is eligible for payments, and state licensure boards' acceptance of AMA credits awarded by institutions accredited by the ACCME. Although, on one hand, accreditation is voluntary, the loss of this status can be detrimental to an organization and the constituencies that it serves.

Guidance documents issued by federal agencies do not establish legally enforceable responsibilities. Instead, these statements describe current thinking on a topic and function only as recommendations, unless specific regulatory or statutory requirements are cited. The use of the word *should* in guidance documents means that something is suggested or recommended. The Office of the Inspector General's Guidance for Pharmaceutical Company Compliance Programs is one such example.[23] While it is certainly prudent to adhere to the principles of guidance documents, failure to do so may not necessarily result in adverse consequences. In some cases, guidance is eventually used as the basis for laws and regulations.

Governmental laws, regulations, and codes (compendia of laws or regulations) are legally binding and carry risk for civil or criminal actions if violations exist. It is critically important that CME professionals discriminate among professional guidelines, accreditation requirements, and governmental requirements, in order to understand the risks of noncompliance, including potential consequences. Recent suits and compliance agreements, such as the example noted above related to the promotion of off-label uses of gabapentin, serve as sobering examples of the seriousness with which both state and local governments are addressing the impact of commercial influence on prescribing habits.

Future Trends

What does the future hold for the regulation of CME? Given the increasing emphasis on maintenance and assessment of professional competence, evidence-based practice, and cost containment, the question is certainly not whether regulation will continue but rather how stringent it will become and who will administer it. Regardless of whether commercial support of CME remains, there will undoubtedly be ongoing concern at the federal and state levels about the influence of industry on the balance and validity of educational content. The US Senate Finance Committee's staff report document *Use of Educational Grants by Pharmaceutical Manufacturers* is an excellent example of government concerns that enforcement of the ACCME Standards for Commercial Support is not sufficiently rigorous to prevent abuses.[24] It is likely that some form of mandatory disclosure of payments to physicians from industry will also be a part of health-care reform legislation. There are increasing efforts to encourage commercial supporters to provide grants to independently controlled CME funding "pools," from which specific program grants would be distributed to accredited providers based on needs assessments not always directly related to the therapeutic categories currently supported by pharmaceutical and device manufacturers. The concept has come from sources other than industry and the provider community, e.g., the Institute of Medicine (IOM) and officials of the OIG, and therefore its adoption in some form is in doubt.[25]

The forces defining CME—ACCME, government, medical specialty certifying boards, IOM, and others—are now promoting education as a strategy for improving patient and population outcomes, rather than an end in itself. The ABMS Maintenance of Certification program has been a major driver in this regard, and there is considerable debate about the level of coherence between lifelong learning (Part II) and performance in practice (Part IV). Similarly the state licensing boards are trying to determine mechanisms for documenting and assessing ongoing competence. The Federation of State Medical Boards (FSMB) has recommended that its members examine the use of specialty certification as a means of assuring competency in a field of practice; this, the FSMB states, would be a better basis for maintenance of relicensure than hours of CME.[26] Politically, it may take time for such boards to act in cooperation with their state legislatures. But someday, it is likely that state boards will become part of this process. In addition the Joint Commission standards for hospital accreditation require CME that is closely aligned with the privileging and credentialing requirements of the medical staff; here, too, certification may replace CME as a requirement.

The IOM, a quasi-public agency, has gone even further. A 2009 report from an IOM committee recommends the formation of a public-private institute for continuing professional development (CPD), to coordinate content and knowledge of CPD, regulation across states and national providers, a new system of financing, and development of a scientific basis for the practice of CPD.[27] Whether the United States will ever adopt such a national approach to what has been a state and professional province is open to question.

Health-care reform will also have a profound impact on CME. It is likely that Pay for Performance (P4P) will be a tangible outcome of a reformed health-care system in desperate need of money. Paying for quality not quantity care will be inevitable for the system to survive. Such pressure creates a financial incentive for physicians to be up to date with clinical practice guidelines, practice performance measures, and standards of care—the bases for performance measures that will drive P4P. The future CME curriculum will be replete with emerging guidelines, performance measures, and other metrics to ensure and sustain high-quality patient care. These metrics will provide much-needed quantitative information for CME needs assessment, identification of practice gaps, and outcomes assessment.

Regulation, therefore, has had, and will continue to have, a significant impact on CME, physician participants, and health outcomes. Regulation is bringing about a shift in emphasis from CME to continuing professional development (CPD), which is also implicit in the ABMS standards. Educators will therefore not only focus on more than presenting evidence-based clinical data but will strive to move the physician to participation in team-based learning and practice, including the patient as a member of the team. They will integrate practice improvement in systems and data management. They will measure results in not only physician satisfaction and knowledge change, but also in changes in physician performance, patient outcomes, and population health outcomes. Without the pressure of regulation—within and without the profession— these changes may not have occurred or may not have done so in the space of some 15 years. The jury is still out, however. We do not know how successful educators will be in accomplishing these significant objectives, nor do we know how physicians will respond to their efforts.

Conclusions

With the rapid growth of knowledge and technology, as well as the need to implement the best possible evidence in practice, CME is an increasingly essential part of the continuum of medical education. Professional organizations advance their mission by creating standards that assure educational quality and create metrics to determine how much and what type of professional development physicians should undertake. Similarly, the regulatory sector protects the interests of the public by overseeing the quality, effectiveness, safety, and affordability of medical care. The relationships among voluntary efforts of physicians, standards imposed by professional organizations, and governmental requirements will continue to evolve, hopefully achieving equipoise that balances the needs of professional fulfillment and responsibility, the best interests of patients, and the needs of the public at large.

Notes

1. S. R. Ell, "Five Hundred Years of Specialty Certification and Compulsory Continuing Medical Education. Venice 1300–1802," *Journal of the American Medical Association* 251, no. 6 (1984): 752–753; S. Flexner and J. T. Flexner, *William Henry Welch and the Heroic Age of American Medicine* (New York: Viking Press, 1941).

2. Roland McGovern, *William Osler, the Continuing Education* (Springfield, Ill.: Charles C. Thomas, 1969).

3. E. Freidson, *Profession of Medicine: A Study of the Sociology of Applied Knowledge* (Chicago: University of Chicago Press, 1988); R. S. Fisher, "The Role of the AMA in Accreditation of Medical Education" (report of the Council on Medical Education, report 1, 1979), 1–79.

4. W. C. Rappleye, *Graduate Medical Education: Report of the Commission on Graduate Medical Education* (Chicago: University of Chicago Press, 1940); C. R. Brown and H. S. M. Uhl, "Mandatory Continuing Medical Education: Sense or Nonsense?" *Journal of the American Medical Association* 213, no. 10 (1970): 1660–1668; H. Jeghers and others, "An Experiment in Making the Hospital a Graduate Medical Education Center," *Journal of the American Medical Association* 158: 245–252; P. Starr, *The Social Transformation of American Medicine* (New York: Basic Books, Inc., 1982); R. K. Richards, "CME Accreditation: An Overview with Two Challenges," *Jour-*

nal of Continuing Education in the Health Professions 12, no. 2 (1992): 77–81; J. Schrock and R. K. Cydulla, "Lifelong Learning," *Emergency Medical Clinics of North America* 24, no. 3 (2006): 785–795.

5. A. L. Fritschler, *Accreditation's Dilemma: Serving Two Masters—Universities and Government* (Washington, DC: Council for Higher Education Accreditation, 2008).

6. N. L. Davis and C. E. Willis, "A New Metric for Continuing Medical Education Credit," *Journal of Continuing Education in the Health Professions* 24, no. 3 (2004): 139–144.

7. D. K. Wentz and G. Paulos, *Journal of Continuing Education in the Health Professions* 20 (2000): 181–187; C. H. Ruhe, "Continuing Education Courses for Physicians," *Journal of the American Medical Association* 181, no. 6 (1962): 115–118; R. K. Richards, "CME Accreditation: An Overview, with Two Challenges," *Journal of Continuing Education in the Health Professions* 12 (1992): 77–81.

8. Ruhe, "Continuing Education Courses."

9. "ACCME Annual Report Data," Accreditation Council for Continuing Medical Education Web site, http://www.accme.org/index.cfm/fa/home.popular/popular_id/127a1c6f-462d-476b-a33a-6b67e131ef1a.cfm (accessed November 28, 2009).

10. Ibid.

11. P. E. Mazmanian and D. A. Davis, "Continuing Medical Education and the Physician as a Learner: Guide to the Evidence," *Journal of the American Medical Association* 288 (2002): 1057–1060; Agency for Healthcare Quality and Research, "Effectiveness of Continuing Medical Education" (publication #07-E006, 2007).

12. "Society for Academic CME Biennial Surveys," SACME Web site, http://www.sacme.org/index.cfm?id=1028 (accessed November 26, 2009).

13. Ibid.

14. Institute of Medicine, "Conflict of Interest in Medical Research, Education, and Practice," Institute of Medicine Web site, http://www.iom.edu/Reports/2009/Conflict-of-Interest-in-Medical-Research-Education-and-Practice.aspx (accessed December 4, 2009).

15. Starr, *The Social Transformation*.

16. "Guidance for Industry: Industry-Supported Scientific and Educational Activities," Food and Drug Administration Web site, http://www.fda.gov/downloads/RegulatoryInformation/Guid ances/UCM125602.pdf (accessed December 19, 2009).

17. "Compliance Program Guidance for Pharmaceutical Manufacturers," US Health and Human Services Web site, http://oig.hhs.gov/fraud/docs/complianceguid ance/042803pharmacymfgnonfr.pdf (accessed December 18, 2009).

18. S. A. Steinman and others, "Narrative Review: The Promotion of Gabapentin: An Analysis of Internal Industry Documents," *Annals of Internal Medicine* 184 (2006): 284–293.

19. *Rx Compliance Report* 3, no. 3 (2004): 3.

20. "Physician Payments Sunshine Act of 2009," Policy and Medicine Web site, http://policymed.typepad.com/files/physician-payment-sunshine-act-2009-1-22-09.pdf (accessed October 12, 2009).

21. Fisher, "The Role of the AMA," 1–79.

22. T. A. Brennan and others, "Health Industry Practices that Create Conflicts of Interest: A Policy Proposal for Academic Medical Centers," *Journal of the American Medical Association* 295 (2006): 429–433; "Industry Funding of Medical Education, 2008," Association of American Medical Colleges Web site, http://services.aamc.org/publications/showfile.cfm?file=version114.pdf&prd_id=232&prv_id=281&pdf_id=114 (accessed December 1, 2009); "PharmFree Scorecard," American Medical Student Association Web site, http://www.amsascorecard.org/ (accessed December 2, 2009); Institute of Medicine, "Conflict of Interest."

23. "Compliance Program Guidance for Pharmaceutical Manufacturers, 2003," Office of the Inspector General Web site, http://www.oig.hhs.gov/fraud/docs/com plianceguidance/042803pharmacymfgnonfr.pdf (accessed December 4, 2009).

24. "Committee Staff Report to the Chairman and Ranking Member, Use of Educational Grants by Pharmaceutical Manufacturers, April 2007," US Senate Committee on Finance Web site, http://finance.senate.gov/press/Bpress/2007press/prb042507a.pdf (accessed December 4, 2009).

25. "Redesigning Continuing Education in the Health Professions," Institute of Medicine Web site, http://www.iom.edu/~/media/Files/Report%20Files/2009/Redesigning-Continuing-Education-in-the-Health-Professions/RedesigningCEreportbrief.ashx (accessed December 18, 2009); L. Morris and J. K. Taitsman, "The Agenda for Continuing Medical Education—Limiting Industry's Influence," *New England Journal of Medicine* 361, no. 25 (2009): 2478–2482.

26. "Federation of State Medical Boards Special Committee on Maintenance of Licensure Draft Report on Maintenance of Licensure," Federation of State Medical Boards Web site, http://www.fsmb.org/pdf/Special_Committee_MOL_Draft_Report_February2008.pdf (accessed December 18, 2009).

27. "Redesigning Continuing Education," IOM Web site.

Robert F. Orsetti, Susan Alpert,
Maureen Doyle-Scharff, and Michael Saxton

CHAPTER 23

Industry Support of Continuing Medical Education and Continuing Professional Development: A Perspective on the Past and Implications for the Future of Pharmaceutical and Device Company Support

In recent years the pharmaceutical and medical device industries have adopted new procedures and policies such as the PhRMA and AdvaMed codes to support continuing medical education (CME) activities that contribute to physician knowledge, application of skills, improved patient care, and the advancement of medical science. Despite such efforts, some view commercial support of CME as a disguised extension of marketing and promotion that is reflected in inappropriate, biased, subjective, and often scientifically unsupported influence on CME participants at considerable cost to the public in the form of high-cost medications and procedures.

Bowman and Pearle[1] were among the first to question the appropriateness of commercial support of CME, in 1988. They expressed concern about the steady and increasing rate of commercial support of CME in the absence of regulation from the mid-1970s through the late 1980s. Prior to that time the pharmaceutical and later the device industries earmarked product support funding primarily for marketing and sales campaigns, with occasional and modest support of academic medical education.

This chapter traces the evolution of industry policy and practice in support of CME from the early 1970s through to the present, while also describing the introduction and strengthening of regulations that have improved and standardized the development and delivery of CME. Prominent policy-making organizations and projections about the future direction and form of CME are discussed.

The Pharmaceutical Industry in the 1970s

The pharmaceutical industry entered the 1970s with then blockbuster cardiovascular, central nervous system, anti-infective, and anti-inflammatory medications, and some of the major pharmaceutical companies used ever-increasing marketing budgets to expand their product outreach through educational offerings for physicians. That was a time largely without regulations pertaining to medical education. Still in its infancy, the Accreditation Council for Continuing Medical Education (ACCME), under the guidance of Richard Wilbur, MD, focused on setting standards and guidelines to upgrade and demonstrate the accountability of the medical education enterprise in the United States.[2] The ACCME along with the American Medical Association (AMA) wished to ensure that individual physicians were keeping up to date in their medical practices and, as such, paid little attention to industry activities. As long as industry remained in compliance with the advertising and promotion components of the Food, Drug, and Cosmetic Act (FDCA),[3] it could self-sponsor and support medical education at will.

Because of the rapid release of new and unfamiliar classes of medications, physicians welcomed the opportunity to be educated by the pharmaceutical industry, its clinicians, and its research scientists. Prior to the growth of industry-supported live educational activities, symposia, clinical papers, scientific exhibits, and other activities at nonsupported, annual association meetings, occasional monographs, newsletters, and sales representatives were the main sources of physician education.

Physicians, especially high-volume prescribers, were key targets of industry education, with few programs designed for other health-care professionals. To that end, industry sought to build and strengthen relationships with clinical thought leaders and recognized authors and faculty. These individuals assisted their industry colleagues in planning and staffing educational programs designed, for the most part, to convey messages tied directly to product marketing campaigns. In virtually all instances, funds were allocated from marketing product budgets, with product managers and directors intimately involved in the planning process.

Selection of subject areas, content, faculty, and location were typically within the purview of the marketing department. In a few companies, the units responsible for these activities and other forms of medical communications (such as publications) reported to the medical department; but, in this setting, marketing had the final word. Medical, regulatory, and legal staffs reviewed and approved content for release to ensure compliance with Food and Drug Administration (FDA) advertising and promotion requirements. Education became an extension of the marketing effort without much concern for independence, objectivity, fair balance, or scientific method.

The current benchmarks for validation of best practices in CME—needs assessment, learning objectives, adult learning principles, and outcome evaluation—were years away from being required in supported activities. Few staff members were trained educators. Many had meeting planning and medical writing and communication experience, and some simply learned by doing.

While most educational activities were live and didactic, in some companies there was a concurrent establishment of publication, communication, and medical writing units. These groups were also arms of the marketing department with the goals of publishing educational material in the form of ghostwritten manuscripts and scientific exhibits based on the results of company-funded phase IV clinical trials in support of current product campaigns.

Often, clinical investigators agreed to lend their names as authors to papers written by company staff. The investigators reviewed the papers prior to publication and suggested changes for accuracy. Companies often submitted the manuscripts to medical journals on behalf of the authors and worked with the journal editors to make required changes. Peer-reviewed journals in carefully selected therapeutic areas were the primary targets for publication, but pay-for-publication journals also were used commonly. Following publication, companies ordered reprints in quantities sufficient for author use and sales force distribution. Often publication content was repurposed to develop scientific exhibits for display at national medical association conferences. Occasionally, scientific exhibits provided content for manuscript development. Scientific exhibits were usually staffed by the pharmaceutical staff writer and one of the participating investigators.

The content of both live educational activities and publications was generally heavily specific to the company's product, with little mention made of other available medications or treatment options, and was subject to weakly supported claims, e.g., based on these findings, X is clearly the drug of choice for patients with Y. Although delivered without regard for therapeutic balance, the content was based on statistically validated research and clinical investigation results.

During those years, the Upjohn Company, under the leadership of its president Theodore Cooper, MD, established its Medical Science Liaison (MSL) program to bridge the research and information exchange gap between academic medical centers, community hospitals, and corporate medical research divisions. Cooper had been the assistant secretary for health in the US Department of Health, Education, and Welfare and then the FDA commissioner. Out of the new MSL group, the first foray into education was the creation of the MSL education program that originally consisted of a small group focused exclusively on graduate medical education (GME) curriculum support. Resources were developed in support of faculty needs like the Scope Monograph Series of publications on different topics, along with educational method support. An example of the latter was the Patient-Oriented Problem Solving (POPS) booklets intended to support small group learning. Dave Lichtenauer and others helped to develop and lead the early MSL education program.

The Pharmaceutical Industry in the 1980s

Funds allocated for CME increased substantially, though educational regulations remained nonexistent. The increase came about as the companies began to appreciate the many benefits of using educational activities to complement and supplement promotional campaigns, coupled with revenue realized from successful product launches. With readily available and substantial budgets in hand, company meeting planners were given free rein to be as innovative and extravagant as possible to attract key physicians to planned conferences. At its height, such behavior became quite competitive among pharmaceutical companies.

What began as perhaps a half-day, company-sponsored conference or dinner meeting in a local hotel or restaurant soon escalated to multiday, all-expenses-paid events at five-star, offshore resort locations. Caribbean and European venues

were popular meeting destinations in the 1970s and 1980s. Ski resorts were also favored meeting locations, with participants hitting the slopes from 10 AM to 4 PM and attending educational offerings from 7 AM to 9 AM and 5 PM to 7 PM.

Funding included payment for transportation, lodging, meals, and recreation for the physician and his/her spouse or guest. Physician attendance required no proof of participation. Additionally, attendees often received gifts (e.g., paintings by local artists, wine, gift certificates, or moderately priced sport or jewelry items) for their participation. Sales and marketing representatives often attended the educational programs and interacted freely with physician attendees. Typically, daily classroom education encompassed half of the day, with the remainder dedicated to recreational or sight-seeing activities. It was not required that educational time take precedence.

As the industry gained sophistication in conducting activities of the type described, many companies sought to ensure that those selected as faculty were capable speakers when it came to implanting and implementing conference themes and messages. That requirement gave rise to special sessions on platform speaking skills. Sessions were often videotaped for speaker critique by colleagues and hired professional trainers. Physician attendees at the company-sponsored programs usually were hand-picked by company sales representatives and product managers. These select physicians were, for the most part, key opinion leaders, researchers, investigators, specialists, leading academics, or authors with specific ties to the drug or disease being featured. Often, invitations were extended directly by sales representatives or product managers. Many such physicians attended multiple programs on the same or similar topics. Only available budgets limited attendance. Faculty was often the same from venue to venue (road shows) and received handsome honoraria.

Product management and sales also suggested program content and faculty. Needs assessment was limited to determining what physicians needed to know about the use of the company product rather than about filling knowledge or patient care gaps. Learning objectives were not stated, per se, but faculty were instructed to present on-label clinical or experiential evidence to show why the host company's product was the first line of therapy in a treatment while minimally discussing competitive products. Usually, content was designed so that one speaker complemented another in delivering the company message. This content was captured in newsletters and other print material and delivered to participants post-meeting to reinforce the message. In this setting, head counts and participant testimonials served as the only forms of meeting evaluation. Sparse attention was paid to the quality of education, and CME credit was not offered for company-sponsored activities.

Industry has never been one monolithic block in terms of how it supported CME in the past or present. An alternative model to the commercial unit support of large national meetings is represented by expansion in the 1980s of the Upjohn Company's original MSL education group to support CME in the community setting. ACCME-accredited organizations primarily funded CME at the local and regional level. Funding came from an external medical affairs department, initially called Community Affairs, that was separate from the commercial organization.

After several years without regulation, the medical education landscape changed dramatically and for the better in response to the FDA 1997 Final Guidance on Medical Education.[4] In the years immediately prior to the FDA guidance, the industry modified its practices somewhat in response to investigations by Senator Ted Kennedy and others into how and in what amounts industry was spending its marketing and educational budgets. While company-planned educational activities became less extravagant, frequent, and costly in those years, it was not until issuance of the FDA guidance that industry made major adjustments. During those years and im-

mediately afterward, change in industry medical education practices was fostered and supported by the involvement and leadership of certain key chief executive officers, (i.e., Douglas Watson of CIBA-Geigy; Charles Saunders, MD, of Wyeth; Theodore Cooper, MD, of the Upjohn Company; Robert Ingram of Glaxo; and Fred Lyons of Marion Merrell Dow).

The pharmaceutical industry, like the medical profession, was squarely against possible government regulation of medical education and gradually changed past practices that violated the FDA requirements of balance, objectivity, independence, and scientific rigor in educational activities supported by industry. Throughout the 1980s, real change escalated toward compliance as the FDA rules were more fully and clearly understood.

Those initial efforts also generated eventual development, acceptance, and implementation of the AMA Gifts to Physicians from Industry Ethical Policy under the leadership of AMA President James Todd, MD, and Senior Vice President M. Roy Schwarz, MD, along with Dennis K. Wentz, MD, who later assumed responsibility for the AMA continuing medical and professional education unit. Under the leadership of Frances Maitland, the ACCME continued to set standards and regulations for professional performance in CME by strengthening its Guidelines for Commercial Support to become Standards of Commercial Support. Industry soon followed with its adoption of the PhRMA Code.[5] Other national CME leaders who helped to initiate change included Dave Lichtenauer; Kathy Lucas; Bob Orsetti; Peter Rheinstein, MD, JD; Marty Shickman, MD; and Lee Yerkes.

The Alliance for Continuing Medical Education (ACME) witnessed the first representation by industry on the ACME board of directors during this period. John Benjamin of the Upjohn Company was the first appointed representative, followed by Lichtenauer of Upjohn and Orsetti of CIBA-Geigy. Years later, Mike Saxton would become the first elected industry representative to the ACME board. In 2008, Maureen Doyle-Scharff became the first industry representative elected as an ACME officer.

Lichtenauer, Lucas, Orsetti, and Yerkes were instrumental in aligning the pharmaceutical industry's changing educational model with policies, programs, and practices endorsed by the ACME. In 1991, the ACME board accepted a proposal to permit the newly formed Pharmaceutical Association for Continuing Medical Education (PACME) to meet in conjunction with its annual conference. In 1998, PACME became the first fully affiliated section of ACME.

Meaningful change in CME policies and practices did not occur rapidly; but with the new ethical and commercial support regulations, continuance of past policies and practices was not an option. Internal implementation of the new requirements took time as companies sought to change their organizational, marketing, and financial structures and strategies for compliance. Change was particularly difficult to implement among sales representatives. Some companies adapted to these changes sooner than others, but as the 1980s drew to a close, self-supported and endorsed educational activities and by-invitation and all-expenses-paid programs to lavish locations were being eliminated and gifts to physicians were reduced to the AMA allowable $100 maximum. In a few companies, medical departments gradually began to assume responsibility for educational programs with oversight provided by legal and regulatory departments. In general, however, marketing departments remained in control of CME budgets.

The Medical Device Industry in the 1980s

Education and training requirements for the medical device industry differ significantly from the pharmaceutical industry. A major contributor to the effectiveness and performance of products is linked to the proper use of the device by a well-trained professional. Proper patient selection, the correct operating or procedural environment, skilled nursing support, appropriate adjunctive care, and patient education additionally contribute to the safe use and best patient outcomes for many device therapies. Device companies, therefore, have long been engaged directly with professional health-care provider training and education.

Often, in the early days of the device industry, surgeons designed the products and trained users on what often were handheld and operated devices, e.g., scalpels, sutures, and orthopedic hardware. As the industry evolved and products became more sophisticated in design and manufacture (e.g., implantable mechanical heart valves, lasers for cutting and annealing, and active cardiac implants with various programming options), the industry and the regulators recognized the need for device users—no matter how senior and well-trained in their specialty—to have device-specific training to achieve appropriate outcomes. These needs have been exacerbated by the fact that each manufacturer, even for similar devices, has incorporated unique design and operations in their specific product. For many of the highest-risk novel technologies, the FDA and other regulators have added to their approval the requirement that the manufacturer provide training to each potential user prior to the user purchasing the devices.

In this environment, the support of medical education from the device industry has evolved in multiple directions. The device-specific training needs have led to the development of training and education units within the larger companies and the evolution of independent entities that provide training on behalf of companies. Given that technologies are continually being created to address unmet patient needs and to treat well characterized conditions in new ways, a need to educate the health-care community on available treatment options has grown as these therapies evolve. This type of education (i.e., on disease states and the many diagnostic and therapeutic options available for them) resembles the types of education provided by the pharmaceutical industry and has evolved in parallel in many ways.

Like the pharmaceutical industry, the device industry has struggled to keep a separation between marketing and education. In the early years, marketing focused on education. The device industry advertised primarily by describing the new product and training early adopters on its use so they would, in turn, train and educate others, thereby stimulating sales. This often led to local promotional materials that were not regulated, serving as a means of education but also of marketing. The device industry has struggled to limit training and education to on-label uses (i.e., approved uses) for these products. Once products are introduced into the market, health-care providers have identified and expanded uses well beyond those approved by the FDA. In some cases, off-label uses become more common than the initial use for which the product was approved. Keeping a distance between the manufacturer, who is not allowed by law to discuss or promote uses beyond the labeled ones, and the professionals who are legally allowed to use, train, and discuss such therapies, including in the context of CME, has been difficult. As it became clear that medical education was a path to broader user knowledge and attention, the industry began to participate in these larger educational efforts.

Medical education efforts, including those that grant CME credits, have been a focal place for participation by the medical device industry on both the diagnostic and therapeutic sides. Industry has worked with education and CME providers from both the professional and educational arenas to develop materials and support educational events. In addition, companies have distributed materials developed by themselves and others to train and educate product users. As medical education regulation has evolved, many of these relationships are no longer appropriate, and industry is working to comply with these new requirements. AdvaMed, the largest device industry trade association, has developed as part of its code of conduct for members[6] the appropriate way for companies to engage in the support of CME and comply with FDA regulations and ACCME guidelines.

The Pharmaceutical and Medical Device Industries in the 1990s

In the 1990s, the pharmaceutical and medical device industries continued to support CME but within the parameters of a new paradigm. Independence, objectivity, and balance in planning and delivery of CME became the watchwords of the day, and a real revolution in CME began in terms of industry recognizing its role as supporter rather than sponsor of CME.

This era also saw a shift from a local focus on CME support to national-level programs based on national epidemiologic needs assessments. Often, these programs focused on establishing a scientific concept new to medical training that formed the foundation of knowledge necessary to understand the treatment options based on emerging science. The CME activities were still better described as programs in the traditional sense of didactic lectures to largely passive audiences. This era saw increasing efforts to recruit an audience, and focus was paid more to venue, meals, and other incentives to attract an audience than to the quality of the education as measured by educational effectiveness.

At the same time, a major shift in provider types funded by industry occurred. For-profit medical education and communications companies started receiving accreditation in the late 1980s and saw explosive growth in the 1990s as they increasingly received a larger share of commercial support. Their portion of commercial support peaked around 50 percent early in the new millennium.

While the early 1990s represented an era of reform, those reforms were largely process driven and did not address some of the underlying, his-

Box 23-1
History of Commercial Support Changes Big Pharma

Organizational Development and Decision Level	External Relationship	Average Date
1. Decentralized brand driven	Promotional high touch	1970s–2002
2. Compliant grant administration	Confused	2002–2005
3. Decentralized process driven: transactional	Grant review assembly line	2003–Current
4. Centralized process driven: tactical	Education vendor	2003–Current
5. Centralized education driven: strategic	Education supporter	2005–Current
6. Center of excellence for healthcare provider education	CPD supported	2006–Current
7. Center of excellence for healthcare quality performance	Org PI supporter	2009–Future

toric issues related to conflict of interest that have yet to be addressed. Educational support, for the most part, remained embedded in the commercial division of companies. Additionally, the model of supporting medical education companies who were often owned by the same ad agencies of record for a brand, created its own set of conflict of interest issues that went largely unresolved.

The Pharmaceutical and Medical Device Industries in the New Millennium

As the new century began, medical departments within industry assumed responsibility for CME. Gone were the marketing-driven methods of years past.

In 2002, industry funding of nationally accredited providers passed 50 percent of the providers' total income for the first time. Combined with concerns emanating from the 1990s model of industry support, this fact led to a significantly elevated level of public and professional scrutiny that has been healthy for the profession. The 2003 publication of the Office of Inspector General Health and Human Services Compliance Program for Pharmaceutical Manufacturers established compliance as a primary driver of commercial support. Box 23-1 represents a general overview of a rapidly evolving landscape inside pharmaceutical companies. After several decades of largely commercial decision making with respect to educational support, organizations were developed that focused first on compliance and then on increasing educational quality.

Starting in the early 1970s and continuing in some companies through 2002, commercial support was largely decentralized and brand driven. Various departments within the company provided funding linked to specific product interests. In the years that followed, companies sought to administer educational grant applications in accord with newly promulgated regulations and requirements. While this represented a more compliant approach, much confusion arose as to whether and how to apply the regulations. The process often varied greatly from company to company and lacked consistent application.

From 2003 and continuing to the present, companies have established formal grant review processes using grant review committees and other procedures to evaluate grant applications for funding approval. In 2003, educational vendors known as medical education and communication companies (MECCs) began to plan and develop CME activities independent of company influence and control. Within two years, as the CME paradigm continued to change in response to new regulations and public critique, pharmaceutical companies formed centralized,

Box 23-2
The Evolving CME Environment: Regulation, Policy, and Public Opinion

1992 Original ACCME Standards for Commercial Support
1997 Final FDA Guidance on Industry-Supported Scientific and Educational Activities
2002 PhRMA Code on Interaction with Health Care Professionals
2003 OIG HHS Compliance Program Guide for Pharmaceutical Manufacturers
AdvaMed Code of Ethics on Interactions with HealthCare Professionals
2004 Updated ACCME Standards for Commercial Support;
Conjoint Committee CME Task Force Recommendations
2006 Health Industry Practices That Create Conflicts of Interest: A Policy Proposal for Academic
Medical Centers (T. A. Brennan and others, *Journal of the American Medical Association* 295
[2006]: 429–433)
ACCME Revised Accreditation Standards
2007 Senate Finance Committee Report on Use of Educational Grants by Pharmaceutical
Manufacturers
Macy Report: Continuing Education in the Health Professions; recommends phasing out
support for CME
2008 Senate Finance Committee investigation of special societies such as the American College of
Cardiology, etc.
Journal of the American Medical Association publishes editorial calling on professional
organizations and CME providers not to "condone or tolerate" input from for-profit
companies
Senator Grassley (R-Iowa) reintroduces Physician Payments Sunshine Act requiring public
disclosure of gifts to physicians; industry-supported CME is a form of payment
AMA House of Delegates refers back proposal by Committee on Ethical and Judicial Affairs to
purge industry funding from CME
AAMC Task Force report on industry funding
ACCME Call for Comments: Should Industry Support CME?
2009 IOM Report on COI in Medical Research, Education, and Practice

education-driven units to support independent and compliant CME, with no direct involvement in topic, content, and faculty development or with other aspects of the educational planning process.

The movement toward support of quality education expanded in 2006 and continues today as companies place greater emphasis on activities that offer excellence in provider health-care education and quality performance.

Following in rapid progression, a series of additional guideline and policy changes occurred that placed the viability of future commercial support in question, culminating in the first formal report calling for commercial support to cease.[7] Box 23-1 provides a summary of these changes and the dates of release or implementation.

These questions increasingly spotlighted the degree of dependency on commercial support, conflict-of-interest issues, and the overall minimal effectiveness of the traditional model of medical education support. Today, commercial support, like the CME profession, remains largely linked to educational activities of far less value to patients than the model now emerging to address professional practice gaps. There are increasing calls for a new model that could help ameliorate lingering concerns about the presence of com-

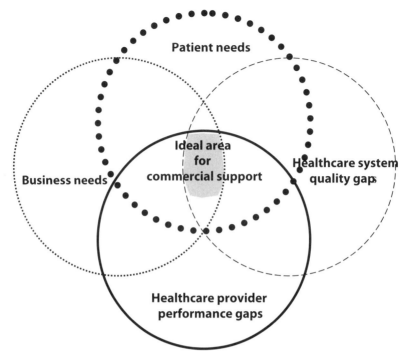

Figure 23-1 A Convergence of Interests Model for Foundation of Commercial Support. The area represented in gray indicates overlapping zones of mutual value.

mercial support. Such a model will require fundamental changes in perspective and procedures by both industry and CME providers. Many believe commercial support is at a tipping point beyond which it should either transform or cease to be available. If it is to transform into the golden age of commercial support, measured by effectiveness rather than dollars, then this new age needs to recognize the convergence of interest that all stakeholders appropriately have in the system. As with much of history that is cyclic in nature, it is also recognized that educational support needs to return to its historic roots of being available at the local level closer to the point where care is delivered.

A View of the Future

What are the role, value, and risk of commercial support to CME as we look to the future? This question is asked more frequently in light of what

is perceived to be an increasingly restrictive environment for commercial support of CME. To answer this question, one must recognize the tremendous and accelerating pace of change in the medical education and health-care environments. Some of these changes are associated with CME and the fact that interventions that include learning are being used as strategic components within health-care systems for accelerating health-care performance improvement efforts focused on improving patient safety.

Where does industry support for CME fit in this emerging framework? Figure 23-1 may illustrate one future model. The intersection of zones of interest representing patient needs, health-care system quality gaps, and health-care provider performance gaps defines the boundaries within which the fourth circle of overlapping industry business needs can be appropriately placed. The appropriate business need that aligns with CME support most often occurs where a company recognizes market expansion as a core strategy. It is never appropriate for industry to consider independent medical education a strategy to enhance market share. Industry support needs to be free of proprietary bias, and the CME forum must remain an environment that allows for the open exchange of research findings and the best available evidence.

What will not change is that the public benefits by any model of commercial support that supports effectively using the right treatment plan at the right time for the right patient. This model requires many health-care provider competencies that characterize the overlap of these four interests. They include patient care, medical knowledge, practice-based learning and improvement, interpersonal and communications skills, professionalism, and systems-based practice. This paradigm—espoused and increasingly being embraced by agencies and groups concerned with health-care quality and professional education (e.g., Joint Commission, AHRQ, AAMC, and IOM)—is being adopted by leading organizations providing CME. The change represents an opportunity for industry to move away from its limited focus on a largely ineffective meetings-based CME economy that has higher compliance risks and offers little mutual value based on the data indicative of what works in CME. The only beneficiaries are those that prosper from this outdated meetings-based model of support. Industry, along with the medical profession and patients, sees valuable and increasingly scarce resources wasted. This recognition has led to calls for change that will likely lead to profound changes in the commercial support model over the next several years.

Fully adopting this convergence-of-interests model of industry support can reshape commercial support of CME. Applying this model can improve the quality of grants awarded while facilitating improvement in other operational aspects of commercial support. Policies and procedures can be simplified, compliance risk mitigated, and overhead costs reduced. One example of change

using this model might be industry adoption of a pooled-funding-with-a-purpose approach that may lead to block grants as the norm within several years. By forgoing one-grant-at-a-time decisions in favor of a more accountable and effective approach, industry may find that opportunities will increase for re-engaging the medical community in strategic health-care improvement level discussions where the compliance concern of individual grant making bias is removed. In many companies, CME support has become so frozen in place by compliance issues and other policy requirements that dialogue between industry and providers intended to benefit patients no longer occurs. The Convergence of Interests Model can be the foundation for a new dialogue and transformation of commercial support of CME. With a better model for managing conflict of interest and preventing the potential introduction of commercial bias, the future state could lead to improved patient-centric collaboration. We are at a fork in the road where we either adopt a model in defense of the status quo or we transform the way commercial support is used and viewed. If history shows the former to be the path taken, future commercial support of CME will be limited. If, however, the latter is the path taken, then the golden age of industry support as measured by patient benefits rather than dollars available may yet lie ahead.

Future optimal effectiveness of CME activities (or, perhaps more properly, continuing professional education) will depend on providers recognizing the importance of the entire health-care team in patient care and, as such, developing content to satisfy the needs of nonphysician practitioners (i.e., nurses, pharmacists, physician assistants, technicians, etc.). These individuals must be exposed to relevant material and qualified faculty with whom they can discuss important matters of patient care in much the same way as they would do in a hospital or office setting. Progress has been made in the advancement of this goal, but additional integration is needed and possible.

Medical education depends on academic institutions, and they should be encouraged to play a greater role in CME by collaborating to a greater degree with industry and MECCs to sponsor a greater number of CME activities without the total exclusion of commercial support or in detriment to nonacademic providers. CME has traditionally benefited from integration, innovation, and diversity; as partners, academia and private industry can contribute immensely to the advancement of CME. Each organization offers unique attributes and possibilities and in combination will provide a more solid best-practices foundation for CME.

As commercially supported CME continues to evolve and improve to meet 21st-century requirements of physicians and patients, the challenges of old and new maladies, new treatment modalities and technical advances, and educational quality and performance improvement methodologies will be of paramount importance. Consumers of CME will expect those who design activities do so in a manner most conducive to demonstrable behavior change and performance improvement among health-care providers, resulting in verifiable patient benefits. These goals will be secured by the application of proven quality assurance and performance improvement methods and techniques designed to address knowledge and performance gaps and decision-making processes over time, and upon changes in the health of their patients as identified by physician self-evaluation and self-study. Methods and practices will emerge to process, implement, and apply best practices in quality and performance improvement. To achieve such purposes, carefully conducted and validated needs assessment and directly related learning objectives will remain the pillars of CME activities.

To meet future challenges in medicine, science, and patient care, the key components of the CME process (i.e., needs assessment, learning objectives, content development, evidence-based content, adult learning principles, outcome evaluation, and ongoing knowledge reinforcement)

will become inseparably integrated as an expected and ongoing system of activities supported by multi-media learning opportunities, case vignettes, and greater participant interactivity.

Outcome measurement in a to-be-determined optimally effective form and at assessment levels acceptable to most CME providers will be a focal point to determine that learning has occurred and that knowledge has been transferred, retained, applied, and coupled with meaningful behavior change, resulting in improved patient and health-care statistics. The acquisition of data from patient records to confirm improved disease management and the public health as a result of quality- and performance-based CME activities will require new forms of cooperation among medical institutions, practitioners, and perhaps legislators, while ensuring patient privacy. Advances in computer and telecommunication technology will assist providers in the timely acquisition, analysis, interpretation, application, and storage of outcome and other activity-related data.

As new communication and data transfer technology is perfected and becomes available, health professionals will increasingly expect data on patient records, disease states, drugs and therapeutics, scientific literature, and other information to be instantaneously accessible. Point–of-care CME will continue to gain acceptance as data devices become easier to use and more widely available at lower cost. Device-to-device communication will be an important component.

Global CME has advanced more slowly because of local economics, cost, and differing cultures and regulations. As nations continue to trade and collaborate across borders and create more of a world economy, it is reasonable to expect CME to contribute to and benefit from that process. Multinational pharmaceutical companies will view global CME as part of their corporate missions and obligation to improve patient care worldwide. Support of CME activities will depend on content availability, content focus, and cost. Repurposed US content will not be sufficient in the long term. Content availability, not regulations, will determine the globalization of CME. Electronic transfer of medical education to distant global locations will advance CME growth. It may also be necessary for US-based companies to share the cost of global CME with their foreign subsidiaries.

The future of CME depends on finding the common ground within the plethora of guidelines and regulations so that time, energy, and funding can be devoted to quality and performance improvement and the application of best practices throughout the industry. Balancing the ways and means to fund CME without relying primarily on the pharmaceutical industry in a manner that is acceptable to participants, government, the public, and industry will be essential to the continued availability and advancement of CME. ACCME and other regulatory groups will continue to work together in the best interests of CME to bring stability to the regulation and monitoring of educational activities and provider organizations.

Notes

1. M. A. Bowman and D. L. Pearle, "Changes in Drug Prescribing Patterns Related to Commercial Company Funding of Continuing Medical Education," *Journal of Continuing Education in the Health Professions* 8, no. 1 (1988): 13–20.

2. A. B. Rosof and W. C. Felch, eds., *Continuing Medical Education: A Primer* (Westport, Conn.: Praeger, 1992).

3. "Federal Food, Drug, and Cosmetic Act," Food and Drug Administration Web site, http://www.fda.gov/opacom/laws/fdcat/fdcact5d.html (accessed July 31, 2009).

4. "Guidance for Industry: Final Guidance on Industry-Supported Scientific and Educational Activities," *Federal Register* 62, no. 232 (1997): 64093–64100, http://www.fda.gov/Cder/Guidance/isse.html.

5. "The Code on Interactions with Healthcare Professionals," The Pharmaceutical Research and Manufacturers of America Web site, http://www.pharma.org/come_on_interactions_with_healthcare_professionals/ (accessed July 31, 2009).

6. "Code of Ethics on Interactions with Health Care Professionals," Advanced Medical Technology Association Web site, http://www.advamed.org/Member Portal/About/code/ (accessed July 31, 2009).

7. S. W. Fletcher, *Continuing Education in the Healthcare Professions: Improving Healthcare through Life-Long Learning* (New York: Josiah Macy, Jr. Foundation, 2008).

PART VII

Emerging Themes and Forces in
Continuing Medical Education

CHAPTER 24

Continuing Professional Development: Concept, Origins, and Rationale

The move toward using the term *continuing professional development* (*CPD*) to replace the traditional term of *continuing medical education* (*CME*) is now a global movement and has huge implications for all stakeholders involved in the education of practicing physicians. It is regularly used today throughout the world as the preferred term for adult physician learning and continuing medical education, but its true significance is often obscure. This is the story of how CME is being transformed to being a subset of CPD.

Origin of the CPD Concept

The use of the abbreviation *CPD* for *continuing professional development* received increasing attention in the United Kingdom in 1993 when it was formally proposed for use by a government-sponsored Standing Committee on Postgraduate Medical and Dental Education (SCOPME), chaired by Dame Barbara Clayton, MD. SCOPME was established in August 1988 to advise the UK government on the delivery of postgraduate medical and dental education in that country. The members were appointed by the Secretary of State for Health on advice from the Chief Medical Officer and the Chief Dental Officer. Although the committee was disbanded at the end of March 1999 due to a ministerial decision, during its term of operation it found that the educational

needs of practicing doctors and dentists were more complicated than expected.

Early on, SCOPME realized that the traditional CME approach no longer covered the whole of a doctor's or dentist's educational and career development needs in modern health care. It cited examples drawn from experiences within the National Health Service (NHS) where the following new learning needs were among several identified:

- Managers of NHS trusts want changes in skills or practice to underpin new service developments.
- Shared care across the primary/secondary care interface and between NHS trusts and general practice makes teamwork essential.
- Clinical audit—another new activity—is by nature multi-professional and presents new challenges.
- General practitioners are increasingly expected to understand areas such as information technology, population medicine, management, and communication skills.

In its final report, SCOPME wrote:

These requirements do not correspond, however, with the traditional specialist definition of continuing medical education. Change, whether rapid, discontinuous or incremental, more often than not means altered responsibilities for doctors and dentists. Wider roles, changing professional responsibilities and career development become important. Professional functions evolve or are adapted, but even more extensive role changes—sometimes even whole new career directions—may be needed. The prudent professional has to be responsible for mapping the clinical, organizational and social changes and negotiating a way through them.[1]

The SCOPME report was a working paper titled "Continuing Professional Development for Doctors and Dentists." Leading up to its publication, SCOPME carried out "a wide-ranging consultation about CPD, of which CME is an important part." The committee concluded that traditional specialty-based CME does not meet all of the needs of doctors and dentists. It stressed that use of the term *CPD* would have major advantages, and that within CPD there should be "(a) strategies for personal coping and professional growth, career development, and role adaptations, (b) [education in] ability to manage, and (c) [education and training in] multidisciplinary and multi-professional working and learning."[2]

Also important to this story was a special conference—"Continuing Medical Education in Europe: The Way Forward through European Collaboration"—held at the Royal College of Physicians in London, in March 1995. The conference was chaired by Sir Leslie Turnberg, president of the Royal College of Physicians, and brought together 31 faculty members and 149 delegates from most countries in Europe as well as the United States and Canada. Clayton, representing SCOPME, presented the recommendations brought forward by the committee, and these were debated by a subgroup of the attendees led by R. D. Atley of the Royal College of Obstetricians and Gynaecology in the United Kingdom. One of us (Dennis K. Wentz) served as the working group secretary and reported, "In

conclusion, we feel that the term CPD best encompasses the total development of the individual doctor from medical student to retirement. It includes all that was in the term CME, in fact CME should and will remain a very important part of CPD, but CPD goes beyond to encompass self-appraisal, career development, personal coping and professional growth. And we believe the profession should take the lead in enunciating its commitment to the concept of CPD with cognizance of what the future holds."[3]

But not all were persuaded. M. C. T. Morrison, MD, of the United Kingdom rose to say:

> The medical profession has a great propensity for contemplating its own navel. It is worth asking why this meeting is here, why there is this interest in CME or CPD . . . whilst I think it is fine that people should talk about CPD, in the current climate, certainly in the UK, it is useful to confine ourselves to CME because managers will perceive CPD as something different, and I think it is. CME may mean keeping up to date within one's own sphere of practice, whereas professional development is perhaps learning new skills to practice in a different way in one's specialty, or even a different specialty, and particularly in management. In the UK, managers are very happy to spend money on management courses, and less happy on medical courses. They control, at present, the financing of their career-grade doctors who will require time for CME.[4]

Implementation of the CPD Concept

Regardless of Morrison's skepticism, this concept of CPD gained quick and important support in the United Kingdom, and other parts of the globe have adopted the term and the concepts. The concept of CPD thus spread quickly from the United Kingdom to continental Europe.

Instrumental for the development in Europe were the initiatives taken by the different organizations dealing with education established within the medical profession in Europe. Among the cornerstones for development of CME and later

CPD were the Charter on CME of Medical Specialists in the European Union by the Union Européenne des Médecins Spécialistes (UEMS) from 1994,[5] the establishment of the European Accreditation Council for CME (EACCME) in 1999, and the UEMS Charter on CPD known as the Basel Declaration from 2001.[6] A new consensus statement on CPD was introduced at the conference "CPD: Improving Health Care," which took place in Luxembourg in December 2006.[7]

The Medical Directive of the European Union, introduced in 1975 and later published with only minor changes (the latest publication being 2005[8]), only deals with basic and postgraduate medical education. However, the Advisory Committee on Medical Training, set up to promote harmonization of medical education in the European Union, and which worked from 1977 to 1997, also contributed to the development.[9]

Change in medical education comes slowly and usually for good reason. The traditional three phases of medical education have been (a) undergraduate or basic medical education; (b) graduate or postgraduate medical education, comprising preregistration training, vocational or professional training, specialist and subspecialist training, and other formalized training programs for defined expert functions; and (c) CME. Each phase has a defined audience, and most of us know what is meant when these terms are used today. But there has been confusion, both in North America and globally, over the terms used to define these phases. Often forgotten is the precedent set in 1959 by the American Medical Association (AMA) House of Delegates (the policymaking body of the AMA) when it took action to strongly urge that the term *continuing medical education* immediately replace the term then in use for education directed at practicing physicians, *postgraduate medical education* (*PGME*). And the term *CME* slowly replaced *PGME*, became a global reality, and obviously continues to exist today.

Then 40 years after that precedent-setting decision, the AMA Division of Continuing Medical Education—now realizing the need for a broader context—again changed the designation, this time accepting the concept of CPD. The change was based upon the SCOPME report and other learned conferences. However, the AMA slightly altered the term *CPD* in an effort to emphasize that physicians were the primary focus of their CME efforts. Thus it chose to add the word *physician,* thereby creating the term *continuing physician professional development* (*CPPD*). A concise statement of the reasons for this decision was published by Wentz and Greg Paulos in 2000.[10] However, the term *CME* is still used by the Accreditation Council for Continuing Medical Education (ACCME) that accredits providers who in turn designate AMA Physician's Recognition Award credit.[11]

Another important step in the direction toward the new name of CPD was the publication of a book in 2003 examining the process of CME from research to knowledge translation to practice. The editors—Dave Davis, MD; Barbara Barnes, MD; and Robert Fox, EdD—decided that the book should represent a forward look at the field of physician learning, discarding the term *continuing medical education* (which they noted all too frequently connotes only lecture presentations) in favor of the concept of CPD. Hence the book's title became *The Continuing Professional Development of Physicians,* and hereby another important milestone was passed in the United States and Canada.[12]

The authors open their argument by citing a holistic definition of CME authored by Nancy Bennett, PhD, on behalf of the Association of American Medical Colleges (AAMC): "Continuing medical education is a distinct and definable activity that supports the professional development of physicians and leads to improved patient outcomes. It encompasses all the learning experiences that physicians engage in with the conscious intent of regularly and continually improving their practices."[13] Yet, despite such a definition, the authors write, "It seems to us, that, perhaps of the commonplace nature in medicine of the acronym CME, it is the 'gestalt' or the picture of the term CME that truly carries the day. Physicians most often see CME in quite narrow and constraining ways, usually as the lecture-based experience in a resort or hotel. As a result, most physicians still conjure up images of darkened meeting rooms with slides presented by a speaker."

And then they make the case for CPD:

Apart from the still-pervasive narrower picture of CME described earlier, we prefer the term CPD for three reasons. First, it establishes greater content depth, encompassing not only the narrower clinical dimensions of cardiology or infectious disease (what Miller calls a categorical content model[14]) but also the broader field of practice management, ethical decision-making, evidence-based care, managed care principles, and other, broader aspects of medical practice. Second, the formats conjured by the phrase CPD appear to us to be more comprehensive than those that arise from considering CME. Perhaps because of the relative newness of the term, we see CPD as being the umbrella for all sorts of interventions, not just the traditional conference or mailed material. In this area, CPD more easily encompasses other learning formats such as reminders, audit and feedback, academic detailing, and Web-based guidelines. Third, the difference between CME and CPD for us resides in the venue of the learning or setting of the educational intervention. CME, still in its traditional mode, makes us think of the lecture hall or conference room, often miles, both physically and symbolically, from the real practice setting. . . . The phrase (CPD) more accurately reflects this observation: the theme in adult learning that has emerged over the past 25 years, beginning with Knowles,[15] that adults learn independently of teachers and in a manner that is closely tied to their experience. The term CPD ties the study and practices of facilitating learning to the broader concepts of CPD and adult learning. In that sense, it situates the learn-

ing in the learner, perhaps the ultimate venue in which CPD may occur.[16]

Global Standards

Among the early adopters of CPD was the World Federation of Medical Education (WFME). WFME was founded in 1972 as the global organization concerned with the education and training of medical students and medical doctors at all levels. In 1997, the WFME announced a project— known as WFME Global Standards for Quality Improvement in Medical Education—to define global standards to outline not only minimum requirements but also standards for quality development of medical education institutions worldwide.[17] It subsequently convened panels of international experts from all six World Health Organization (WHO)/WFME regions of the world to cover each the three areas of medical education: basic medical education, postgraduate or specialty medical education, and CPD. The first documents released dealt with WFME global standards for basic medical education, first presented as a discussion document in the journal *Medical Education*,[18] and for postgraduate medical education. In October 2002, the Task Force on Definition of International Standards for CME/CPD was convened in Copenhagen to complete the third and final part of the project. Although spirited debate occurred on many of the standards proposed by an earlier 2001 working party, task force members unanimously agreed that the former document title of "CME/CPD" should be replaced by "Continuing Professional Development of Medical Doctors." The task force wrote the document using the following definition:

CPD includes all activities that doctors undertake, formally and informally, in order to maintain, update, develop and enhance their knowledge, skills and attitudes in response to the needs of their patients. Doctors are autonomous and independent, i.e., they act in the best interest of the patient without undue external influence. Engaging in CPD is a professional obligation but also a prerequisite for enhancing the quality of health care. The strongest motivating factor for continuous professional life-long learning is the will and desire to maintain professional quality.[19]

The CPD document is structured in nine areas with a total of 36 subareas. The nine areas cover the universe (structure, process, content, educational environment, and outcome) of CPD: mission and outcomes; learning methods; planning and documentation; the individual doctor; CPD providers; educational context and resources; evaluation of methods and competencies; organization; and continuous renewal. For each subarea, standards are specified at two levels of attainment: basic standards, meaning that the standard must be met and fulfillment demonstrated during evaluation of CPD; and quality development standards, the implication of which is that the standard is in accordance with international consensus about best practice of CPD and that fulfillment of—or initiatives to fulfill—some or all such standards should be documented.

Examples of more essential statements in the document are that:

- CPD is an obligation of the individual doctor, who will be the first of the principal stakeholders in formulation of mission and outcomes.
- CPD must be tailored to the needs of the individual doctor, and needs assessment will serve as the basis for planning of CPD activities.
- CPD should take advantage of a variety of learning modalities with emphasis on self-directed and active learning.
- CPD must serve the purpose of enhancing the professional and personal development of doctors.
- CPD must be recognized as an integral part of medical practice reflected in budgets, resource allocations, and time planning and not subordinate to service demands.

- Funding of CPD must be part of the expenses of the health-care system.

Medical schools must provide leadership in improving the quality of CPD. At the March 2003 World Congress on Medical Education held in Copenhagen, the final document was released as part of the WFME Trilogy of Global Standards.[20] It was given immediate and wide circulation. The implementation process, which followed the broad international endorsement[21] of the Global Standards Program at the Congress, included translations, testing in pilot studies, disseminating information at several national and international meetings and workshops, as well as a large number of publications, specifications for individual disciplines (e.g., family medicine), and use of the CPD standards as benchmark and in formulation of national standards (e.g., in China, Egypt, France, Georgia, Russia, and Ukraine). The WFME standards also became the basis for Project Globe, which aims at enabling excellence for physicians in primary care services.[22] In 2007, WFME and the Association of Medical Schools in Europe jointly published European specifications to the WFME Trilogy as part of the Thematic Network MEDINE, sponsored by the European Commission and the WHO Regional Office for Europe.[23]

Rationale for the Concept of CPD

Why are we seeing a departure from the conventional term *CME*, embodied in the conceptualization of the three phases of medical education, undergraduate (basic), graduate (postgraduate), and CME? Words *are* important, and in today's world there is an urgent need for CME to evolve in a new direction and to new relevance for practicing physicians. The term *CPD* provides a clear signal to everyone involved in the global enterprise of learning by practicing physicians. Above all, the term *CPD* best reflects the direction in which medical education for the practice years should move: *continuous* education along the reality of a continuum of lifelong learning. CPD speaks to an overlap between the traditional phases of medical education. In the definition of CPD used by WFME, it is emphasized that "although CPD designates the period commencing after completion of postgraduate training, CPD has much further ramifications. CPD activities have a basis in the life-long continuing process, starting when the student is admitted to the medical school and continuing as long as the doctor is engaged in professional activities."[24]

CPD differs in principle from the preceding two phases of medical education; whereas these are conducted according to specified curricula and defined criteria, CPD mainly implies self-directed and practice-based learning activities. The responsibility to conduct CPD rests with the profession and the individual doctor; law and regulation could hardly regulate CPD. Where regulations do exist, these are flexible, even in countries demanding relicensure or re-registration of doctors in practice.[25]

A new concept for CME has arrived, and the entire field is faced with a change in expectations coupled with a change in purpose. To veteran observers, the message is to focus on new concepts. Providers of CME must take deliberate steps to broaden their base, to expand their relevance to practice, to demonstrate that CME or CPD in fact makes a *difference* for doctors and the quality care of patients.

Many formal definitions of *CME* exist in the United States but none of *CPD*. Perhaps new definitions are unnecessary. The AMA, the steward of the major US CME credit system, uses a long-standing definition of *CME* that is in conformance with the new term *CPD*:

CME consists of educational activities which serve to maintain, develop or increase the knowledge, skills, and professional performance and relationships that a physician uses to provide services for patients, the public, or the profession. The content of CME is the body of knowledge and skills generally recognized and accepted by the profession as within the basic medical sciences, the discipline of clinical medicine, and the provision of health care to the public.[26]

For CPD to succeed, it will still need to be proven that the new concepts within CPD provide a positive return on investment for physician participants, patients, faculty, and external financial supporters. CME will be articulated in a vastly broader context, focusing more clearly on the cumulative lifetime learning needs of physicians as they deal with radical changes in their practice environment.

Has current CME been relevant to physician needs? Did physicians learn about the changing environment facing their medical practices via the current system? Did the current system assist physicians in balancing their primary purpose of providing optimal patient care to a single patient versus the challenge of better use of societal resources? Did traditional CME alert physicians to the need and relevance of medical informatics in their lives? Did the current CME system teach physicians to be involved in designing, implementing, and using systems that offer feedback to them about their patient care and patient outcomes? Has current CME helped physicians to understand the value of regularly setting aside sufficient time to adequately reflect on their practice of medicine? Did CME or the entire continuum of medical education help physicians in training or in practice design systems for focused, personalized learning in order to catch up in a clinical management area of which they are unaware or deficient in? A move to the term *CPD* may help us to reconceptualize the role of CME and provide new direction for enhancing lifelong learning.

Arnold Relman has written of three revolutions in medicine. He calls the third revolution "The age of accountability."[27] The implications of this third revolution resonate with the concepts inherent in the new term of *CPD*. A physician's performance in practice is the end result of his or her professional development; and society is increasingly holding physicians and all health-care professionals accountable.

The concepts of CPD can be helpful as physicians deal with other external initiatives. The maintenance of certification (MOC) initiative of the American Board of Medical Specialties and its 24-member medical specialty boards is such an initiative. To remain board certified in the United States, a physician will now be evaluated at least every seven years on the following six general competencies:

- Patient care
- Medical knowledge
- Interpersonal and communication skills
- Professionalism, including adherence to ethical principles
- Systems-based practice
- Practice-based learning and improvement[28]

Certainly the concepts of CPD match the individual practitioner's needs and requirements under MOC far better than the concepts behind traditional CME.

What are other opportunities that fall within CPD? Physicians must learn the principles of leadership, and these most likely will be learned during their practice years. They need help in equipping themselves with the skills needed to integrate their roles as physicians with other health professionals as part of multiprofessional teams. Physicians should become aware of (a) the increasing cultural diversity of their patients and (b) their own assumptions and personal biases that might distort their care of individual patients or dishonor the cultural heritage of individual patients. Physicians can be made aware that it is acceptable for them as practitioners to consider, understand, seek help, and then cope with their own personal needs, including the management of personal stress or other feelings such as anger, inadequacy, and hopelessness, as well as lack of knowledge. CPD should open up a continuing reflective process.

Wentz and Paulos wrote, "Successful organizations in today's environment have moved from the development of plans that are too narrow in focus, or that concentrate on singular areas that in the long run prove to be ineffective in driving correct business decisions. Our discipline of CME is no different. Successful organizations choose to think and plan strategically. Thus they 'create the future.' The concept of a process of CPPD can creature the future for our discipline."[29]

As stated in the WFME CPD standards document,[30] motivation for CPD, from the perspective of the individual doctor, derives from (a) a professional drive to provide optimal care for the individual patient, (b) the obligation to honor the demands from employers and society, and (c) the need to preserve job satisfaction and prevent burnout.

The concepts of CPD reflect education throughout a lifetime. The process of becoming a compassionate and well-educated doctor begins well before the college years and progresses through medical school, residency, and fellowship to continue into the 40 or more years of medical practice. If the goal is *continuous* learning, the concepts of CPD must be planted early.

Implementation Challenges

Although some progress has been made, obstacles remain before the move to CPD can be completed. In the United States and Canada, many medical schools and medical specialty societies have renamed their departmental units to include the term *CPD*, signaling acceptance and adoption of the concept. In Europe, under the leadership of the WFME, UEMS, and EACCME, many entities embed the concept of CPD by referencing the continuous education of physicians with a combined CME/CPD designation. But many entities, including those that have been at the forefront of the CPD movement, appear to be reluctant to make a more formal commitment to the terminology, especially when referencing educational activities, credit systems, and accreditation activities. The AMA, credited with an initial push to CPD in the United States, still predominately references *CME* as the standard term rather than *CPD* (with the exception of the name of its division of CPPD).[31] The ACCME continues the term CME in its name, perhaps understandably, but has a virtually complete lack of reference to CPD on its Web site and in its accreditation materials. The EACCME, which does reference the concepts and terms associated with CPD, also still has CME in its name.[32] These are a few examples of the inconsistent adoption of the CPD terminology. These entities, as well as other leading educational organizations, are the primary influencers of the CME/CPD movement and help set the rate of adoption for changes.

In addition to the organizational or institutional efforts associated with the change in terms, individual physician's usage and acceptance of the concept of CPD needs further encouragement. As indicated earlier, if the goal is *continuous* physician learning, the seeds and concepts of CPD must be planted early. The pendulum has begun to swing as the understanding of physicians about the concepts and value of CPD increases, perhaps more rapidly in Europe than in the United States. The time will come when institutions, physicians, and society will be as cognizant of the term *CPD* as they are of *CME*.

Conclusion

This story cannot end without raising the major question, from where will the funding for this enlarged view of CME come? Many current CME offerings depend heavily on funding from the pharmaceutical and medical device industry. Unless industry buys into this broadened agenda for CME, can the concepts espoused in CPD move forward? Can CME providers and educators articulate these new needs well enough to attract support? If industry does not accept the concept, is there another solution?

In 1987, when CME was viewed as the frontier of medical education, Phil Manning and Donald Petit proposed three approaches to CME.[33] Their concepts for CME, re-articulated within this new concept of CPD, have never been more relevant or important. They pointed out that physicians would always need broad education to keep them informed *in general* about the current state of medical knowledge. The second area of CME outlined by these authors was education directed toward the specialty-specific aspects of the physician's individual learning needs. CPD could add to that by assisting physicians in studying the patients they actually cared for as well as analyzing the outcomes of that care. The third area addressed by Manning and Petit was the challenge to deliver on-the-spot and just-in-time information to effectively answer questions arising from practice. We believe the term *CPD* encompasses all of these areas, but funding of such a comprehensive approach may be difficult.

It is also our belief that the concept of CPD becomes especially useful as the profession works globally toward worldwide application of quality standards, as espoused by the WFME, and enters into an era of inter-professional education. While the globalization of medical education is a foregone conclusion, it lags far behind the business world and other global enterprises. But eventually medicine will and can be no different. We believe that within the concepts of CPD no geographic or political boundaries exist and the profession will achieve a new level for itself.

Notes

1. Standing Committee on Postgraduate Medical and Dental Education, "Consultation on Continuing Professional Development for Doctors and Dentists" (working paper, London, United Kingdom, 1994).

2. Standing Committee, "Consultation on Continuing Professional Development."

3. R. D. Atlay and D. K. Wentz, "CME or CPD?" *Postgraduate Medical Journal* 72, suppl. 1 (1996): S61.

4. Atlay and Wentz, "CME or CPD?" S65.

5. European Union of Medical Specialists, "Charter on Continuing Medical Education in the European Union," UEMS Web site, http://www.uems.net/ (accessed March 24, 2009).

6. European Union of Medical Specialists, "Basel Declaration: UEMS Policy on Continuing Professional Development," UEMS Web site, http://www.uems.net/ (accessed March 24, 2009).

7. Standing Committee of European Doctors, "Continuing Professional Development Improving Health Care Quality, Ensuring Patient Safety" (consensus statement, Continuing Professional Development Conference, Luxembourg, December 14, 2006).

8. "EU Directive 2005/36/EC of 7 September 2005 on the Recognition of Professional Qualifications," European Commission Web site, http://europa.eu.int/comm/internal_market/qualifications/future_en.htm (accessed March 24, 2009).

9. Advisory Committee on Medical Training of European Commission, *Report and Recommendations on Continuing Medical Education* (ACMT Document XV/E/8414/94, Brussels, 1994).

10. D. K. Wentz and G. Paulos, "Is Now the Time for Continuing Medical Education to Become Continuing Physician Professional Development?" *Journal of Continuing Education in the Health Professions* 20 (2000): 181–187.

11. "ACCME Standards for Commercial Support," Accreditation Council for Continuing Medical Education Web site, http://www.accme.org/dir_docs/doc_upload/68b2902a-fb73-44d1-8725-80a1504e520c_uploaddocument.pdf (accessed April 9, 2009).

12. D. Davis and others, *The Continuing Professional Development of Physicians: From Research to Practice* (Chicago: American Medical Association, 2003).

13. N. L. Bennett and others, "Continuing Medical Education: A New Vision of the Professional Development of Physicians," *Academic Medicine* 75 (2000): 1167–1172.

14. G. E. Miller, "Continuing Education for What?" *Journal of Medical Education* 42 (1967): 320–346.

15. M. D. Knowles and others, *The Adult Learner: The Definitive Classic in Adult Education and Human Resource Development* (Houston, Tex.: Gulf Publishing Company, 1998).

16. Davis and others, *Continuing Professional Development*.

17. The Executive Council of the World Federation for Medical Education, "International Standards in Medical Education: Assessment and Accreditation of Medical Schools' Educational Programmes, A WFME Position Paper," *Medical Education* 32 (1998): 549–558.

18. WFME Task Force on Defining International Standards in Basic Medical Education, "Report of the Working Party, Copenhagen, 14-16 October 1999," *Medical Education* 34 (2000): 665–675.

19. "Continuing Professional Development (CPD) of Medical Doctors: WFME Global Standards for Quality Improvement," World Federation for Medical Education Web site, http://www.wfme.org (accessed March 24, 2009).

20. "Basic Medical Education: WFME Global Standards for Quality Improvement," World Federation for Medical Education Web site, http://www3.sund.ku.dk/Activities/WFME%20Standard%20Documents%20and%20translations/WFME%20Standard.pdf (accessed March 24, 2009); "Postgraduate Medical Education: WFME Global Standards for Quality Improvement," World Federation for Medical Education Web site, http://www.fmh.ch/files/pdf4/wfme.pdf (accessed March 24, 2009); "Continuing Professional Development (CPD) of Medical Doctors: WFME Global Standards for Quality Improvement," World Federation for Medical Education Web site, http://www3.sund.ku.dk/Activities/WFME%20Standard%20Documents%20and%20translations/WFME%20CPD.pdf (accessed March 24, 2009).

21. J. P. de V. van Niekerk, "WFME Global Standards Receive Ringing Endorsement," *Medical Education* 37 (2003): 585–586.

22. "Making the World a Healthier Place," Project Globe Web site, http://www.globecpd.org/pdfs/PGCbrochurefunds.pdf (accessed March 24, 2009).

23. Quality Assurance Task Force, "MEDINE: WFME Global Standards for Quality Improvement in Medical Education European Specifications," World Federation for Medical Education Web site, http://www.anemf.org/IMG/pdf_MEDINE_WFME_standards_for_Quality_Improvement.pdf (accessed March 24, 2009).

24. "Continuing Professional Development (CPD) of Medical Doctors," WFME Web site.

25. Ibid.

26. American Medical Association, "House of Delegates Policy #300.988, A Definition of Continuing Medical Education," The Physician's Recognition Award and Credit System (Chicago: American Medical Association, 2006).

27. A. S. Relman, "Assessment and Accountability," *New England Journal of Medicine* 319 (1988): 1220–1222.

28. "MOC Competencies," American Board of Medical Specialties Web site, http://abms.org/Maintenance_of_Certification/MOC_competencies.aspx (accessed March 24, 2009).

29. Wentz and Paulos, "Is Now the Time?" 181–187.

30. "Continuing Professional Development (CPD) of Medical Doctors," WFME Web site.

31. American Medical Association, "AMA Continuing

Medical Education," AMA Web site, http://www.ama-assn.org/ama/pub/education-careers/continuing-medical-education.shtml (accessed March 30, 2009).

32. "Furthering Globalization, Reciprocity and the Substantial Equivalency of Systems of Accreditation and Credit in Continuing Medical Education and Continuing Professional Development," European Union of Medical Specialists Web site, http://admin.uems.net/uploaded files/492.pdf (accessed March 30, 2009).

33. P. R. Manning and D. Petit, "The Past, Present and Future of Continuing Medical Education," *Journal of the American Medical Association* 258 (1987): 3542–3546.

Steven Minnick, Nancy L. Davis,
Charles E. Willis, and Errol R. Alden

CHAPTER 25

Contemporary Developments in Continuing Medical Education and Continuing Professional Development

"All experience is an arch wherethro' gleams that yet untravel'd world, whose margin fades for ever and for ever when I move," wrote Tennyson in his poem about the travels of the ancient Greek hero Ulysses. It is a passage that beautifully captures the transition from current experience to the untraveled world of the future always beyond our reach. This chapter explores some of the newer developments in continuing medical education (CME) and continuing professional development (CPD), developments that will likely serve as structural supports for the arch wherethro our current experience in CME and CPD, as part of its odyssey, will pass.

From a general and conceptual perspective, change appears to be emanating from the following major trends: (1) changes occurring in physician specialty certification and recertification, credentialing, and licensure processes; (2) advances occurring in learning and communication technologies; and (3) the movement by society, insurers, and the federal government toward transparency in health-care delivery. The first trend regards the emergence of a set of physician competencies, broader than just medical knowledge, that can be applied across the continuum of undergraduate, graduate, and continuing medical education and will form the framework of many of the future CME and CPD activities. Examples of the second trend include sophisticated tech-nologies that extend beyond the lecture hall and printed page, creating opportunities to more fully explore the use of images, video, and sound; new and advancing clinical simulation capabilities; and real-time clinical information at the point-of-care that also captures and records the associated physician learning for CME and CPD purposes. The emphasis on transparency for the third trend has increased the expectation to demonstrate improvement in the quality of health care and patient safety. When and where appropriate, these quality and patient safety goals offer expanded opportunities for CME and CPD professionals. Examples include the Joint Commission's set of national patient safety goals, various payer-driven quality-of-care initiatives, such as Medicare's heart failure index, and increased public reporting of hospital and physician quality-of-care measures (the Leapfrog Group, etc.).

With these trends in mind, this chapter will focus on three important developments in CME and CPD: performance improvement CME (PI CME), Internet point-of-care (PoC) learning, and the growing use of simulation in CME and CPD.

PI CME

In 2001, the American Medical Association (AMA) convened a group to examine the quality improvement (QI) activities physicians were engaged in and to determine what construct would most efficiently and accurately permit CME credit to be awarded for participation in these activities. QI and better patient care have always been intended outcomes of CME; the trick was to determine how some form of QI CME could demonstrate improvement, especially if linked to clinical data and embedded in the physician's practice.

Why should physicians not be rewarded for activities that would have the most impact in their practice? Much of the literature signals that individual, frequently isolated, traditional CME activities have a limited effect on practice.[1] Yet, that is how the majority of CME has been delivered: remote from practice, usually lecture-based, and built around the global aggregation of perceived needs rather than developed with data abstracted from a physician's practice.

In the late 1990s, radiologist Robert Pyatt, MD, a hospital CME committee chairman, informed Dennis K. Wentz, MD, then director of the AMA's Division of Continuing Physician Professional Development (CPPD), that he was awarding AMA Physician's Recognition Award (PRA) Category 1 credit for physicians participating in quality assurance work. He had described his program at the Alliance for Continuing Medical Education (ACME) annual meeting.

Pyatt found that while the program led to improved practice, it did not fit the standard criteria for assembling a CME activity, making credit difficult to award under the current system. Wentz and others had a "long-standing dream that CME credit would be awarded for something doctors should be doing in their daily work." So Wentz and Pyatt worked on a simple experiment, based on Pyatt's program, that suggested something bigger was at hand.

More work remained to describe this type of CME and to sort out a system for allocating CME credit for these activities. Wentz presented the concept to the CME Advisory Committee of the AMA Council of Medical Education, who liked the idea. The committee appointed a working group and called on Steven Minnick, MD, director of medi-

cal education at St. John Hospital and Medical Center (Detroit, Michigan), to chair the working group. Minnick was a past chair of the Accreditation Council for Continuing Medical Education (ACCME), a member of the AMA's section on medical schools, and a member of the Michigan State Medical Society's committee on CME.

The AMA Division of CPPD, one of the thought leader organizations for CME, experienced a more immediate pressure to articulate how quality and CME could be brought under the same umbrella. One driver was the Physician Consortium for Performance Improvement, already underway and sited at the AMA. The consortium actively developed performance measures, employing the best available evidence and working across specialties and with multiple stakeholders. CME, if it was to become CPD, could ill afford not to join and integrate with the quality revolution. Otherwise, we risked becoming irrelevant.

Under Minnick's leadership, the AMA CME/CPPD Performance Measurement Pilot Project was launched in June 2001. The steering committee membership consisted of experts in CME and quality improvement: Barbara Barnes, MD, MS, associate dean of CME at the University of Pittsburgh Medical Center; William Golden, MD, director general internal medicine at the University of Arkansas College of Medicine and former chair of the AMA Council on Medical Education; Richard Horowitz, MD, FACP, AMA Physician Consortium for Performance Improvement; Thomas Knabel, MD, national medical director at United Healthcare; Edward Langston, MD, AMA Council on Medical Education; and Pyatt, chief executive officer of Chambersburg Imaging Associates (Pennsylvania). Additionally, Nancy Davis, PhD, director of CME for the American Academy of Family Physicians (AAFP), was invited to serve on the project to engage the AAFP and ensure that any new policies would be congruent with the AAFP CME credit system. Staff leadership for the project was provided by the AMA Division of CPPD and included Dennis K. Wentz, MD, division director; Charles Willis, MBA, PRA director;

Greg Paulos, associate division director; Rebecca DeVivo, MPH, MSW, director of accreditation and certification activities; and Tina Blair, MPH, research associate. Other AMA staff participants included Karen Kmetic, PhD, program director of the division of clinical quality improvement, and Joanne Schwartzberg, MD, director of the division on aging and community health.

The first meeting of the Performance Measurement Pilot Project steering committee occurred on August 16, 2001. Wentz reviewed the environmental issues that spurred interest in the project. The AAFP was moving toward an evidence-based approach to CME content. The CME field was moving away from traditional, lecture-based programs. The AMA had approved nontraditional activities for AMA PRA Category 1 credit, e.g., being published in refereed journals, presenting peer-reviewed posters, or publishing abstracts. The Royal College of Physicians and Surgeons of Canada had implemented standards for mandatory CME and singled out practice audits as an important component of physicians' professional development.

After a call for proposals and a review of applications, the steering committee initially chose to examine four pilot programs in an effort to gain a sense of the initiative, physician and nonphysician roles, outcomes, mechanisms for documenting participation, and changes in practice. The four programs included the Accreditation Association for Ambulatory Health Care Institute for Quality Improvement (AAAHC-IQI); US Department of Veterans Affairs—Employee Education System (EES); University of Pittsburgh Medical Center; and Iowa Foundation for Medical Care. At a later date, two more programs were also included: American College of Physicians (ACP) and Arkansas Foundation for Medical Care. By participating in the pilot, the organizations were able to offer AMA PRA Category 1 credit to physicians who participated.

Over a period of three and a half years, the steering committee heard reports from the pilot initiatives, reviewed their progress, queried constituent physicians, and formulated a process for documenting and awarding CME credit for these activities. Although not a seated member of the steering committee, the ACCME was apprised throughout of the project's activities.

During this period, the AAFP not only participated in the work of the steering committee, it also actively prepared to make similar provisions and implement a common process into its CME credit system.

At the August 2002 meeting, the steering committee debated whether its mission was performance measurement or improvement. Measurement (with data) was instrumental to improvement, but the ultimate purpose for the CME community was and remains demonstrated PI. Consequently, the project reorganized itself around PI CME, the currently accepted moniker for this type of CME activity.

Components of PI CME

The steering committee agreed on the following guiding principles for PI activities appropriate for AMA PRA Category 1 credit: measurement of the practice based on evidence-based guidelines, feedback or analysis provided to learner, implementation of practice change intervention, remeasurement of the practice, and evaluation or evidence of learning. After evaluating the pilots against these guiding principles, the steering committee arrived at a consensus description of an appropriate PI CME activity. It included three stages:

- *Stage A, Learning from Current Practice Performance Assessment:* Assess the current practice using identified performance measures, either through chart reviews or some other appropriate mechanism; participating physicians should be actively involved in data collection and analysis.
- *Stage B, Learning from the Application of Performance Improvement to Patient Care:* Implement an intervention based on the

performance measures selected in Stage A, using suitable tracking tools (e.g., flow sheets); participating physicians should receive guidance on appropriate parameters for applying an intervention and assessing performance change, specific to the performance measure and the physician's patient base (e.g., how many patients with a given condition, seen for how long, will produce a valid assessment?).

- *Stage C, Learning from the Evaluation of the Performance Improvement Effort:* Reevaluate and reflect on performance in the practice (Stage B) by comparing against the assessment from Stage A; summarize any practice, process, and/or outcomes changes that resulted from conducting the PI activity.

Assigning Credit to PI CME

For PI CME activities, the questions still remained regarding how to assign credit and how much credit to award. To encourage participation and reward physicians appropriately for the volume of work and learning involved, a significant amount of credit was assigned to such activities. Using the rationale that 50 annual credit hours marked the upper bound for state licensure requirements and the requirement for AAFP membership, the steering committee concluded that PI CME should fill a significant portion of that requirement. Another consideration was an AMA recommendation, current at that time, that single activities be limited to 50 credit hours.

Based on those premises, this group of experts decided on 20 credits for PI CME. To complement that total credit allocation for successfully completing the PI activity, the group also believed an option for partial credit should be available to physicians who were unable to complete the entire project or who joined late. This structure permitted enhanced credit for those who completed the entire project, an arrangement that resulted in assigning five credits per stage and an additional five credits for completing the whole proj-

ect, for a maximum of 20 credits. (The option to offer partial credit is at the provider's discretion.)

While the steering committee recognized that QI was done in practice and outside the CME office, it also fundamentally believed that patient care and physician professional development would be better served by linking them as a CME certified activity approved, managed, and documented through the CME office. In other words, physicians would not randomly self-report their projects and retrospectively request CME credit. PI CME set a higher standard through the controlled deployment of evidence-based measures in practice assessment with documented participation.

Launching PI CME

PI CME was approved by the AMA Council on Medical Education in fall 2004, with Internet PoC CME adopted in spring 2005. The AMA publicized the new criteria in the CPPD newsletter, other publications, and presentations but did not widely disseminate the information until the 2006 revision of the AMA PRA booklet.

CME providers showed interest in the new format but were not typically involved in QI activities and lacked the skills to develop and promote this new type of CME. They did not have working relationships with the quality initiatives in their organizations. Those involved in QI efforts were either unaware of CME credit or failed to see the value in awarding credit for these activities. Adding CME credit increased administrative burden and cost. The barriers these departmental rigidities present, along with the lack of a shared vocabulary to describe how and what PI CME can do for a hospital, clinic, or practice, have lessened but continue to this day.

At the same time PI CME was being developed, the American Board of Medical Specialties (ABMS) was ramping up its maintenance of certification (MOC) program. The ABMS serves as the parent organization for the 24 medical specialty certifying boards. Until 2001, certifying boards had either lifetime certification or time-limited certification of six to 10 years. MOC imposed four components, including demonstrated PI in practice (Part IV), which closely matched the PI CME requirements.

By 2010 all specialty certifying boards must implement all four components of MOC. The ABMS has further heightened interest in PI CME by announcing required performance improvement modules (PIMs) in patient safety and patient communications in 2010 (with peer-to-peer communications added in 2012). This move to documented practice assessment and performance improvement will continue to drive collaboration between CME and MOC.

Further validation of the PI CME concept came from the ACCME. In 2006, it adopted updated accreditation criteria. The revised model represented a change in emphasis for the ACCME, focusing on rewarding accredited CME providers for moving through levels of accreditation while changing and improving their practice of CME. Practice improvement became the goals for both learners and CME providers.

The Future of PI CME

The correlation with MOC will continue to drive PI CME. The physician's natural impulse for excellence will find a vehicle through PI activities (eligible for CME credit and MOC points), which demonstrably improve practice. Additionally, these activities may qualify for various pay-for-performance programs adopted by both private and government payers. The ultimate goal should be to reward high quality performance in practice.

PoC CME

The ACCME began tracking Internet usage by accredited providers and physicians for CME purposes in 1998. The 1998 ACCME Annual Update reported Internet enduring material usage by accredited providers to be 733 activities, offering 2,023 credits, and involving 21,100 physician participants.[2] By 2002, the numbers had grown substantially, with the ACCME Annual Update reporting accredited providers offering 23,365 activities, 15,387 credits, and engaging 154,542 physician participants—a more than 30-fold increase in offerings and a 10-fold increase in physician participants.[3]

However, another use of the Internet—one closer to their day-to-day patient care needs—was evolving among physicians. The Internet was becoming an effective mechanism to search quickly for information related to patient care. A 2004 article on physician Internet information-seeking behaviors compared survey data collected in December 2002 through January 2003 to a survey conducted in June and July 2001. The comparison showed that the average time physicians used the Internet for clinical information had doubled (4.4 times per month to 8.6 times) and that physician use of the Internet increased from 29 percent to nearly 57 percent (when used to search for information related to a specific patient's care).[4]

The AMA recognized the educational format evolving from the growing use of the Internet for patient care information and also recognized the Internet as an important source of physician learning. In light of such, the AMA Division of CPPD formed a steering committee to lead a pilot project that would assess Internet PoC learning, defined as follows:

> Internet point of care (PoC) CME describes structured, self-directed, online learning by physicians on topics relevant to their clinical practice. Learning for this activity is driven by a reflective process in which physicians must document their clinical question, the sources consulted, and the application to practice.

Errol R. Alden, MD, executive director of the American Academy of Pediatrics, chaired the steering committee. Alden brought extensive CME experience to the task (during this period he would ascend to chair of the ACCME council), and his organization had already implemented *Pedia*Link®, one of the earliest and best physician learning portals. The steering committee first met on December 20, 2000, and its members included Kent Anderson, publishing editor of the *New England Journal of Medicine;* James L. Borland, Jr., MD, AMA Council on Medical Education; Norman Kahn, MD, vice president of education and scientific affairs at AAFP; Kenneth Melmon, MD, chief medical officer of Skolar, Inc.; K. M. Tan, MD, assistant physician-in-chief of the Permanente Medical Group; and John R. Windle, MD, of the health informatics program at the University of Nebraska Medical Center.

The late Ken Melmon, MD, sparked the pilot project. Melmon had been chair of medicine and then associate dean for CME at Stanford. He contacted CPPD to ask whether the AMA would permit AMA PRA Category 1 credit to be awarded to physicians using the university's new PoC system Stanford E-Scholar. As CPPD director, Wentz funneled the concept through the Council on Medical Education. The Council recommended other entities working on similar learning platforms be consulted and evaluated to ensure that any credit system parameters developed for this type of activity were adequately inclusive.

Murray Kopelow, MD, executive director of ACCME, participated in the first meeting, and the ACCME was kept informed as the pilot project evolved the concepts that eventually crystallized as Internet PoC CME. The CPPD staff who served on the Performance Measure Pilot Project also worked on this new project.

Kahn, and later Davis, assumed responsibility for representing and coordinating AAFP input into the development of these CME standards. At their initial meeting, the steering committee members grappled with natural tension between their role as conservators of medical education's traditions (i.e., scholarship, dialogue, and critical thought) and their obligation to manage and integrate highly disruptive technologies; as Melmon put it, "What you want to do is *not have* [emphasis added] to live within the traditional framework of CME."

Looking back across nearly 10 years, the technology has moved through several generations but the challenges of knowledge management remain largely the same. The Medical Matrix project, referenced in the minutes of that first meeting, offered criteria that describe principles for good on-line CME that apply today:

- *Peer review*: Previously evaluated, verifiable, endorsed, dated, current, referenced
- *Application*: Ability to enhance the knowledge database of the target clinician or specialist at the point of care
- *Media*: Text, hypertext, or use of multimedia: images, video, sound in the context of the resource database
- *Feel*: Search features, navigation tools, composition, advanced HTML tools, and integration within a larger database
- *Ease of access*: Clinical content, reliably and intuitively available, across a rapid link (bytes to the page)
- *Dimension*: Size, effort, and importance scaled to the discipline
- *Adult learning principles applied*: Must be self-directed

The Self-Directed/Self-Initiated Internet CME Pilot Project began with the Stanford SHINE project as the first participant; AMA PRA Category 1 credit was awarded under the aegis of the pilot project. Stanford subsequently spun off this initiative, which now operated independently as SKOLAR, MD. Other organizations applied for the project, and three were selected to participate:

- The ACP Physicians' Information and Education Resources (PIER) featured a database of peer-reviewed, evidence-based information, with credit awarded once a clinical decision was made.
- MerckMedicus, which worked as a content aggregating portal under the direction of regional medical directors, offered fairly comprehensive reference materials for

selected specialties; physicians claiming credit under the pilot participated in a brief on-line interview regarding their clinical inquiry.

- UpToDate took its proprietary and independently generated content—fully referenced, brief reviews of the most recent literature, built to quickly answer questions faced by practicing clinicians—and awarded Category 1 credit for the time subscribers spent consulting the database.

Over the several years of the pilot, data accumulated and the steering committee continued to grapple with the issues of what constitutes learning and what should be the metric for this learning modality. In parallel with the experience of the Performance Measure Pilot Project, the group was attempting to determine whether learning should be measured by time invested. Time's role was energetically debated at the outset, and disagreements continued to the end; however, it was Kelley M. Skeff, MD, PhD, a Stanford educator and internist, who stepped in after Melmon's death and parsed the issue and described the group's ultimate consensus:

Time is perhaps a physician's most scarce resource, and an essential one for education, but what I can't escape is how I teach my residents: How did the patient present? What does the literature tell you? *What did you do with the patient?* I just don't know how it can be learning without the last question.

In the end, AMA PRA Category 1 credit and AAFP Prescribed Credit would be awarded not for time on task but for searching on a clinical question and indicating the application to practice. At the pilot's conclusion, this type of CME activity was renamed from SDSI Internet CME to Internet PoC CME. The new name served as an easier handle while still emphasizing the online and clinical care elements that the steering committee believed represented its strength and avenue for future growth. The final AMA PRA

rules were published in January 2006 (the AAFP adopted identical guidance):

Internet point of care (PoC) CME describes structured, self-directed, online learning by physicians on topics relevant to their clinical practice. Learning for this activity is driven by a reflective process in which physicians must document their clinical question, the sources consulted, and the application to practice. To award AMA PRA Category 1 Credit for this activity, accredited providers must assure that they:

- Establish a process that oversees content integrity, with responsibilities that include, but are not limited to, the appropriate use and selection of professional, peer-reviewed literature, and keeping search algorithms unbiased.
- Provide clear instructions to the physician learners on how to access the portal/database, how their online activities will be tracked, and how the provider will award credit for their participation.
- Verify physician participation by tracking the topics and sources searched. Implement reasonable safeguards to assure appropriate use of this information.
- Provide access to some mechanism by which participants can give feedback on overall system effectiveness, and evaluate whether the activity met the participant's learning objectives, or resulted in a change in knowledge, competence, or performance as measured by physician practice application or patient health status improvement.
- Establish a mechanism by which participating physicians may claim AMA PRA Category 1 Credit for this learning cycle, if they:
  Review original clinical question(s).
  Identify the relevant sources from among those consulted.
  Describe the application of their findings to practice.

The credit allocation makes no reference to time spent but does permit an asynchronous relation between the clinical encounter and the learning cycle: "Physicians conducting structured online searches on clinical topics may claim a half (0.5) AMA PRA Category 1 Credit for documented completion (either at the point of care or later) of the three step learning cycle defined above."

As physician-referenced Internet sites grow increasingly sophisticated, the ease with which these resources can assist physicians looking for patient care information has also grown along with the ability to capture PoC CME credits. When PoC CME first joined the ACCME Annual Report in 2005, only one activity (providing one credit) was reported by an accredited provider.[5] By 2007, ACCME accredited providers reported a rapid expansion in PoC CME: 15,556 activities, offering 10,439 credits, with 103,135 physicians participating.

Assigning Credit for PI CME and PoC

As previously mentioned, a major issue in the credit discussions for these new CME formats was whether and how to eliminate the existing time metric for assigning credit. Traditionally, the amount of CME credit was determined by the amount of time it took for a physician to complete an activity. For live, lecture-based CME activities, this was simple. Credit was assigned commensurate with the time it took to complete the activity (subtracting breaks, meals, etc.).

But this was impractical for PI CME and PoC CME. A PI project might take months to complete and a meaningful Internet search less than 15 minutes. Many argued it does not matter how much time it takes, only what practice improvement or improvement in patient care occurs. Even with support to eliminate hours, some harmonization of this new credit type with the state legislated CME requirements in 41 states was needed. The solution: AMA and AAFP agreed to replace the term *credit hours* with *credits*.

Advanced Simulation

Simulation, in one form or another, has always been a part of clinical education. This chapter, however, refers to newer developments in simulation and its usage. Simulation laboratories are growing in number across the country, appearing in medical schools and teaching hospitals, and the American College of Surgeons Division of Education has established standards and criteria for accredited education institutes whose purpose is to enhance patient safety through simulation. Advanced simulators are evolving rapidly and offering better capabilities for recreating complex clinical scenarios and a variety of procedures.

The advanced simulators and simulation laboratories will move CME beyond individual physician assessment. They will create significant potential for improved evaluation of physician and health-care team functioning and communication skills. The ability for enhanced team training during mock operating room procedures, cardiovascular interventions, C-arrests, etc., will allow teams to practice responses to various scenarios, especially those unexpected clinical scenarios.

The developing labs and advanced simulators will allow new opportunities for CME and CPD to explore higher-order clinical reasoning and decision-making. Educators will have new opportunities to develop physician knowledge, skills, and/or attitudes. Advanced simulation will allow the capability to study "reasoning-in-transition," the clinician's ability to recognize and reason about changes in a patient's baseline condition and act upon it; "response-based practice," the ability to apply medical knowledge and respond to the patient within the immediacy of the situation at hand; and "perceptual acuity and skill of involvement," referring to the ability to identify, define, and frame the problem(s) being faced in the patient/simulation scenarios.[6]

At this time, the enhanced capabilities of simulation coupled with the growing availability of simulation laboratories are leading to greater discussion among the accrediting agencies and the specialty boards about the use of simulation in physician training and for MOC requirements. Unlike PI CME and PoC CME, which have their initial guidelines in place, advanced simulation remains a work in progress.

Conclusion

PI CME, PoC CME, and simulation are newer developments in CME and CPD. They offer an exciting, expanded horizon to the CME and CPD professional going forward—which leads us to the question, using Tennyson's verse, What of the yet untravel'd world whose margin moves for ever and for ever when we move?

Notes

1. D. A. Davis and others, "Changing Physician Performance: A Systematic Review of the Effect of Continuing Medical Education Strategies," *Journal of the American Medical Association* 274, no. 9(1995): 700–705.

2. Accreditation Council for Continuing Medical Education, "1998 ACCME Annual Report Data," ACCME Web site, http://www.accme.org/dir_docs/doc_upload/dc316660-2a48-46d4-916f-60334f7527ba_uploaddocument.pdf (accessed July 30, 2010).

3. Accreditation Council for Continuing Medical Education, "2002 ACCME Annual Report Data," ACCME Web site, http://www.accme.org/dir_docs/doc_upload/f94000bf-a188-438f-ad8a-d28aa506d5b0_uploaddocument.pdf (accessed July 30, 2010).

4. N. L. Bennett and others, "Physicians' Internet Information-Seeking Behaviors," *Journal of Continuing Education in the Health Professions* 24, no. 1 (2004): 31–38.

5. Accreditation Council for Continuing Medical Education, "2005 ACCME Annual Report Data," ACCME Web site, http://www.accme.org/dir_docs/doc_upload/9c795f02-c470-4ba3-a491-d288be965eff_uploaddocument.pdf (accessed July 30, 2010).

6. P. Benner and others, "Clinical Wisdom and Interventions in Critical Care; A Thinking-in-Action Approach," in *Clinical Simulation: Operations, Engineering, and Management*, R. R. Kyle, Jr., and W. B. Murray, eds. (Burlington: Elsevier, 2008), 37.

Madeline H. Schmitt, DeWitt C. Baldwin, Jr.,
and Scott Reeves

CHAPTER 26

Continuing Interprofessional Education: Collaborative Learning for Collaborative Practice

This chapter traces the development of continuing interprofessional education (CIPE) and illuminates present challenges and opportunities. Interprofessional education (IPE) in the United States occurred first as informal CIPE, emerging and re-emerging in various forms up to the present day in response to the changing needs of practitioners and, only subsequently, finding its way into undergraduate, graduate, and formal CE. A major question explored in this chapter is why consideration of formal CIPE has been delayed until recently. Some of the forces driving CIPE as an essential component of continuing medical education (CME) for the future are described. In addition, some recent efforts to locate CIPE within the broader arena of IPE and lifelong learning in the health professions are outlined. Finally, CIPE educational and research needs are highlighted.

We prefer the term *interprofessional education* because it is widely used in the fields that we cover, where collaborative learning is practice-based. We reserve *interdisciplinary education* for learning and research between academic disciplines but recognize that the two terms often have been used interchangeably. Where *interdisciplinary* appears in this chapter, it reflects use in its original context.

We use the term *continuing interprofessional education* within the wider definition of *interprofes-*

sional education, defined as "two or more health professions learning with, from and about each other to improve collaboration and the quality of care," widely adopted globally.[1]

The Guild Model of Medicine's Professional Development: Building Silos

Any discussion of the late recognition of the need for formal CIPE in CME must recognize that some of the forces delaying this recognition are the same ones that have delayed, for so long, the acceptance of the very concept and practice of interprofessional collaboration and teamwork in health care. Prominent among these has been the development of specialization and professionalization of health occupations during the past century. Much of this has been influenced by the guild model of professional development. Occupational guilds have a long history of developing and controlling knowledge on behalf of their members' interests. Examples of such guild structures are found in medicine as early as 1505, when the Barber Surgeons of Edinburgh were formally established to restrict the practice of the "craft" of surgery. Guild models were preserved during the professionalization of medicine and its segmentation into specialties in the early twentieth century.[2]

As Garfield has pointed out, at the beginning

of the twentieth century, most physicians practiced by themselves, often in their homes, in a traditional one-to-one relationship with a patient and almost never in concert with other physicians or health workers. Flexner's report established the primacy of the hospital for medical education, where physicians could conduct research to advance the science of medicine simultaneous with the clinical care of patients.[3] With the advent of scientific medicine, practitioners were able to do more for their patients and began to associate and to specialize, with the hospital and medical societies becoming logical places where they could meet and exchange emerging knowledge and skills. The increasing success of hospital-based specialists led to numbers of them congregating into specialty societies, each of which had its own set of knowledge and skills, which they sought to constantly upgrade through postgraduate and continuing education. The idea of certifying qualified members followed. However, providing and/or requiring systematic continuing medical education and certification has firmly established itself only in the past 60 years.

Adoption of Guild Structures by Emerging Professions: The Creation of Educational Silos

Like medicine, other health professions have occupational beginnings extending back in time. However, the growth of hospitals in the twentieth century, coupled with scientific and technological advances, led to an extended range of health services provided, with a concomitant need for the skills and contributions of other health workers. As the latter increased in number, they began to seek greater recognition through enhanced professional status. In their professional development, other occupations emulated the guild model of medicine, including opportunities for advanced, specialized education and CE.[4] Although each health profession and each nation has had a unique trajectory of professionalization and specialization, characteristics of a college or university-based education, identification of an

autonomous scope of practice, and the development of a distinctive knowledge base developed through research have been indicators of professional status shared in common.

Other Factors Impeding Interprofessional Practice and Education

Processes of professionalization and specialization were not the only barriers to the acceptance of interprofessional collaboration and teamwork in health care. A more egalitarian social structure was promoted through movements such as unionism, suffrage, civil rights, feminism, consumerism, and patient rights.[5] Feminism and civil rights challenged the gender and race segregation in the health-care professions, which were mostly homogeneous: Caucasian men in medicine and women in nursing, social work, and most of the allied health disciplines. Although this has been changing, at least in medicine, the former dispositions still frequently obtain at the leadership level. These social movements emphasized an empowering egalitarianism that was also implicit in the underlying philosophy of interprofessional collaboration. This philosophy was quite correctly perceived as a significant threat to medicine's control of health care.

Finally, one of the most powerful and obstinate of all forces in human interaction—professional culture—must be recognized. Educated separately, usually in complete isolation from each other, by teachers firmly dedicated to guarding and preserving the traditions of their field against the claims and inroads of practitioners of the other healing arts, it is no wonder that powerful professional cultures were (and still are) so firmly established by the time health professions students enter the practice arena.

Early Teamwork

As early as 1903, Richard Cabot of the Massachusetts General Hospital expressed concern about the move into hospitals and toward specialization in medicine, which he believed would result in a withdrawal from the community and from the intimate knowledge of patients' lives. To counter the community disconnect, Cabot introduced the role of the social worker into the hospital outpatient clinic in order to insure the continuing knowledge of and contact with the patient's family and community. He spoke enthusiastically of "the teamwork of the doctor, the educator, and the social worker."[6] Through Walter Cannon, the noted physiologist, he met and worked with Ida M. Cannon, a nurse and graduate of Boston (Simmons) School of Social Work, to establish the first hospital medical social work department, at Massachusetts General Hospital.

Cabot's Boston contemporaries, Davis and Warner, also were interested in "the functional interrelations of physician, nurse, social worker, administrator, and others" in medical dispensaries and agreed that, in the shift to hospital centered care, there was "the missing social component," leading them to support the idea of the teamwork of the physician and the social worker.[7]

The unfolding of professional relationships between nursing and medicine requires a separate treatment, but as hospitals expanded, they became the central workplace for nurses. Until after the mid-20th century, preparation for nursing was largely hospital-affiliated. The close working relationship between doctors and nurses led to articles in nursing journals describing the need for teamwork in the hospital. In the beginning, however, those outside of nursing often viewed the rhetoric as less substantive than ideological. In commenting on the early interprofessional teamwork movement in nursing, as well as on the widespread movement of other occupational groups, including social work, toward professional recognition, Brown viewed these as efforts by "ambitious allied fields . . . [using the rubric of teamwork] as a device to level hierarchic distinctions and to make for more egalitarian inter-professional relations."[8]

Some specialties, like surgery, have always re-quired the assistance of others in their work, and these took on some of the characteristics of teams and teamwork. These developments, starting in the 1940s, led to the beginning of multi-professional teams organized around special conditions or diseases, such as cleft palate or diabetes, that clearly called for (and benefited from) the input of multiple specialists. These teams, however, were based primarily in hospitals and clinics where the specialists were located and frequently were hierarchical in nature, seldom developing truly interactional, interprofessional teamwork.

The idea of working more interprofessionally in teams to deliver needed complex specialty care emerged in rehabilitation medicine in the 1940s. One of the first published reviews of outcomes of interprofessional team-based care, spanning 25 years, was by a rehabilitation physician.[9] About the same time, the mid-1970s, Rosalie Kane, a social worker, published her classic review of interprofessional teamwork in the health field. She reviewed 229 published articles and books on the topic, 41 percent of them interprofessional in authorship. She was strongly critical of the use of the terms *interdisciplinary* and *team*, proposing in their place the terms *interprofessional* and *teamwork*.[10]

Interprofessional Teams and Ambulatory Care

The issue of providing care that was more integrated with social needs and community context, identified early in the century as being problematic by Cabot, led to a number of post–World War II initiatives to respond to needs related to comprehensive health care for families, patients with long-term chronic conditions, and the underserved. In 1949, Martin Cherkasky, based in a group medical practice at the Montefiore Hospital in New York City, described sending teams of physicians, nurses, and social workers on home visits into the community to care for their chronically ill patients. George Silver also utilized teams of physicians, nurses, and social workers to provide care for patients enrolled in his Family Health Maintenance Demonstration Project. With the support of the Commonwealth Fund, the idea of promoting such comprehensive care was adopted by 32 leading academic health centers by 1959.[11]

Team Care of the Urban and Rural Underserved: The Beginnings of CIPE

The late 1960s and 1970s marked what Brown has referred to as the period of "high tide" for health-care team initiatives.[12] Under President Johnson's "War on Poverty" program, community health centers were created to meet primary health care needs in urban and rural underserved areas. The concept of primary health-care teams working together interprofessionally, adding newly created community health outreach workers, was central to the program. Stating that "ways should be sought to develop, train and utilize a health team," the Office of Economic Opportunity sponsored four team seminars in Washington, DC, in the winter of 1968–1969.[13]

Lack of experience with working in primary care teams led to an initial sense of frustration. Harold Wise of the Martin Luther King Health Center in New York City consulted with Richard Beckhard of the Sloan School of Management at MIT, whose group began to write extensively on the subject and came up with specific modules for team training and a new vocabulary, inherited from the emerging fields of organizational development and group dynamics. These modules offered specific directions for training teams to deal with issues like leadership, decision-making, task definition, and role conflict, surely a nascent form of CE in this new method of health-care delivery. Simultaneously, David Kindig and his group at Montefiore Hospital started the Institute for Health Team Development, which began to provide consultation, conferences and a newsletter for aspiring teams. This work included the

creation of a prototype private practice featuring a practicing interprofessional team.[14]

Many other developments to address the growing problem of access to community-based primary and comprehensive care were also occurring. From 1960 to 1980, 40 new medical schools were developed, many responding, at least in part, to the need to educate more physicians to provide primary care. New professional roles, designed to partner with physicians to extend physician resources and to provide health promotion and disease prevention in the community, were being created. Eugene Stead, MD, worked with Thelma Ingles, a nurse educator at Duke University, to promote advanced educational programs in nursing. When this failed, Stead then succeeded in the creation of the physician assistant role through the advanced training of ex-military corpsmen. Henry Silver, MD, and Loretta Ford, a public health nurse educator at the University of Colorado, created the nurse practitioner role.[15] These programs began as CIPE programs.

Sparked by the community health center movement, the period of the 1970s marked a groundswell of what might be thought of as early CIPE, with a number of books, articles, and training manuals proliferating on the subject of the dynamics of interdisciplinary health delivery teams. These served as an emerging new format for CE for practitioners. Notable among these was the monograph by Alberta Parker, which described diverse models for primary care teams and discussed methods for their implementation.[16]

The Emergence of Undergraduate IPE

One specific outgrowth of the ferment in interprofessional practice in primary care during this period was to focus attention on training future generations of health professionals for interprofessional teamwork. In 1972, the Institute of Medicine (IOM) convened a conference on "Educating for the Health Team: The Interrelationships of Educational Programs for Health Professionals." Chaired by Edmund Pellegrino and an 11-member steering committee representing nursing, medicine, pharmacy, dentistry, and allied health, the conference, in its report, arrived at the first limited definition of *interdisciplinary education*: "an educational experience can be interdisciplinary at the level of students, at the level of faculty, or at both levels."[17]

Concurrently, David Kindig established the Office of Interdisciplinary Programs in the Bureau of Health Manpower in Washington, DC, where separate programs funded family practice trainees, nurse practitioners, physician assistants, and others, including expanded funding for allied health professions. Between 1974 and 1979, 20 university medical centers were funded specifically for training pre-professional and health professions students in interdisciplinary team training programs. Unfortunately, federal funding for these efforts dried up by 1980, and these kinds of programs virtually ceased, except for a few. However, through several Part D, Title VII programs in the Public Health Service Act, HRSA developed and continues to fund a number of interdisciplinary, community-based programs directed at increasing the number of health professionals caring for vulnerable and underserved rural and urban populations. These include the Area Health Education Centers (AHECs), the Health Education Training Centers, the Geriatric Education Centers, Allied Health Special Projects, and the Burdick Program for Rural Interdisciplinary Training. Many of these programs developed their own curricula and training manuals.

In the 1970s, as AHECs evolved, some institutions opened CE offices for the health professions. For example, the University of Illinois at Urbana-Champaign served physicians, nurses, pharmacists, social workers, and librarians throughout the state in federally supported programs in underserved areas. Many health professionals shared common educational activities, but a collaborative, team-based educational program was not a focus during this time.[18] As funding streams for higher education declined, by the 1980s many of these university-based programs closed. However, to this day, evidence of CE programming remains a criterion for funding the AHECs.

The Annual Interdisciplinary Health Care Team Conferences

The earlier HRSA funding for interprofessional health professions education programs led to another development. In 1976, attendees at a landmark conference at Snowbird, Utah, heard first reports from a number of these programs. The success of this conference led to a second conference in 1979, which was followed by a series of national, annual conferences that broadened the focus of the previous two and came to be known as the annual Interdisciplinary Health Care Team Conferences.[19] Operating with a volunteer national steering committee, these conferences continued for 23 years, providing a place for health professionals interested in interprofessional health-care teams to meet and present papers each year on their teamwork and team training experiences. The attendees and specific presentations reflected the cycles of interest emerging from practice. The bulk of presentations were focused on the methods and processes of team delivery of care, and often were hospital-based, with a vast majority of papers being focused on practitioners.

Until 1994, these papers were published as uncopyrighted proceedings and probably constitute the single largest compilation of information concerning the beginnings of this field in the United States. Although these annual conferences cannot be considered formal CIPE in the current sense, they were in fact the major method by which persons and institutions interested in IPE and collaborative practice from 1980 to nearly the present were able to learn from the experience of others in this field.

Interprofessional Teamwork in Geriatrics

Over time, the literature reflects recurring cycles of interest in interprofessional teams emerging in mental health, intensive care, geriatrics, and hospice and palliative care, to name a few, based on a recognition of the contributions of a variety of health professions to addressing the clinical needs of patients and families. Geriatrics is one of the medical specialty areas where interprofessional practice is viewed as fundamental to the comprehensive and often complex chronic care needed for this vulnerable population. In the late 1970s and early 1980s, the Veterans Health Administration (VHA) initiated the first large-scale team-based care in hospital settings when it created the "Interdisciplinary Team Training in Geriatrics" (ITTG) program and appointed team trainers at 12 hospital demonstration sites, each of which was to provide training resources to other VHA hospitals as well as its own. Team-based geriatric care was provided in Geriatric Evaluation and Management Units, nursing homes, hospital-based home care (now home-based primary care), and adult day health-care programs using protocols developed and monitored by the VHA Central Office. Based on their experience, trainers collaborated to produce the first book-length compendium of measures to assess team performance in health care.[20] Although the ITTG program per se no longer exists, it provided impetus for the evolution of team-based care and workplace team training throughout the Department of Veterans Affairs health-care system (e.g., the home based primary care program).[21] These team-based programs throughout the system served as training sites for VHA-sponsored interprofessional student training.

Other team-training efforts in geriatrics followed the VHA experience. Starting in 1995, the John A. Hartford Foundation supported a national eight-site demonstration project—Geriatric Interdisciplinary Team Training (GITT)—to introduce geriatric team training outside the VHA system. Training materials were developed by the demonstration sites. Although GITT was designed primarily to prepare health professions students, some of the demonstration sites trained practitioners who would be role models for students. In 2000, the John A. Hartford Foundation directed its training efforts specifically to practitioners in the five-site Geriatric Interdisciplinary Teams in Practice Program to test innovative models of team-based geriatric care.[22]

Some Factors Contributing to a Lack of Mainstreaming of Early CIPE and IPE

It is clear that CIPE training efforts repeatedly emerged in informal fashion in practice settings, but by the late 1990s such training had yet to be formalized. The cyclical emergence of interest in and use of health care teams during the latter half of the 20th century without mainstreaming CIPE or IPE attests to the difficulty of overcoming the centripetal forces of professionalization and specialization in the education of health professionals. A number of other factors are also important to consider in this lack of mainstreaming.

In the larger arena of CME, professional silos in practice were solidified further in the late 1970s and 1980s with the mandatory continuing education movement. Two forces created this regulatory environment for health professionals. Rapidly increasing scientific research findings with implications for professional practice was referred to as the *knowledge explosion*, bringing recognition that one half of knowledge acquired during professional education would be obsolete in five years. For the first time, professionals could no longer be considered competent for life, and the concept of formal CE for all professionals gained favor.

Second, by the 1970s, a general mistrust of traditional institutions, public services, and professional expertise was taking hold as a result of events such as the Watergate scandals and the end of the Vietnam War. This increased scrutiny of professional performance created an environment for more regulation of institutions, occupational groups, and professions, including in health. During this era, state legislatures passed mandatory licensure requirements, often 15 hours of formal CE annually. Many professional societies followed suit in the certification arena. New infrastructures in academic institutions and professional associations codified the continuing education unit (CEU).

These regulations had several impacts. Continuing education became a business and industry rather than an informal activity of an individual profession, further decoupling education and clinical practice performance. Professionals were rewarded for *seat time*, most often equated with passive listening to experts updating new information in conferences and other meetings. Physicians, nurses, pharmacists, and other health professionals sought their educational opportunities where they were rewarded in their own separate professional venues.

Also during this time, a few academic programs in adult education at research universities invested in the nascent scholarly field of professional CE. The Kellogg Foundation funded research in adult and CE as well as centers for adult learners on university campuses. Doctoral programs in this field evolved in universities such as the University of Illinois at Urbana-Champaign, the University of Wisconsin–Madison, the University of Georgia, the University of Oklahoma, and Pennsylvania State University. Scholars at these institutions partnered with professionals to generate theory and research regarding educational strategies for professional performance. In 1979, these programs were highlighted in a seminal text by Kockelmans as part of a larger consideration of interdisciplinarity in higher education. In 1980, Houle published *Continuing Learning in the Professions*, a seminal contribution to guide the design of professional CE.[23]

In the 1980s, the Kellogg Foundation refocused away from CE and adult learners. As state and national funding for higher education declined, colleges of education focused more narrowly on education at the K–12 level, diverting funding away from many adult and CE programs. Mandatory CE requirements did not reward innovation in educational design. Therefore, the number of scholars in professional CE who were academically prepared and university based declined. The most robust area of scholarship that endured over time focused on CME, either situated in or closely aligned with university and professional association CE.

Another factor was that, with the exception of the hospital-based work in the VHA, early CIPE efforts occurred largely outside of the hospital, in underserved rural or urban communities. Physicians in these practice settings involved in participating in and advocating for interprofessional training had limited internal professional political leverage. Undergraduate medical education was primarily hospital-based and taught by basic scientists and medical specialists who valued clinical education less as their research moved them more and more into laboratory settings.[24] Additionally, to the extent that the development of the primary care nurse practitioner role was associated with the interest in IPE, including CIPE, there was a predictable push-back from medical organizations. None of the early IPE efforts appear to have impacted a large or powerful enough sector of the health-care system or health professions educational programs to grab the attention or the resources necessary to institute formal IPE at any educational level more widely.

Another factor in the lack of mainstreaming was the limited evidence of outcomes of team-based care. Following emergence of interprofessional practice in primary care during the 1960s and 1970s, teamwork in health care entered what Brown called the "period of re-evaluation."[25] Practice in interprofessional teams required considerable effort with no professional preparation; workplace training was ad hoc and generally not administratively supported. Documenting the outcomes of interprofessional practice was challenging.[26] Practitioners who engaged in team training to improve their delivery of care made a personal investment and frequently sacrificed recognition and advancement in their own profession. And, health professions students who received team training found themselves, after graduation, practicing in settings that were not designed to foster teamwork and team-based practice in the delivery of care.

One fateful consequence of the erratic funding and volunteer approach to CIPE, IPE, and team-based practice was the failure to develop an overarching national organization with a recognized professional voice, such as a journal. In fact, participants at the Interdisciplinary Health Care Team Conferences took some pride in being a part of a minimalist organization, governed only by a steering committee, with hosts at a different university each year and, eventually, a volunteer site planner to provide continuity from one meeting to the next.

Finding journals whose mission encompassed IPE or team-based care was problematic. To address this issue the attendees at the Interdisciplinary Health Care Team Conferences circulated their uncopyrighted proceedings among participants until 1994, when the *Journal of Interprofessional Care*, based in the United Kingdom, was identified as a place to submit papers for publication consideration. In contrast, in 1967, the allied health professions established the Association of Schools of Allied Health Professions, with the *Journal of Allied Health* following in 1972.

Finally, a major factor has been the lack of recognition of the importance of educating practitioners and health professions students in the processes of teamwork and collaborative care delivery. All of the health professions have a clear focus on the rapidly changing scientific knowledge and the technical skills related to specific disease conditions for which they claim care responsibility and feel obliged to maintain and update themselves through CE. There are books and courses on specific conditions about which practitioners can be tested and expected to be current.

In interprofessional practice, clinical input to the team is expected to come from the participating professionals.

Although interprofessional care delivery is also driven by a clinical focus, such as primary or geriatric care, teamwork and team approaches to care are primarily a philosophy and set of methods for working together. The focus is on andragogical, or adult, learning strategies and methods; more on process and relationships than on content and techniques. The work of the team is to coordinate, integrate, and utilize knowledge and skills in new, more creative, and efficient ways. This requires interaction and reflection about the issues of primary interest to teamwork processes, such as leadership, shared goals, role definition, conflict resolution, and shared decision-making. In early training efforts this was the stuff of time-consuming and labor-intensive group process and was mediated by workshops and in-service learning, under the guidance of trainers and consultants.

The early guidance for team training, then, was embedded in limited distribution conference reports and proceedings, consultations, workshops, group discussion and decision-making, personal and professional observations, training manuals and exercises, books, and book chapters. In the early period of intense interest in interprofessional team-based delivery of health care, between 1969 and 1975, some 18 books appeared in the United States with titles bearing the terms *team* or *teamwork* in health care.

Re-Emergence of CIPE and IPE in the Context of Quality and Safety Issues

In the 1990s, another round of reports called for transformation of health professions education, which included recommendations to incorporate interprofessional learning.[27] However, it has been quality and safety issues emerging from practice that, by all appearances, have done what no other cycle of interest in interprofessional practice and education has done in the past; bring the professions, the health-care system, the business and financial communities, the government, and the public together in a search for ways to improve quality of care and prevent and mitigate medical errors, in part through improved teamwork and team-based care models.

Quality and safety are different and competing problems, which are often conflated. Quality "is a health care state to be achieved" and "is associated with evidence regarding how to carry out care to achieve the best health outcomes and high patient satisfaction." Safety, on the other hand, is an "emergent process . . . associated with awareness and anticipation of more or less latent flaws in otherwise apparently 'good' processes (whether intra- or inter-professional, devices and technologies, or policies and procedures, etc.)"[28] However, ensuring each has been identified as requiring effective communication and teamwork within and across the health professions.[29]

This present cycle, which continues to unfold, has similarities to previous ones, but also differences that suggest we are in an era of fundamental change in how the health professions deliver health care and are educated across the continuum from undergraduate to CE. Compared to earlier, clinically specific cycles, issues of quality and safety are broad concerns highlighted in numerous IOM reports.[30] Unlike earlier periods, the quality and safety agendas have been introduced by powerful medical leaders focused on hospital settings, such as the leaders of the Institute for Healthcare Improvement, the Joint Commission, and the National Quality Forum, who have created voluntary learning opportunities, regulatory expectations, and standards for improvement in areas related to communication and teamwork.

Frameworks, theories, empirical data, research, and teamwork interventions have been drawn from business, aviation, organizational development, and group dynamics, education, and relevant academic disciplines, such as psychology and sociology. Efforts to develop evidence for the links between team-based care,

teamwork processes and outcomes of care, costs, and patient and provider satisfaction have multiplied and have produced important evidence for best practices, especially in hospital settings, providing the basis for targeted workplace CIPE for quality and safety.

There is overlap with, as well as significant expansion of, the content related to team functioning with earlier CIPE initiatives and research. However, the amount of attention currently being given to the creation of national, accessible training programs, such as the Medical Team Training Program in the VHA; the IHI Open School for health professions students; and the Agency for Healthcare Research and Quality and Department of Defense–developed TeamSTEPPS for practitioners (and increasingly for health professions curricula), and widespread university-based initiatives suggest a "sea-change" in the role of IPE and CIPE for the future. Intensive effort is being devoted to identifying outcomes that are sensitive to teamwork improvements.[31]

From an interprofessional perspective, two key outcomes of the attention to quality and safety have been (1) the acceptance of the importance of health professions education focused on the processes of care delivery as well as clinical care and (2) the examination of interprofessional team-based learning in the context of large and complex health-care institutions. This has led to new ways of thinking about teamwork processes at the microsystem level as well as larger organizational culture change.[32] The implications of these two differences are playing out not only in workplace learning, but across the educational continuum, with CIPE generated from these practice issues creating demands for change in both undergraduate and graduate health professions education, as well as within their many oversight bodies.

There is no doubt that health-care quality and safety are compelling agendas for IPE and CIPE. However, as history indicates, there are other compelling agendas for IPE going forward—in primary care including prevention; in comprehensive care for chronic illness; in a myriad of medical specialties; and in addressing access to care needs for the rural and urban poor. The care problems that propelled interprofessional practice and CIPE in the first place have not disappeared, and some are worse now than they were 40 to 50 years ago.

There is another difference in this cycle. The methods for effective IPE have expanded greatly, and there is mounting evidence for best practices. Health professions educators need to become proficient at pedagogies and andragogies that facilitate effective integration of the knowledge and skills related to teamwork and team-based health care across the continuum of learning, with undergraduate interprofessional learning providing fundamental knowledge and skills that are applied in beginning practice—e.g., for medicine, during residency and fellowship training. Refinements take place in workplace CIPE, with applications appropriate to the settings and specific models of interprofessional care.

Recent CIPE Developments in the United States

Learning side by side (i.e., with, but not from or about, each other) has become more common in CE and gives recognition to the relevance of the same clinical content to practitioners in multiple professions. However, because of educational silos, this has meant that multiple CE accreditors need to accredit the same continuing education events, making for unnecessary duplication. Since the late 1990s, continuing education accreditors across three health professions—medicine, nursing, and pharmacy—have been considering collaboration, seeing if there are ways they can align requirements and systems.[33] These efforts have created the context for more complex discussions related to CIPE.

The Role of Accrediting Bodies in Fostering CIPE and Interprofessional Competency Assessment

In the IOM's report on quality in health care, a section dealing with regulation of the professions focused mostly on licensure and scope-of-practice issues as limiting a variety of innovations to improve care, including the use of interprofessional teams.[34] However, there was also consideration of the lack of consistent methods for ensuring continuing competency.

Another IOM report on integrating five core competencies into all health professionals' education, including working in interdisciplinary teams, emphasized health professions oversight processes as critical to ensuring these competencies at the pre-licensure, initial licensure, and, to some extent, the graduate level.[35] Discussion about ensuring continuing competence included not only maintenance of licensure issues, but also certification and the role of CE in competence assessment. A problem highlighted was that program faculty, and a myriad of oversight bodies across educational levels, work separately, redundantly, with varying effectiveness and, sometimes, at cross-purposes. This led to the following recommendation:

accreditation bodies should move forward expeditiously to revise their standards so that programs are required to demonstrate—through process and outcome measures—that they educate students in both graduate and continuing education programs in how to deliver patient care using a core set of competencies. In so doing, these bodies should coordinate their efforts.[36]

Following the preparation of a white paper with a set of recommendations to improve health professional education and practice, The Joint Commission and Joint Commission Resources, Inc., held a national symposium in 2005: "Transforming Health Professions Education." This was the first national "follow-up" meeting recommended at the IOM health professions education summit (Recommendation 10).[37] The purposes of this meeting were to engage educators, practitioners, regulatory and accrediting bodies, and professional associations in four health professions—medicine, nursing, pharmacy, and health systems leadership/administration—as well as payers, in a consensus-building process around the IOM core competencies, and enlist participants as change agents in implementation of the core competencies at all educational levels. One session by leaders of the four professions was focused on creating a learning continuum. A change objective for that session was "incorporat[ing] the interdisciplinary approach in continuing professional development."[38]

The Role of the Accreditation Council for Continuing Medical Education

In 2002, coincident with the IOM health professions education summit, the Accreditation Council for Continuing Medical Education (ACCME) appointed a Task Force on Competency and the Continuum. ACCME was represented at the educational summit, as were many health professions organizations involved with licensure, accreditation, and certification.

As a result of this overlap, the ACCME Task Force recommendations included a variety of proposed collaborative activities with the American Nurses Credentialing Center (ANCC) and Accreditation Council for Pharmacy Education (ACPE). These activities included identification of common terms, definitions, and shared values/standards, and exploration of the feasibility of a pilot project involving joint accreditation of "interdisciplinary/multi-professional CE."[39] Recommendations also included possible joint research on the effectiveness of accreditation for fostering effective CE. The ACCME board of directors accepted these recommendations.

In 2005, the ACCME was one of the participants in the Joint Commission and Joint Commission Resources cosponsored symposium where the ACCME work related to joint accreditation was presented in the session on creating a learning continuum. In late 2006 and early 2007, both the ACPE and the ANCC adopted the ACCME Standards for Commercial Support.[40]

Early in 2009, ACCME, ANCC, and ACPE published a process for joint provider accreditation of CE for health-care teams that had been approved by all three organizations.[41] Drawing from the Pew Health Professions Commission, this approach had been suggested in the IOM report on health-care quality in order to create an additional level of oversight "in which teams of practitioners, in addition to individuals, would be licensed or certified to perform certain tasks."[42]

The Josiah Macy, Jr. Foundation Recommendations for Reform in CME

In 2007, the Josiah Macy, Jr. Foundation sponsored the conference "Continuing Education in the Health Professions: Improving Healthcare through Lifelong Learning." Nursing was explicitly included with medicine—and education—because "all health professions are facing similar or analogous problems."[43] CIPE was introduced in a section on "Education in the Practice Years: Using Continuing Education to Improve Collaboration and Teamwork." It was noted that physicians and nurses already often learn side by side in CE that is focused on clinical care issues and that both formal CE and informal workplace CE present ideal opportunities for learning interprofessional care management. Several CE formats were suggested, as well as that the interprofessional learning should be judged by improvements in quality and safety of health care in systems of care. In her conference summary, the chairman noted that currently CE does not promote teamwork, interprofessional collaboration in practice, or efforts to improve systems of care. Conclusions drawn from the conference relevant to CIPE included that CE must address the special learning needs of the health-care team; that quality improvement efforts and CE activities overlap and reinforce one another, including CIPE; that accrediting bodies across the professions need to partner to create opportunities for CIPE; that a national interprofessional institute should be created to advance the science of CE, including discovering and fostering effective and efficient ways to conduct CIPE; and that the ACCME and ANCC should develop "a vision and plan for a single accreditation organization for both nursing and medicine."[44]

Two additional events have followed from this major report. The Josiah Macy, Jr. Foundation funded the follow-up conference "Promoting Lifelong Learning in Medicine and Nursing: From Research to Practice" early in 2009, co-organized by the Association of American Medical Colleges and the American Association of Colleges of Nursing. The purpose was to discuss how the findings of the 2007 conference might be formulated into recommendations and strategies for implementation. The conference focused on four major themes: CE methods; workplace learning, with special attention to point-of-care learning; CIPE; and lifelong learning. This conference was preceded by draft white papers and was followed by reformulation of those in the context of a second report titled "Lifelong Learning in Medicine and Nursing."[45] Report recommendations included (1) the integration of IPE at all levels of learning, including design and implementation of CIPE programs specific to work settings; (2) the development and assessment of interprofessional competencies by oversight bodies in conjunction with health professions organizations; (3) creation of outcomes-oriented CIPE learning strategies by CE providers, faculty members, and certification and CE accreditation bodies; and (4) incorporation of CIPE experiences, including performance feedback, into standards and policies of health-care institutions' accrediting and regulatory bodies.[46]

One recommendation to emerge from the first Macy conference was to create a national interprofessional CE institute to advance the science of CE. Subsequently, this recommendation was considered by an international, interprofessional IOM committee, which has recently released its report. The IOM committee noted that continuing professional development is an ideal context for interprofessional learning for practice and that it can play a role in transforming practice cultures toward more collaborative care. Four goals for a Continuing Professional Development Institute related to CIPE would be to (1) provide a clear rationale for CIPE, (2) promote it from the perspective of patient-centered care, (3) address differences among the professions while emphasizing collaborative competencies, and (4) work with credentialing agencies to enhance evaluation of interprofessional activities in the credentialing process for each of the health professions.[47]

Locating CIPE within the Broader Arenas of CME, IPE, and Lifelong Learning

In these recent reports, the nature of what CME and health professions education will be for the future is being re-conceptualized to broaden the types of learning methods and locations for learning—such as the workplace and point of care—as well as incorporate interprofessional learning.[48] The models being proposed formalize the type of informal learning that characterized the early period of CIPE, that is, practitioners from different professions learning how to work in teams collaboratively in the workplace to improve their delivery of care. Increasingly, the education needed is being conceptualized as a continuum of learning from pre-professional through CE for practitioners in a lifelong learning model.[49] CIPE should be built on and complementary to the interprofessional training provided at undergraduate and graduate levels. Until this is achieved, much of CIPE will remain basic and remedial, making up for what was not provided earlier rather than refining basic knowledge and experience in its specific applications to varying workplace settings and models.

CIPE Considerations Going Forward

In this last part of the chapter we explore a range of CIPE trends that have emerged that will need to be addressed to formalize, standardize, and expand CIPE. For this part of the chapter, we draw primarily on a special collection of CIPE papers published in 2009 in the *Journal of Continuing Education for the Health Professions*.

A Clear Conceptualization for CIPE

Despite the publication of increasing amounts of IPE, CIPE, interprofessional collaboration (IPC), and teamwork articles, chapters, and texts, a lack of conceptual clarity remains about these different terms. It appears that authors continue to blur CIPE (as a learning activity) with IPC (as a practice-based activity) into a single interprofessional phenomenon. Although the division between learning and practicing can, at times, be difficult to establish, collapsing these activities with little regard for the differences that exist between them is problematic. This poor conceptualization is particularly challenging when attempting to distinguish the different outcomes each of these different interprofessional activities can produce.[50]

Recent work by Barr provides a helpful anatomy of CIPE. He outlined how different approaches have been employed and compared them with different forms of pre- and postlicensure IPE.[51] He discussed the roles formal CIPE (e.g., university-based workshops) and informal CIPE (e.g., quality improvement initiatives) have played. He also described the variety of formats in which CIPE can be delivered, such as in seminars and conferences, as well as the range of learning methods (e.g., self-directed, distance, or e-learning) that can be drawn upon in the delivery of CIPE.

Goldman et al. have explored these conceptual issues but expanded their focus to help illuminate the nuances that exist between CIPE and IPC.[52] Drawing upon the findings of a review of more than 100 different interprofessional invention studies, these authors described how they categorized them into three separate interprofessional interventions—education-based, practice-based, and organization-based—to help improve the clarity of distinctions between these inter-

related activities. In their categorization, they also developed a framework to distinguish the nature of the different interventions, participants, objectives, and outcomes. They argued that greater clarity of the design, development, and implementation of these different interprofessional interventions will result in a better understanding of the role and effectiveness of CIPE as well as IPE and IPC.

The Increasing Role of Theory in CIPE

The use of theory can provide a more complex understanding of phenomena that are not easily explained, such as why organizations function and how professionals in teams interact in certain ways. Despite these benefits, CIPE has tended not to draw explicitly upon theory in its design and development. This situation is beginning to be addressed. There are a number of theoretical approaches that can be useful incorporated into the design and development of CIPE programs. Recent work by Sargeant has helpfully demonstrated how the application of social and educational theory can generate insightful accounts for CIPE. Sargeant discussed how systems' approaches (complexity theory in particular) and educational theory (reflective learning and situated learning) can illuminate the nature of CIPE and provide tools to inform and guide the development of CIPE programs. Wilcock and colleagues[53] have applied social learning theory to health-care improvement and CIPE.

The Use of Information Technology in CIPE

In the past 20 years we have seen an expansion in the use of information technology systems across public and private sectors. This expansion has led to the development of several forms of electronic media with the potential for delivering education in innovative ways. Like other forms of education, the use of these technologies offers important potential for CIPE. They can support health care practitioners to work and learn together over both time and space in a more flexible, open, and creative manner. Many recent examples exist of how CIPE programs have embraced information technology to ensure it can be delivered in a variety of interactive synchronous and asynchronous formats. A helpful recent example is offered by Luke et al., who describe how they employed a Web-based online CIPE format to encourage virtual interaction between practitioners, which in turn fostered the creation of an interprofessional learning community.[54]

The Assessment of CIPE

Despite the central importance of the assessment of learning within CIPE, it has received relatively little serious attention. As a result, while a range of assessment approaches have been employed (e.g., team presentations, team posters, written assignments), most have little validity, reliability, and documented educational impact. It is, therefore, encouraging to see that this shortfall is being addressed, and, as a result, a small number of more comprehensive assessment approaches and tools are beginning to be created. Reviewing these recent developments in the assessment of CIPE, Simmons and Wagner have argued that a number of key issues need to be included when developing a valid CIPE assessment.[55] For example, the use of assessment blueprints can enhance the rigor of the assessment. They also discuss the use of multiple assessment methods and how simulation can be a key method to assess CIPE.

The Need for Faculty Development

Throughout the earlier high water mark of IPE for health professions students in the 1970s, attention was focused on faculty development and training.[56] However, in general, the IPE and CIPE literature has concentrated on describing and discussing a range of learner-focused issues.[57] As a result, although the literature can provide detailed accounts of learners' experiences, relatively little is known about faculty perspectives. Importantly, there is limited knowledge about how to support faculty in order to prepare them for facilitating CIPE programs. Indeed, as interprofessional friction can emerge within CIPE faculty when professional boundaries are infringed, for example, faculty require effective preparation for this role. A recent article provides a helpful account of the issues related to faculty development for CIPE.[58] These authors argue that faculty development is needed to enhance skills to facilitate CIPE in an effective manner. They offer a planning guide, and suggestions for a curriculum, teaching strategies, and tools for planning CIPE faculty development, including use of a theoretically informed approach to curriculum design.

Summary and Conclusions

Continuing interprofessional education is the earliest form of IPE and emerged informally in response to the desire of practitioners to improve their ability to work together across the professions in the delivery of health care. Many factors, reviewed in this chapter, have worked against its integration into CME. The emergence of the quality and safety movements in health care, and the recognition of the role of improved interprofessional teamwork in both of these arenas, have drawn attention to the importance of integrating IPE into preparation for the delivery of health care. New paradigms for and approaches to CE, in the context of lifelong learning, are creating opportunities for the formalization of CIPE as part of IPE and CME going forward. Some key issues needing consideration as part of this formalization include greater clarity about what CIPE is, the preparation of faculty to offer CIPE, the development of the knowledge base related to CIPE through greater integration of theory and evidence of effectiveness, how the effectiveness of CIPE can be assessed, and how the use of educational technologies can contribute to the effectiveness of CIPE.

Notes

1. "Interprofessional Education: The Definition, 2002," CAIPE Web site, http://www.caipe.org.uk/about-us/defining-ipe/ (accessed January 19, 2010); J. Yan and others, "World Health Organization Study Group on Interprofessional Education and Collaborative Practice," *Journal of Interprofessional Care.* 21 (2007): 588–589; World Health Organization, *Framework for Action on Interprofessional Education and Collaborative Practice* (Geneva, Switzerland: WHO Press, 2010).

2. S. Reeves and others, "Leadership within Interprofessional Health and Social Care Teams: A Socio-Historical Analysis of Key Trials and Tribulations," *Journal of Nursing Management* 18 (2010): 258–264; L. Barker, "The Specialist and the General Practitioner: Teamwork in Medical Practice," *Journal of the American Medical Association* 78, no. 11 (1922): 773–779.

3. S. Garfield, "The Delivery of Medical Care," *Scientific American* 222 (1970): 15–23; A. Flexner, *Medical Education in the United States and Canada: A Report to the Carnegie Foundation for the Advancement of Teaching* (New York: Carnegie Foundation for the Advancement of Teaching, 1910); M. Cook and others, "American Medical Education 100 Years after the Flexner Report," *New England Journal of Medicine* 355, no. 13 (2008): 1339–1344.

4. J. Gilbert, "Abraham Flexner and the Roots of Interprofessional Education," *Journal of Continuing Education in the Health Professions* 28, no. S1 (2008): 11–14.

5. D. Baldwin, "Territoriality and Power in the Health Professions," *Journal of Interprofessional Care* 21, no. S1 (2007): 97–107.

6. R. Cabot, *Social Service and the Art of Healing* (New York: Moffart, Yard and Company, 1915).

7. M. Davis and A. R. Warner, *Dispensaries, Their Management and Development* (New York: The Macmillan Company, 1918).

8. T. Brown, "A Historical View of Health Care Teams," in *Responsibility in Health Care*, ed. G. J. Agich (Boston: D. Reidel Publishing, 1982).

9. L. Halstead, "Team Care in Chronic Illness: A Critical Review of the Literature of the Past 25 Years," *Archives of Physical Medicine and Rehabilitation,* 57 (1976): 507–511.

10. R. Kane, *Interprofessional Teamwork* (Manpower monograph no. 8: Syracuse University Press, 1975).

11. M. Cherkasky, "The Montefiore Hospital Home Care Program," *American Journal of Public Health* 39 (1949): 163–166; G. Silver, "Beyond General Practice: The Health Team," *Yale Journal of Biology and Medicine* 31

(1958): 29–38; G. Silver, *Family Medical Care: A Design for Health Maintenance* (Cambridge, Mass.: Ballinger Publishing Co., 1974); G. Reader and R. Soave, "Comprehensive Care Revisited," *Milbank Memorial Fund Quarterly* 37 (1976): 391–414.

12. Brown, "Health Care Teams."

13. Office of Economic Opportunity, *An Introductory Guide to Training Neighborhood Residents in Comprehensive Health Service Programs* (OEO Pamphlet 6128-7, 1970).

14. H. Wise and others, eds., *Making Health Teams Work* (Cambridge, Mass.: Ballinger Publishing Co., 1974); R. Beckhard, "Optimizing Team Building Efforts," *Journal of Contemporary Business* 1, no. 3 (1972): 23–32; I. M. Rubin and others, *Improving the Coordination of Care: A Program of Health Team Development* (Cambridge, Mass.: Ballinger Publishing Co., 1975); D. Kindig, "Interdisciplinary Education for Primary Care Team Delivery," *Journal of Medical Education* 50 (1975): 97–110.

15. J. Schofield, *New and Expanded Medical Schools, Mid-century to the 1980s,* (Washington: Jossey-Bass Publishers, 1984); "Biographies: Eugene A. Stead Jr., MD (1908–2005)," Physician Assistant History Center Web site, http://www.pahx.org/steadBio.html (accessed February 7, 2010).

16. A. Parker, *The Team Approach to Primary Health Care* (Berkeley: University of California, 1972).

17. Institute of Medicine, *Educating for the Health Team* (Washington, DC: National Academy of Sciences, 1972).

18. D. K. Bloomfield, *Keys to the Asylum: A Dean, a Medical School and Academic Politics* (Champaign, Ill.: New Medical Press, 2000).

19. D. Baldwin and B. Rowley, eds., *Interdisciplinary Health Team Training: Proceedings of a Workshop* (Lexington: University of Kentucky Center for Interdisciplinary Education, 1982); D. Baldwin and others, *Interdisciplinary Health Care Teams in Teaching and Practice* (Seattle: New Health Perspectives, 1980).

20. M. Schmitt, "USA: Focus on Interprofessional Practice, Education, and Research," *Journal of Interprofessional Care* 8 (1994): 9–18; D. Baldwin, "Some Historical Notes on Interdisciplinary and Interprofessional Education and Practice in Health Care in the USA," *Journal of Interprofessional Care* 10 (1996): 173–187; D. Baldwin and R. Tsukuda, "Interdisciplinary Teams," in *Geriatric Medicine*, vol. 2, *Fundamentals of Geriatric Care,* ed. C. Cassel and J. Walsh (New York: Springer-Verlag Inc., 1984), 421–435; M. H. Schmitt, "The Team Approach in the Elderly," in *The Practice of Geriatrics*, ed. E. Calkins and others, (Philadelphia: W. B. Saunders Co., 1986); G. D. Heinemann and T. M. Zeiss, *Team Performance in Health Care: Assessment and Development* (New York: Kluwer Academic/Plenum Publishers, 2002).

21. "Home-based Primary Care Program," VHA Handbook 1141.01, United States Department of Veterans Affairs Web site, http://www1.va.gov/vhapublications/ViewPublication.asp?pub_ID=1534 (accessed February 3, 2010); "Home-based Primary Care," United States Department of Veterans Affairs Web site, http://www1.va.gov/HCBC/page.cfm?pg=68 (accessed February 3, 2010); J. L. Beales and T. Edes, "Veterans Affairs Home Based Primary Care," *Clinics in Geriatric Medicine* 25 (2009): 149–154.

22. "Geriatric Interdisciplinary Team Training Prepares Students in the Health Professions to Care for Older Patients," The John A. Hartford Foundation Web site, http://www.jhartfound.org/pdf%20files/GITT.pdf (accessed February 22, 2010).

23. J. J. Kockelmans, ed., *Interdisciplinarity in Higher Education* (University Park, Pa.: Pennsylvania State University, 1979); C. O. Houle, *Continuing Learning in the Professions* (San Francisco: Jossey-Bass Publishers, 1980).

24. M. Cook, "American Medical Education," 1339–1344.

25. Brown, "Health Care Teams."

26. M. H. Schmitt and others, "Conceptual and Methodological Problems in Studying the Effects of Interdisciplinary Geriatric Teams," *The Gerontologist* 28 (1988): 753–764.

27. Pew Health Professions Commission, *Contemporary Issues in Health Professions Education and Workforce Reform* (San Francisco: University of California Center for Health Professions, 1993); Pew Health Professions Commission, *Critical Challenges: Revitalizing the Health Professions for the Twenty-first Century, Third Report* (San Francisco: University of California Center for the Health Professions, 1995).

28. S. Sheps, "Reflections on Safety and Interprofessional Care: Some Conceptual Approaches," *Journal of Interprofessional Care* 20 (2006): 545–548.

29. President's Advisory Commission on Consumer Protection and Quality in the Health Care Industry, *Quality First: Better Health Care for All Americans* (Washington, DC: US Government Printing Office, 1998); Institute of Medicine, *To Err Is Human: Building a Safer Health System* (Washington, DC: National Academy Press, 2000); Institute of Medicine, *Crossing the Quality Chasm* (Washington, DC: National Academy Press, 2001); Institute of Medicine, *Keeping Patients Safe* (Washington, DC: National Academies Press, 2004).

30. Institute of Medicine, *To Err Is Human*; Institute of Medicine, *Crossing the Quality Chasm*; Institute of Medicine, *Keeping Patients Safe*.

31. "Medical Team Training Using Crew Resource Management Principles Enhances Provider Communication and Stimulates Improvements in Patient Care," Agency for Healthcare Research and Quality Web site, http://www.innovations.ahrq.gov/content.aspx?id=1809 (accessed February 23, 2010); "IHI Open School for Health Professions," Institute for Health Care Improvement Web site, http://www.ihi.org/IHI/Programs/IHIOpenSchool/ (accessed February 24, 2010); "Team-STEPPS: National Implementation," Agency for Healthcare Research and Quality Web site, http://teamstepps.ahrq.gov/ (accessed February 22, 2010); "Outcome Measures for Effective Teamwork in Inpatient Care (Santa Monica: RAND Corporation, 2008).

32. J. Mohr and others, "Integrating Patient Safety into the Clinical Microsystem," *Qual. Saf. Health Care* 13 (2004): ii34–ii38; J. Gittell, *High Performance Healthcare* (New York: McGraw-Hill, 2009).

33. "Joint Accreditation for Providers of Continuing Healthcare Education," Medicexchange Web site, http://www.medicexchange.com/Imported/imported-2875.html (accessed January 19, 2010).

34. Institute of Medicine, *Crossing the Quality Chasm.*

35. Institute of Medicine, *Health Professions Education: A Bridge to Quality* (Washington, DC: National Academies Press, 2003).

36. Ibid.

37. Ibid.

38. Joint Commission on Accreditation of Health Care Organizations, "Transforming Health Professional Education: Core Competencies, Microsystems, and New Training Venues," (conference program, Chicago, 2005).

39. "Final Report from the ACCME Task Force on Competency and the Continuum," Accreditation Council for Continuing Medical Education Web site, http://www.accme.org/index.cfm/fa/news.detail/news_id/cfefdccd-10f5-44c3-8a9f-b4e1d0b809dc.cfm (accessed January 25, 2010).

40. "Standard 5: Standards for Commercial Support," Accreditation Council for Pharmacy Education Web site, http://www.acpe-accredit.org/pdf/SCS_Standard%205_February%202009_update.pdf (accessed January 24, 2010); "Standards for Disclosure and Commercial Support," American Nurses Credentialing Center Web site, http://www.nursecredentialing.org/ContinuingEducation/Accreditation/How-to-Apply/CommercialSupport.aspx (accessed January 25, 2010).

41. "Joint Accreditation for the Provider of Continuing Education for the Healthcare Team Now Available," Accreditation Council for Continuing Medical Education Web site, http://www.accme.org/index.cfm/fa/news.detail/news_id/a71d122c-0a81-45c1-ad90-b71af47739c3.cfm (accessed January 25, 2010); "Joint Accreditation for the Provider of Continuing Education for the Healthcare Team is Now Available," American Nurses Credentialing Center Web site, http://www.nursecredentialing.org/

ContinuingEducation/Accreditation/Joint Accreditation Announcement.aspx (accessed January 19, 2010); "Joint Accreditation Process for Health Care Professionals," Accreditation Council for Pharmacy Education Web site, http://www.acpe-accredit.org/ceproviders/application .asp (accessed January 25, 2010).

42. Pew Health Professions Commission, *Contemporary Issues*; Pew Health Professions Commission, *Critical Challenges*; Institute of Medicine, *Crossing the Quality Chasm*.

43. M. Hager and others, eds., "Continuing Education in the Health Professions: Improving Healthcare through Lifelong Learning" (conference proceedings, Josiah Macy, Jr. Foundation, Bermuda, November 28–December 1, 2007).

44. Ibid.

45. American Association of Colleges of Nursing, "Lifelong Learning in Medicine and Nursing" (conference report, Association of American Medical Colleges and the American Association of Colleges of Nursing, Washington, DC, 2010).

46. Ibid.

47. Institute of Medicine, *Redesigning Continuing Education in the Health Professions* (Washington, DC: National Academies Press, 2010).

48. American Association of Colleges of Nursing, "Lifelong Learning."

49. Ibid.

50. M. Zwarenstein and S. Reeves, "Knowledge Translation and Interprofessional Collaboration: Where the Rubber of Evidence Based Care Hits the Road of Teamwork," *Journal of Continuing Education in the Health Professions* 26 (2006): 46–54; S. Reeves, "An Overview of Continuing Interprofessional Education," *Journal of Continuing Education in the Health Professions* 26 (2009): 142–146.

51. H. Barr, "An Anatomy of Continuing Interprofessional Education," *Journal of Continuing Education in the Health Professions* 29 (2009): 147–150.

52. J. Goldman and others, "Improving the Clarity of the Interprofessional Field: Implications for Research and Continuing Interprofessional Education," *Journal of Continuing Education in the Health Professions* 29 (2009): 151–156.

53. H. Barr and others, *Effective Interprofessional Education: Argument, Assumption and Evidence* (London: Blackwell, 2005); J. Carpenter and H. Dickinson, *Interprofessional Education and Training* (Bristol, United Kingdom: Policy Press, 2008); J. Sargeant, "Theories to Aid Understanding and Implementation of Interprofessional Education," *Journal of Continuing Education in the Health Professions* 29 (2009): 178–184; P. M. Wilcock and others, "Health Care Improvement and Continuing Interprofessional Education: Continuing Interprofessional Development to Improve Patient Outcomes," *Journal of Continuing Education in the Health Professions* 29 (2009): 84–90.

54. R. Luke and others, "Online Interprofessional Health Sciences Education: From Theory to Practice," *Journal of Continuing Education in the Health Professions* 29 (2009): 161–167.

55. B. Simmons and S. Wagner, "Assessment of Continuing Interprofessional Education: Lessons Learned," *Journal of Continuing Education in the Health Professions* 29 (2009): 168–171.

56. S. F. Eichhorn, "Faculty Training for Interdisciplinary Education," in *Interdisciplinary Health Team Training: Proceedings of a Workshop*, ed. D. Baldwin and B. Rowley (Lexington: University of Kentucky Center for Interdisciplinary Education, 1982); J. Takamura and others, "Health Team Development Program" (John A. Burns School of Medicine, University of Hawaii,1979).

57. H. Barr, *Effective Interprofessional Education.*

58. I. Silver and K. Leslie, "Faculty Development for Continuing Interprofessional Education and Collaborative Practice," *Journal of Continuing Education in the Health Professions* 29 (2009): 172–177.

CHAPTER 27

The Maintenance of Certification Program from the American Board of Medical Specialties and Its Member Boards

The American Board of Medical Specialties (ABMS) is the umbrella organization for 24 medical specialty certifying boards. The ABMS mission is to maintain and improve the quality of medical care by assisting its member boards in their efforts to develop professional and educational standards for the certification of physician specialists. The intent of certification, including initial certification and maintenance of certification (ABMS MOC®), is to provide assurance to the public that a physician specialist certified by an ABMS member board has successfully completed an approved educational program and an ongoing evaluation process designed to assess the medical knowledge, judgment, professionalism, and clinical and communication skills required to provide high quality patient care in that specialty.

ABMS is a not-for-profit organization that oversees US physician certification of more than 750,000 physicians through its 24 member boards. Currently, ABMS member boards certify approximately 80 to 85 percent of licensed US physicians in more than 145 specialties and sub-specialties.[1] Certification by an ABMS member board is used widely as an indicator of higher standards and better care.

History and Evolution of Certification

ABMS can trace its roots to the rise and growth of the medical specialty board movement in the early 1900s. This movement has been associated directly with significant advancements in medical science and the resulting improvements made in medical care delivery. Prior to the specialty board movement, there was no means to assure the public that a physician claiming to be a specialist was indeed qualified; each physician was the sole judge of his or her own qualifications to practice a given specialty. Specialty societies and medical education institutions first encouraged and assisted in the development of boards to define specialty qualifications and to issue credentials that would assure the public of a specialist's qualifications. As the original boards and societies matured, they contributed to the development of a system to provide recognition of qualified physician specialists.

The concept of a specialty board was first proposed in 1908, though it was not until 1916 that the first specialty board, the American Board for Ophthalmic Examinations, was formed. In 1917, the board was officially incorporated, and in 1933, its name was changed to the American Board of Ophthalmology. The board established the guidelines for training and evaluating candidates desiring certification to practice ophthalmology.

The second specialty board, the American Board of Otolaryngology, was founded and incorporated in 1924; the third and fourth boards, the American Board of Obstetrics and Gynecology and the American Board of Dermatology and Syphilology, were established in 1930 and 1932, respectively. These boards developed along the same path as their predecessors and shared common objectives.

At a 1933 professional conference, representatives from these four pioneering specialty boards and the American Hospital Association, the Association of American Medical Colleges, the Federation of State Medical Boards, the American Medical Association (AMA) Council on Medical Education and Hospitals, and the National Board of Medical Examiners agreed that the examination and certification of specialists would best be carried out by the national boards (specialty boards). They also concluded that the efficacy of these boards would be maximized by the formation of an advisory committee or council created by two delegated representatives from each of the official specialty boards currently in existence or in the process of formation. Formal organization of the Advisory Board for Medical Specialties, the forerunner of ABMS, occurred that same year.

Since 1933, official recognition of specialty boards in medicine has been achieved by the collaborative efforts of the Advisory Board for Medical Specialties, its successor the ABMS, and the AMA Council on Medical Education. In 1948, these efforts were formalized through the establishment of the Liaison Committee for Specialty Boards (LCSB). The jointly approved publication "Essentials for Approval of Examining Boards in Medicine Specialties" established standards. This document has undergone several revisions through the years and remains the standard for recognition of new specialty boards.

From 1933 to 1970, the Advisory Board operated as a federation of individual specialty boards. It functioned primarily as a forum for discussion without the benefit of a full-time director or a central office from which to conduct its daily operations. This changed in 1970 when the Advisory Board was reorganized as the ABMS.

The official ABMS member boards are provided in Table 27-1.

TABLE 27-1 *ABMS Member Boards*

Member Board	Year Approved
Allergy and Immunology	1971
Anesthesiology	1941
Colon and Rectal Surgery	1949
Dermatology	ABMS Founding Member
Emergency Medicine	1979
Family Medicine	1969
Internal Medicine	1936
Medical Genetics	1991
Neurological Surgery	1940
Nuclear Medicine	1971
Obstetrics and Gynecology	ABMS Founding Member
Ophthalmology	ABMS Founding Member
Orthopaedic Surgery	1935
Otolaryngology	ABMS Founding Member
Pathology	1936
Pediatrics	1935
Physical Medicine and Rehabilitation	1947
Plastic Surgery	1941
Preventive Medicine	1949
Psychiatry and Neurology	1935
Radiology	1935
Surgery	1937
Thoracic Surgery	1971
Urology	1935

Standards for Initial Board Certification

Within the ABMS overall framework, each ABMS member board is responsible for setting the standards in a given specialty. For initial certification, which typically follows completion of Accreditation Council for Graduate Medical Education (ACGME) accredited residency training, candidates are evaluated in completion of predoctoral medical education, of appropriate residency requirements, and of written and oral examinations; possession of a valid license to practice medicine; and demonstration of clinical competence and professionalism.

Research indicates that initial certification is linked to quality care (e.g., a significant reduction in mortality for acute myocardial infarction and lower mortality and fewer complications for peptic ulcer surgery and colon resection). Certification has been associated with a decrease in complications as well as mortality for other major surgical procedures, including carotid endarterectomy and abdominal aortic aneurysm resection. A review of the evidence from many studies suggests that board certification is associated with positive clinical outcomes and that certification examination results are correlated with other measures of physician competence. Board certified internists demonstrated greater knowledge, communicative skills, and preventive care, among other attributes, than did noncertified internists. Another study found that Medicare beneficiaries who saw board certified internists were significantly more likely to receive appropriate preventive care services (including hemoglobin A1c monitoring, mammography, colorectal cancer screening, and pneumococcal and influenza vaccine) than those whose physicians were not board certified. Furthermore, patients cared for by board certified physicians received recommended care (such as aspirin and beta-blockers) for heart attacks and the recommended number of prenatal visits more often than those who were cared for by noncertified physicians. Also, the lack of anesthesiologist board certification has been associated with poorer outcomes. In general, the lack of board certification has been associated with a greater risk of disciplinary action.[2]

Recertification and MOC

Because of concerns about degradation of medical knowledge over time and lack of incorporation of new knowledge, the boards started moving toward time-limited certification in the 1970s, requiring retesting and certification every 6 to 10 years, depending on the specialty. Although physicians certified before the policy was adopted are not required to recertify, all who became physicians after a specified date (dependent upon the certifying board) must pass the periodic certification examination to remain certified.

Subsequently, the ABMS recognized that assessment of medical knowledge, while necessary, was not sufficient to ensure that physicians provide high quality care over their practice careers. A broad range of skills, abilities, and professional behaviors were essential to the continued delivery of safe and effective patient care. In January 1998, David L. Nahrwold, MD, an ABMS executive committee member, suggested in a white paper that the means for assuring patients that doctors provided high quality care was through certification and recertification.

In March 1998, ABMS created the Task Force on Competence. As part of its work, the task force identified core competencies for physicians, specified the same six core competencies as those developed by the ACGME (see Box 27-1), and proposed the ABMS MOC program.

ABMS committee and task force members worked to formulate the principles and guidelines of the ABMS MOC program, including determination of how to assess the six competencies for MOC. The MOC program, approved by the ABMS in 2000, has four key components: Part I, professional standing; Part II, lifelong learning and self-assessment; Part III, cognitive expertise; and Part IV, practice performance assessment (see Box 27-2). In 2006, all member boards received approval for their MOC program plans.

MOC is a more continuous process then recertification, focusing on assessing and improving practice performance and patient outcomes. The core competencies and MOC program serve as an organizing framework to guide professional development that leads to improved care.

The ABMS MOC program uses evidence-based guidelines, national clinical and quality standards, and best practices along with customized continuing education, self-assessment, patient assessment, and performance feedback to create a culture of lifelong learning.

While the ABMS member boards were contemplating and implementing their MOC programs, several studies were published that reinforced the need for more broad assessment of physician competence and performance and the need to offer educational interventions that targeted skills and behaviors rather than medical knowledge only. The Institute of Medicine's landmark reports "To Err Is Human" (1999) and "Crossing the Quality Chasm" (2001) focused national attention on gaps in the quality and safety of the American health-care system.[3] While system issues clearly contribute to medical errors, physician performance problems are also important factors in medical errors and poor quality health care.[4] A review published in 2005 described declining physician knowledge and performance over time and reinforced the need for periodic assessment of practicing physicians to direct their educational and improvement efforts.[5]

Standards for MOC

In March 2009, ABMS approved the *Standards for ABMS MOC (Parts I–IV)*.[6] These standards will accelerate the pace of implementation of MOC, decrease board-to-board variability, and promote quality health care and patient safety.

Kevin B. Weiss, MD, ABMS president and chief executive officer, stated, "The ability to respond to the needs of the public while keeping pace with the growing field of physician performance measurement requires a dynamic, continuous certification process. These standards, which will define board certified physicians' engagement in continuous professional development and assessment, will need to be continually evaluated and updated. Through these standards,

hundreds of thousands of physicians in this country will be asked to participate in enhanced professional development activities to improve the ABMS lifelong learning evaluation. Ultimately, it's our patients and the public of this country for whom these principles were developed to ensure they are receiving high quality healthcare."[7]

Continuing Medical Education and Self-Assessment Requirements (Part II)

Member boards will document that diplomates (physician specialists certified by an ABMS member board) complete an average of 25 CME credits per year (AMA Physician's Recognition Award [PRA] Category 1, American Association of Family Physicians [AAFP] Prescribed Credit, American College of Obstetrics and Gynecology [ACOG] Cognates, and/or American Osteopathic Association [AOA] Category 1A). At least an average of eight of these credits per year involve self-assessment (e.g., multiple-choice examination or simulation with checklist.) Additionally, the content of continuing medical education (CME) and self-assessment programs will be relevant to the physician's scope of board certification and free of commercial bias and control of a commercial interest as specified in the Accreditation Council for Continuing Medical Education Standards for Commercial Support.[8]

Practice-based Assessment and Quality Improvement (Part IV)

ABMS member boards will require diplomates to provide evidence of participation in practice assessment and quality improvement every two to five years. Boards should base their requirements on a complete cycle of initial assessment, improvement activity, and re-assessment. Currently, the AMA PRA Category 1 practice improvement credits meet this criteria, provided all stages are completed.

Patient Safety and Communication Assessment

As part of MOC Part II self-assessment requirements, member boards will ensure that every diplomate enrolled in MOC will complete an ABMS-approved patient safety self-assessment program at least once per MOC cycle.

Diplomates who provide direct patient care will be required to participate in communication skills assessments by patients and assessment of professionalism by their peers. Member boards will evaluate physicians' communication skills using ABMS-approved surveys, such as the Consumer Assessment of Healthcare Providers and Systems patient survey. Options for peer surveys have not yet been identified.

The ABMS board of directors approved these patient safety and communication assessment requirements as developmental standards; member boards will study the feasibility and validity of available instruments over the next five years before deciding upon and implementing the methods most ideally suited to the practice of their diplomates.

Implementing MOC

The ABMS MOC program, which has been adopted by all 24 member boards, encourages board certified physician specialists to focus on quality and continuous professional development. MOC engages physicians and their teams in self-assessment, lifelong learning, and practice improvement to enhance performance and optimize health care outcomes. Alignment of MOC programs with the six general competencies ensures that learning and improvement efforts focus on the full range of knowledge, skills, and behaviors relevant to optimal patient care. Participation in the various activities of MOC is thus synergistic in identifying gaps and promoting improvement. For example, a Part IV practice performance assessment might identify a gap in a particular area of diabetes care (e.g., blood pressure control). A focused Part II CME or self-assessment activity would provide the physician

with the knowledge and skills necessary to improve blood pressure control of diabetic patients in his or her practice. Re-measurement would likely demonstrate improved outcomes.

Lifelong Learning and Self-Assessment (Part II)

This requirement is designed to help physicians focus on specific clinical areas where they may want to verify that their clinical knowledge and skills are current and consistent with best practices and guidelines. Tools can include take-home and online self-assessment materials (medical knowledge, patient management tests, clinical simulations) on specialty-specific topics as well as general topics applicable to all physicians, including communication, patient safety, quality improvement, and systems-based practice. Some examples include:

- American Board of Internal Medicine (ABIM) offers its diplomates an opportunity to earn MOC self-evaluation points in two categories: self-evaluation of medical knowledge (Part II) and self-evaluation of practice performance (Part IV). For self-evaluation of medical knowledge, diplomates complete ABIM's open-book medical knowledge modules that test clinical and practical knowledge in a particular field. In addition, ABIM has designated several educational self-assessment products from various medical societies (such as the American College of Physicians) and other ABMS member boards that may be used to earn self-evaluation points toward MOC.
- American Board of Family Medicine (ABFM) diplomates can earn Part II credit by completing online self-assessment modules that consist of 60 questions on a particular health topic and correctly answering 80 percent within each subtopic to receive credit. Critiques and references are provided. Once that portion is complete, the physician enters the clinical simulation (ClinSim) segment,

which presents dynamically generated Web-based patient care scenarios corresponding to the topic chosen in the knowledge assessment. The simulated patients respond to the doctor's recommendations and assessments over time, providing the physician an opportunity to demonstrate proficiency in longitudinal patient management skills.

- The ABMS Patient Safety Foundations program can be used by physicians in any specialty to fulfill a Part II patient safety self-assessment program requirement. The Web-based, interactive program provides an educational experience incorporating patient safety scenarios that cut across disciplines (e.g., medical errors, handoffs, and teamwork); patient safety curriculum covering epidemiology, systems, communication, and safety culture; and pre- and post-tests of multiple-choice questions drawn from the curriculum content. A passing score of 80 percent is required in the post-test to complete each section of the course and earn AMA PRA Category 1 credit.

Practice Performance Assessment (Part IV)

Physicians are evaluated in their clinical practice according to specialty-specific standards for patient care. They are asked to assess the quality of care they provide compared to peers and national benchmarks, to implement a quality improvement intervention to address gaps in their practice, and to re-measure to assess improvement. The ideal model for performance assessment and practice improvement may vary with the nature of specialty practice. For physicians practicing primary care, assessment may focus on rates of compliance with evidence-based processes of care or on demonstrable, attributable health-care outcomes. Performance in surgery may best be measured through the application of registries and analytic methods that control for patient- and system-related factors in assessing surgical per-

formance. For physicians not actively engaged with patients (such as pathologists and some radiologists), peer review of diagnostic interpretations and reports may provide an optimal form of performance measurement.

Practice performance assessment begins by understanding and applying quality measurement to practice, using results from the measurement to evaluate the impact of the actions. Practice performance assessment tools offer physicians the opportunity to view their practice as a population of patients with a common condition. The process highlights to physicians that the quality of care provided depends not only on what they know, but also on the system that supports the delivery of care. Some examples include:

- To fulfill Part IV requirements, diplomates of the American Board of Pediatrics (ABP) can complete the comprehensive Education in Quality Improvement for Pediatric Practice (EQIPP) program, an online interactive educational activity offered by the American Academy of Pediatrics. The program includes educational material on a specific disease (e.g., asthma, attention deficit disorder). After completing the educational component, physicians enter data from a review of their patient charts and learn about their performance compared to national standards and benchmarks. After analyzing their performance, physicians identify opportunities for improvement, implement changes in their practice, and then collect data from patients to see if improvement in care has occurred.
- For Part IV of MOC, ABFM offers performance in practice modules (PPMs) directing the physician to survey and gather clinical information on about 10 patients within a particular disease category. The physician enters the patient data and survey information into an online program, which then provides the physician with extensive lists of possible tools and interventions for

developing a quality improvement plan. This plan is followed during the next three to six months, after which physicians are able to study pre- and post-intervention performance, and compare their results to those of their peers. (Other programs, including METRIC developed by the American Academy of Family Physicians, satisfy ABFM's Part IV MOC requirements.) For diplomates who do not have traditional continuity practices, ABFM plans to offer alternative generic methods in medicine modules that will focus on issues, such as information management.

- ABIM offers its diplomates an opportunity to earn MOC self-evaluation points in practice performance (Part IV). Diplomates meet the self-evaluation of practice performance requirement by completing the ABIM Practice Improvement Modules® (PIMs). A PIM is a Web-based tool, using chart data, patient surveys, and a practice system survey that enables physicians to conduct confidential self-evaluations of medical care through analysis of practice data and the development and implementation of targeted improvement plans. There are several categories and types of PIMs, including those focusing on chronic conditions, subspecialty conditions, prevention, care of the vulnerable elderly, hospital-based patient care, communication, and systems-based practice.

- American Board of Surgery (ABS) offers Part IV credit for ongoing participation in a national, regional, or local surgical outcomes database or quality assessment program. Participation in National Surgical Quality Improvement Program (NSQIP), Surgical Care Improvement Program (SCIP), Physician Quality Reporting Initiative (PQRI), or the American College of Surgeons (ACS) Practice Based Learning System (case log system) meets this requirement. (See www.absurgery.org for other acceptable programs.)

ABMS and some of the surgical boards are considering development of a national surgical/procedural outcomes registry that could be used to provide information for Part IV MOC activities.

- Several member boards (e.g., ABFM, ABIM, ABP) have approved structured quality improvement (QI) projects for Part IV MOC credit that take place in the physician's workplace. These projects must meet rigorous standards addressing: project design, results, and sustainability; meaningful physician participation; and Institute of Medicine quality dimensions. They involve teams collaborating across practice sites and/or institutions, guided by coaches experienced in implementing improvement strategies. Approved structured QI projects by the ABP include catheter-associated bloodstream infection collaborative, cystic fibrosis QI care initiative, and Improving Performance in Practice (IPIP), a state-based primary care program.

- 2009, ABFM, ABIM, and ABP began working together in aligning their mechanisms for approved structured QI projects to develop an approach for recognizing institutions that have rigorous internal QI oversight mechanisms and that consistently develop excellent QI projects that cross multiple specialties. The first institution with whom the boards are testing the approach is the Mayo Clinic. Mayo physicians will incorporate MOC into their daily activities, making it part of the culture.

Organizational recognition of MOC would allow these institutions to leverage their existing QI oversight mechanisms to review and approve projects provisionally on behalf of the boards. ABMS Member Boards retain responsibility for ensuring that local programs meet and maintain MOC standards through an initial review and ongoing audit process. This approach should reduce redundancy of effort, providing a way to recognize work that physicians are already doing. It should also encourage healthcare institutions to develop more rigorous oversight and support of their QI projects to advance the quality of care. Furthermore, embedding MOC programs in strong health care systems will provide the infrastructure and support needed for improvement.

Building the Evidence Base for MOC

MOC is a relatively new program, but ultimately studies across multiple ABMS member boards' MOC programs will need to link participation in MOC to improved physician performance and patient outcomes. However, empiric data and a sound rationale exist for framing the current MOC standards around the general competencies. Research studies demonstrate that the domains of medical knowledge, interpersonal and communication skills, professionalism, and patient care are relevant to patient and physician outcomes and/or physicians would benefit from ongoing assessment and improvement efforts targeting these competencies. Additionally, there is evidence that the underpinnings of the MOC program, including effective CME and use of needs assessment, physician cognitive expertise, performance measurement, and feedback about the patient care experience are associated with improved physician competence and/or performance.[8]

Recent studies suggest the value of MOC. Physician cognitive skills, as measured by MOC examination, are associated with better performance on Medicare quality indicators for diabetes and mammography screening.[9] Turchin et al. found a positive association between recent certification/recertification and improved treatment of high blood pressure in patients with diabetes.[10] Two studies demonstrate that physicians who complete ABIM PIMs incorporate significant improvements in practice performance.[11] In addition, 73 percent of physicians who complete PIMs report they have changed their practice as a result.[12]

Many boards are beginning to study or plan to study how participation in MOC activities impacts physician performance and patient outcomes. ABMS and its 24 member boards are in the process of verifying and calibrating their MOC programs as they have previously done for initial certification.

Future Directions

ABMS and its member boards have moved from initial certification with a lifetime certificate, to recertification every 6 to 10 years based primarily on passing a written multiple-choice examination, to MOC, which represents a continuous professional development system requiring maintenance of professional credentials, assessment of competence, demonstration of cognitive expertise, and engagement in practice improvement activities.

As ABMS and its member board MOC programs continue to focus on improving practice performance and health care outcomes, it is important to align these efforts with major initiatives from government, employers, insurers, and other organizations. It is in the best interests of all to work cooperatively to coordinate these activities and to ensure the most appropriate systems are put into place, as well as to avoid duplication of requirements.

ABMS and its member boards are working to tie physician participation in MOC to Medicare and other government-controlled health care initiatives. For example, a new Centers for Medicare and Medicaid Services (CMS) PQRI option would allow board certified physicians participating in a qualified ABMS MOC program and completing a qualified MOC practice assessment to be eligible for PQRI incentive payments.

Other pay-for-performance initiatives are also being linked to MOC. ABFM, ABIM, and ABP have already aligned MOC with health plan reward/recognition programs, and other Member Boards are pursuing similar agreements. There are also efforts to link MOC participation to a reduction in malpractice premiums. ABMS is working with the Federation of State Medical Boards so that participation in MOC may eventually fulfill some new, more stringent requirements for renewing a state medical license (e.g., maintenance of licensure [MOL]).

Future approaches to MOC should continue to meet a high standard for comprehensive assessment, education, and practice improvement of certified physicians, while moving toward continuous, meaningful participation; this will support the recognition of MOC for ongoing credentialing and privileging decisions, re-licensure, pay-for-performance, reduced malpractice premiums, preferred provider identification, and PQRI credit. Furthermore, continued efforts toward increased transparency regarding MOC data should enhance patients' ability to make informed decisions regarding their health care.

Notes

1. American Board of Medical Specialties Web site, http://www.abms.org.

2. J. J. Norcini and others, "Certification and Specialization: Do They Matter in the Outcome of Acute Myocardial Infarction?" *Academic Medicine* 75 (2000): 1193–1198; J. J. Norcini and others, "The Certification Status of Generalist Physicians and the Mortality of Their Patients after Acute Myocardial Infarction," *Academic Medicine* 76 (2001): S21–S23; J. J. Norcini and others, "Certifying Examination Performance and Patient Outcomes following Acute Myocardial Infarction," *Medical Education* 36 (2002): 853–859; J. V. Kelly and F. J. Hellinger, "Physician and Hospital Factors Associated with Mortality of Surgical Patients," *Medical Care* 24 (1986): 785–800; J. B. Prystowsky and others, "Patient Outcomes for Segmental Colon Resection according to Surgeon's Training, Certification, and Experience," *Surgery* 132 (2002): 663–670; W. H. Pearce and others, "The Importance of Surgeon Volume and Training in Outcomes for Vascular Surgical Procedures," *Journal of Vascular Surgery* 29 (1999): 768–776; T. A. Brennan and others, "The Role of Physician Specialty Board Certification Status in the Quality Movement," *Journal of the American Medical Association* 292 (2004): 1038–1043; H. H. Pham and others, "Delivery of Preventive Services to Older Adults by Primary Care Physicians," *Journal of the American Medical Association* 294

(2005): 473–481; J. Chen and others, "Physician Board Certification and the Care and Outcomes of Elderly Patients with Acute Myocardial Infarction," *Journal of General Internal Medicine* 21 (2006): 238–244; J. S. Haas and others, "The Relationship between Physicians' Qualifications and Experience and the Adequacy of Prenatal Care and Low Birthweight," *American Journal of Public Health* 85 (1995): 1087–1091; J. H. Silber and others, "Anesthesiologist Board Certification and Patient Outcomes," *Anesthesiology* 96 (2002): 1044–1052; J. V. Kelly and F. J. Hellinger, "Heart Disease and Hospital Deaths: An Empirical Study," *Health Services Research* 22 (1987): 369–395; P. G. Ramsey and others, "Predictive Validity of Certification by the American Board of Internal Medicine," *Annals of Internal Medicine* 110 (1989): 719–726; R. Rutledge and others, "A Statewide, Population-based Time-Series Analysis of the Outcome of Ruptured Abdominal Aortic Aneurysm," *Annals of Surgery* 223 (1996): 492–502; L. K. Sharp and others, "Specialty Board Certification and Clinical Outcomes: The Missing Link," *Academic Medicine* 77 (2002): 534–542; N. D. Kohatsu and others, "Characteristics Associated with Physician Discipline: A Case-Control Study," *Archives of Internal Medicine* 164 (2004): 653–658; J. Morrison and P. Wickersham, "Physicians Disciplined by a State Medical Board," *Journal of the American Medical Association* 279 (1998): 1889–1893.

3. L. T. Kohn and others, eds., *To Err Is Human: Building a Safer Health System.* (Washington, DC: National Academy Press, 2000); Institute of Medicine, *Crossing the Quality Chasm: a New Health System for the 21st Century* (Washington, DC: National Academy Press, 2001).

4. J. E. Wennberg and M. M. Cooper, eds., *The Dartmouth Atlas of Health Care* (Chicago: American Hospital Association Press, 1999); L. L. Leape and J. A. Fromson, "Problem Doctors: Is There a System-Level Solution?" *Annals of Internal Medicine* 144 (2006): 107–115.

5. N. K. Choudhry and others, "Systematic Review: The Relationship between Clinical Experience and Quality of Health Care," *Annals of Internal Medicine* 142 (2005): 260–273.

6. "ABMS Announces New MOC Standards," American Board of Medical Specialties Web site, http://www.abms.org/News_and_Events/Media_Newsroom/Releases/release_NewMOCStandards_03262009.aspx (accessed May 10, 2010).

7. Ibid.

8. E. A. McGlynn and others, "The Quality of Health Care Delivered to Adults in the United States," *New England Journal of Medicine* 348, no. 26 (2003): 2635–2645; M. K. White and others, *Annotated Bibliography for Clinician Patient Communications to Enhance Health Outcomes* (New Haven, Conn.: Institute for Healthcare Com-

munication, 2005); E. G. Campbell and others, "Professionalism in Medicine: Results of a National Survey of Physicians," *Annals of Internal Medicine* 147, no. 11 (2007): 795–802; D. A. Davis and others, "Impact of Formal Continuing Medical Education. Do Conferences, Workshops, Rounds, and Other Traditional Continuing Education Activities Change Physician Behavior or Health Care Outcomes?" *Journal of the American Medical Association* 282, no. 9 (1999): 867–874; M. Mansouri and J. Lockyer, "A Meta-Analysis of Continuing Medical Education Effectiveness," *Journal of Continuing Education in the Health Professions* 27, no. 1 (2007): 6–15; I. Colthart and others, "The Effectiveness of Self-Assessment on the Identification of Learner Needs, Learner Activity and Impact on Clinical Practice: BEME Guide No. 10," *Medical Teacher* 30 (2008): 124–145; P. E. Mazmanian and D. A. Davis, "Continuing Medical Education and the Physician as a Learner. Guide to the Evidence," *Journal of the American Medical Association* 288, no. 9 (2002): 1057–1060; G. R. Norman and others, "The Need for Needs Assessment in Continuing Medical Education, *British Medical Journal* 328 (2004): 999–1001; R. Tamblyn and others, "Association between Licensure Examination Scores and Practice in Primary Care," *Journal of the American Medical Association* 288, no. 23 (2002): 3019–3026; E. S. Holmboe and others, "Assessing Quality of Care: Knowledge Matters," *Journal of the American Medical Association* 299, no. 3 (2008): 388–340; S. M. Asch and others, "Comparison of Quality of Care in the Veterans Health Administration and Patients in a National Sample," *Annals of Internal Medicine* 141 (2004): 938–945; E. S. Holmboe and others, "The ABIM Diabetes Practice Improvement Module: A New Method for Self-Assessment," *Journal of Continuing Education in the Health Professions* 26 (2006): 109–119; R. S. Lipner and others, "A Three-Part Model for Measuring Diabetes Care in Physician Practice," *Academic Medicine* 82, no. 10 (2007): S48–52; F. D. Duffy and others, "Self-Assessment of Practice Performance: Development of the ABIM Practice Improvement Module (PIM)," *Journal of Continuing Education in the Health Professions* 28 (2008): 39–46; G. Jamtvedt and others, "Audit and Feedback: Effects on Professional Practice and Health Care Outcomes (Cochrane Review)," *The Cochrane Library* 4 (2008); P. D. Cleary and B. J. McNeil, "Patient Satisfaction as an Indicator of Quality Care," *Inquiry* 25 (1998): 25–36; T. D. Sequist and others, "Quality Monitoring of Physicians Linking Patients' Experiences of Care to Clinical Quality and Outcomes," *Journal of General Internal Medicine* 23, no. 11 (2008): 1784–1790; A. Jha and others, "Patients' Perception of Hospital Care in the United States," *New England Journal of Medicine* 359 (2008): 1921–1931; E. H. Wagner and others, "Chronic Care Clinics for Diabetes in Primary C: System-wide Randomized Trial," *Diabetes Care* 24, no. 4 (2001): 695–700; A. M. Fremont and others, "Patient-Centered Processes of Care and Long-Term Outcomes of Myocardial Infarction," *Journal of General Internal Medicine* 16 (2001): 800–808.

9. E. S. Holmboe and others, "Association between Maintenance of Certification Examination Scores and Quality of Care for Medicare Beneficiaries," *Archives of Internal Medicine* 168, no. 13 (2008): 1396–1403.

10. A. Turchin and others, "Effect of Board Certification on Antihypertensive Treatment Intensification in Patients with Diabetes Mellitus," *Circulation* 117 (2008): 623–628.

11. J. Simpkins and others, "Improving Asthma Care through Recertification: A Cluster Randomized Trial," *Archives of Internal Medicine* 167 (2007): 2240–2248; J. Oyler and others, "Teaching Internal Medicine Residents Quality Improvement Techniques Using the ABIM's Practice Improvement Modules," *Journal of General Internal Medicine* 23 (2008): 927–930.

12. ABIM Post PIM Survey, 1/06-12/08, n=approximately 5,000.

CHAPTER 28

The National Commission for Certification of Continuing Medical Education Professionals and Its Certification Program

As with any new field of endeavor, discussion and debate have surrounded the question of raising continuing medical education (CME) to the level of a profession since early in its evolution. Individuals engaged in developing CME have come from a variety of disciplines, including medicine, nursing, adult education, and other related fields. They have brought content, theory, and experience with them, but few attempts have been made to describe the underlying knowledge and competencies needed to develop effective CME programs and content.

CME is as old as Hippocrates, but it entered a more formal era in 1968 with the advent of the American Medical Association (AMA) Physician's Recognition Award. The creation of the Accreditation Council for Continuing Medical Education (ACCME) in 1981 added a layer of regulation that required CME programs to incorporate basic principles of adult learning into certified CME activities. The field generated unique theories and corresponding research through its journal *Mobius,* which evolved into the *Journal for Continuing Education in the Health Sciences.* Critical books like *Changing and Learning in the Lives of Physicians* (published in 1989) and *Physician as Learner: Linking Research to Practice* (published in 1994) linked learning theory with clinical practice and patient outcomes.

An outside observer would likely point to a period somewhere between the mid-1980s and mid-1990s as the time when CME had become sufficiently mature to declare itself a unique discipline. It required another 10 to 20 years to develop and implement professional certification. Along the way, debate has continued as to what it means to be a CME professional.

The Founding of the National Commission for Certification of CME Professionals

In 1980, two icons of the CME community wrote a memo that now resides in the archives of the National Commission for Certification of CME Professionals (NC-CME). The intent of the memo, authored by Lewis Miller, MS, and Richard Wilbur, MD, and addressed to William Felch, MD, executive director of the Alliance for Continuing Medical Education ("the Alliance"), was clear: the CME community could benefit from a certification program that would assess and reward the competence of individuals employed in the CME community. No action resulted from the memo. In 1993, Miller championed the certification concept again. And again, no further activity ensued.

In summer 1997 at the Alliance External Relations Committee meeting in Santa Fe, New Mexico, the topic of certification for CME professionals was on the agenda. The committee adjourned for dinner at a local restaurant famous for its margaritas, and by the end of the evening the members had dubbed themselves "The Margarita Group," dedicated to the proposition that CME professionals deserve a certification program. Members of the venerable Margarita Group were Phil Dombrowski, MBA; Miller; Jackie Parochka, EdD; and Judith Ribble, PhD (chair). The committee formally recommended that the Alliance initiate a certification program for CME professionals; however, once again no action was forthcoming.

In fall 2004, Ribble experienced an "aha" moment when she saw a panel truck bearing the message "Be sure your chimney sweep is certified." The idea that the chimney sweep profession had progressed to the point of having a certification program, but that CME professionals—those individuals responsible for developing, administering, accrediting, marketing, and funding the CME activities that the nation's physicians and physician assistants depend upon—had not, made a powerful impression on her. At a New York City conference, Ribble broached the topic with Minnie Baylor-Henry, JD, then with Johnson & Johnson. On the spot, Baylor-Henry agreed to provide meeting space for a two-day retreat to sort out options. Eighteen CME umbrella organizations received invitations to the retreat asking that each send a representative.

In February 2005, the following eleven colleagues attended a retreat in Lafayette Hill, Pennsylvania: Jann Balmer, RN, PhD; Martin Cearnal; John Kelly, MD; John Kues, PhD; Pam Mason; Miller; Karen Overstreet, EdD, RPh; Phil Puckorius; Ribble; Marissa Seligman, PharmD; and Jon Ukropec, PhD. On the first evening, the attendees examined the certification programs of other health-care organizations. The next day a SWOT analysis was performed to project anticipated strengths, weaknesses, opportunities, and threats. The group accepted the definition of *competence* described on the Alliance Web site: "CME professionals are competent when they use (practice, or apply) the (defined) knowledge, skill, or behavior. . . . This . . . requires assessment and perfor-mance measurements and some form of certification process, which do not exist currently."[1]

By the end of the retreat, a mission statement was adopted and attendees agreed to serve as leaders of the organization they had just founded and named the National Commission for Certification of CME Professionals. The new executive committee, which would become the board of directors, elected Ribble as president and voted unanimously to move forward with the certification initiative. The intent was to pioneer a certification program that assesses and documents competencies deemed essential to the broad spectrum of CME workers. The group consensus was that the CME universe comprised approximately 10,000 individuals working with accredited providers or maintaining formal connections with CME content, implementation, funding, or evaluation.

In July 2005, John Kamp arranged a meeting of an auxiliary advisory board in New York City. The group of 16 focused on recommendations for strategic planning, fundraising, and certification criteria. A timeline was drafted, and the concept of offering a certification program for persons employed in the field of CME became a mandate for implementation.

How does a small group of volunteers with full-time jobs go about creating a valid, reliable, and legally defensible certification program where none existed before? For NC-CME, the answer was to enlist like-minded, enthusiastic volunteers to participate in the project. By the time of the Alliance annual meeting in January 2006, enough groundwork had been laid to attract more than 100 attendees to an ad hoc lunchtime gathering in San Francisco. After the bylaws were adopted, NC-CME was incorporated in New Mexico under the guidance of Incorporators Miller, Cearnal, and Ribble. On February 8, 2006, the IRS approved NC-CME as a tax-exempt 501(c)(3) organization. The Financial Development Committee, chaired by Miller and Cearnal, appealed to the generosity of the CME community for funding to support NC-CME activities and found a groundswell of encouragement that enabled the fledgling organization to create an infrastructure and develop the first certification exam for CME professionals.

After its founding, the NC-CME board of directors met monthly via conference call, and a review team selected a test development company from among 25 companies who answered an online request for information. NC-CME joined the National Organization for Competency Assurance (NOCA, known after 2009 as the Institute for Credentialing Excellence [ICE]) and enlisted the aid of colleagues experienced in certification matters. Volunteers submitted abstracts and presented sessions at national conferences, staffed exhibit booths at conferences, launched a Web site, and gathered a database of interested candidates for the certification exam.

In 2007, Kues assumed the presidency and Ribble was named the volunteer executive director; by third quarter 2009, the board concluded that the organization was sufficiently successful to afford contracting Ribble as the part-time executive director. In 2009, Overstreet succeeded Kues as president, and in 2011 Dennis K. Wentz, MD, succeeded Overstreet. Seligman served as secretary and Laird Kelly as treasurer during the crucial start-up period, which also saw Ellen Cosgrove, MD, Robert Galbraith, MD, Scott Hershman, MD, and Sharyn Lee, RN, MS, named to the board. At the initial retreat, the group had decided against "grandfathering," and from 2009 forward, all board members have been required to have earned their CCMEP credential by submitting an eligibility worksheet and passing the three-hour monitored exam.

The Positioning of CME as a Profession

Persons employed in the CME field had been known to refer to their work as a *job* as opposed to a *profession,* and until 2008, one important characteristic of a profession was indeed missing: the process of certification or licensing. NC-CME has helped to provide this missing element through its Certified CME Professional™ (CCMEP) credentialing program, which assesses and rewards individuals' knowledge of the broad scope of the CME enterprise. This NC-CME effort has contributed significantly to the recognition and value of CME as a profession. As noted by recent recipient of the CCMEP credential Melissa Newcomb, MBA, CCMEP, assistant director for certification, Continuing Professional Education, University of Rochester, New York:

It's hard to pinpoint what it is we do. When people ask, I say we're a little bit medicine, a little bit education, and a little bit business. It's exciting to me that the field has made a commitment to us by offering this exam and saying, instead of being a little bit of all . . . things, we're going to make our own category. I now have a definition for what I do. I am a CME professional. There might be some folks newer to the field who are enticed to stay because it's not just a job—they can make this their career.[2]

A Certification Examination

Following a rigorous request for proposal process, NC-CME contracted with Schroeder Measurement Technologies (SMT) to develop, administer, and validate an examination worthy of CCMEP candidates. NC-CME enlisted enthusiastic volunteers to work with SMT. Prior to the 2008 Alliance annual meeting, a job analysis team spent six hours reviewing the eight competencies and 48 subcompetencies published by the Alliance. The resulting job analysis became the basis of an online survey directed at individuals working in CME. Results from 272 completed surveys identified the following five domains that reflect the relative importance of 75 items requiring specific knowledge and skills: adult learning principles (15 percent), educational interventions (30 percent), relationships with stakeholders (10 percent), leadership/administration/management (25 percent), and the CME environment (20 percent).

The job analysis survey findings guided the

development of an exam that reflects practice-based competencies. During three days, an item writing team composed of 14 subject matter experts wrote and edited more than 200 test items at the SMT office. A validation review team examined each item to verify that the exam captured the domain areas adequately and to ensure that each item was clear in the concept it measures. Finally, SMT psychometricians assisted the validation team in setting the cut score that determines who passes the exam.

Perhaps the most courageous volunteers were those who signed up to be beta testers for the exam. Knowing that they might not pass the exam and paying their own expenses plus a processing fee, 47 candidates sat for the paper and pencil exam in San Francisco and Toronto. Thirty-two candidates served as beta testers for the computer-based test. By July 1, 2008, the CCMEP credential was awarded to 70 individuals, and that count grew to 157 by year's end, resulting in an 86 percent pass rate.

In its drive for continuous improvement, NC-CME launched Form 2 of the CCMEP exam in June 2009. CCMEP-credentialed volunteers for the test writing team submitted more than 200 test items complete with stem, key, distracters, and citations. During a period of three days, an exam review team reviewed the test items and every comment submitted by Form 1 candidates. The validation team gave each item a reality check, and psychometricians calculated a new cut score for Form 2 to ensure that the range of test results would be equal among Forms 1 and 2, in case the exam forms were not equal in difficulty. A similar test development process was undertaken in 2010 and resulted in the writing, reviewing, and posting of an online practice exam available at any time and in the privacy of one's home or office.

Acceptance within the CME Community

The CCMEP certification exam became a reality in June 2008, and within two years nearly 300 CME professionals had achieved the CCMEP credential. Even before NC-CME began working on a certification process, widespread agreement existed that individuals working in CME needed to meet certain standards regardless of their work settings. The closest the CME community came to adopting a measure of competence had been the ACCME Essentials and Standards for accreditation, which applied to organizations wishing to provide *AMA CME Category 1 Credits™* for their continuing education activities. But ACCME accreditation was inaccessible to some segments of the CME enterprise, and even for ACCME-accredited providers the emphasis was on organizations and not on individuals. The Alliance had identified eight competencies and 48 subcompetencies, but no rigorous program was offered to assess and certify the competence of all persons employed in CME settings.

From its inception, the NC-CME board of directors recognized that for a viable certification program to be fully accepted by the broad spectrum of CME professionals, such a program would need to be established in collaboration with other CME organizations whose missions included education and competency development. The board recognized the relatively short window of opportunity that existed to develop and implement a certification program that could survive politically and financially.

Questions from the CME leadership fell into three areas: (1) what is NC-CME and why is it developing this new credential? (2) is a credentialing process the best way to ensure competence within CME? and (3) what are the potential implications for the CME enterprise? In May 2006, an informal meeting was convened by Kues and held in Chicago to discuss these issues. Invitees included key individuals affiliated with the AMA and the Alliance, Society for Academic Continuing Medical Education (SACME), ACCME, specialty societies, and state medical societies. Kues outlined the NC-CME proposal for professional certification as one mechanism to address issues of competency and to promote professional development among individuals working in CME. The meeting marked the first time that a broad contingent of influential individuals discussed the implications of a professional certification program.

In October 2006, the Alliance held a meeting of CME stakeholders to more formally discuss different models of professional development and maintenance of competence within CME. Although NC-CME was not invited, Kues attended as the SACME representative. Ronald M. Cervero, PhD, facilitated the meeting, and the major outcome was a list of three models for addressing continued competence for CME workers: (1) attendance at meetings held by organizations (e.g., the Alliance, SACME, ACCME); (2) development of certificate programs based on a specific curriculum within specialized topics within CME; and (3) implementation of a certification program, such as the one being developed by NC-CME. These three initiatives were considered to be complementary, and further development in all three areas was encouraged. Although the meeting did not convert all certification skeptics, it did open the door to further support and development.

Reactions to the Certification Initiative

While the NC-CME board of directors worried that the certification initiative might not have enough momentum to succeed in the short window of time available, others worried that it *would* succeed. Some feared that the new certification might become a requirement for everyone working in CME and, therefore, require employers to pay certified CME professionals higher salaries that would be too costly for organizations to maintain. Concerns circulated about how pharmaceutical companies might require CME certification to submit grant requests or how ACCME might include certification of providers' CME staff in a future revision of its Essentials for reaccreditation. NC-CME addressed these concerns

through its Web site, personal communications, and presentations at the Alliance annual meeting and similar venues.

Conversely, a growing number of people expressed interest in the credential. At national meetings, presentations about professional certification attracted standing-room-only crowds, and visitors to the NC-CME Web site submitted personal postings to the "What our colleagues are saying . . ." Web page. Results from a NC-CME survey of those professionals receiving CCMEP certification in 2008 indicated that 112 respondents believed they had benefited since receiving certification.

CCMEP Value Propositions: The Public, the Workers, the Employers

Proponents of certification have claimed that having a certification program adds value to the profession as a whole and benefits the general public. Generic benefits of certification posited by ICE have included far-reaching benefits that have accrued to segments of society that have adopted credentialing initiatives. As envisioned by NC-CME, benefits to the public attributable to certification of CME professionals may include providing standards for a self-regulated enterprise that impacts health care; creating an objective, independent program that qualifies persons who develop CME for physicians; offering a measure of assurance that CME activities honor Food and Drug Administration and Health and Human Services–Office of Inspector General guidelines; and encouraging professionalism among persons who migrate into the CME community.

NC-CME has advocated that certification can benefit CME workers (i.e., the individuals who develop, administer, market, and fund CME activities) by positioning CME as a career path, acknowledging excellence, motivating new learning and self-assessment, serving as a rationale for promotion, and providing evidence of competence and portability of skills when job hunting.

Accredited providers and supporters of CME activities may benefit from certification by giving objective evidence of continuous quality improvement within the organization, providing rationale for promoting staff and screening job candidates, encouraging professional development and sharpening skill sets, raising the quality of CME programming, and reducing the risk of noncompliance with national guidelines.

Volunteer Involvement

NC-CME has seen its responsibilities as confined principally to the development of the CCMEP credentialing program, that is, establishing eligibility of applicants, developing test items for certification exams, corresponding with applicants, overseeing the administration of the exams, record-keeping, and creating demand for the credential. Oversight of item writing, psychometric validation of each form of the exam, and online computer-based test administration has been in the purview of the test development company contracted to deliver these program segments.

By 2009, a cadre of more than 80 volunteers had formed committees and teams to accomplish these tasks and to recommend policies and procedures to the board of directors. Committees (and their chairs) in place in 2009 included the following: By Laws (Mason), Exam Development (Hershman), Executive Committee (Overstreet), External Relations (Michael Lemon, MBA, CCMEP), Financial Development (Kues), Marketing (Daniel Guinee, MBA, CCMEP), Standards (Galbraith), and Strategic Planning (Lee).

Initial fundraising efforts by volunteers elicited contributions for start-up funding from charter donors, without whom NC-CME arguably would still be a concept bandied about by various groups. Three organizations pledged and came through with three-year donations. Many more contributed services-in-kind for accounting, marketing, and Web site services. A listing of charter donors and sustaining donors can be found at www.nc-cme.org.

In January 2009, NC-CME received the Alliance for CME Award for Innovation in Continuing Professional Development. In November 2009, the Alliance announced plans to develop educational materials designed to help candidates prepare for the CCMEP exam. This Alliance project represented a positive step toward providing the often requested candidate support that NC-CME had determined was outside of its purview as a certifying organization.

In 2010, the exam development team recommended options for extended certification and recertification for certified CME professionals whose initial certification was timed to expire in June 2011. At the time of this publication, the CCMEP program consists of Initial Certification, which requires candidates to document their professional qualifications and successfully pass a validated, secure, three-hour certification examination; Extension of Certification (EOC), which serves to extend the initial three-year certification to five years for CCMEPs who can fulfill the EOC eligibility requirements; and Recertification, which is available to CCMEPs who have documented additional performance improvement activities and have passed the currently available form of a validated, secure, three-hour certification examination. The ongoing certification program requires sitting for an exam every five years. Details about the NC-CME certification program can be accessed at www.NC-CME.org.

Moving Forward

What does the future hold for the NC-CME and its CCMEP certification program? The ultimate success of this pioneering venture will be acknowledged as a product of the grass-roots acceptance, generosity, and forward-thinking encouragement of the organizations, employers, and individuals who comprise the CME enterprise. Essential to the maturing of CME as a profession, the CCMEP designation will continue to bring a sense of ownership of CME as a career track to those individuals who have taken responsibility for their own continuing professional development, even as they are instrumental in creating continuing education for others. Persons who rely on the services of physicians and other health-care professionals will be the ultimate beneficiaries.

Notes

1. Richard V. King and Sterling A. North, "Competency Areas for CME Professionals," Alliance for CME Web site, http://www.acme-assn.org (accessed February 15, 2005).

2. Martha Collins, "Continuing Medical Education Profession Launches Certification Program," *Medical Meetings* (2008).

Lewis A. Miller, Leonard Harvey,
Bernard Maillet, Alfonso Negri,
Robin Stevenson, and Egle Zebiene

CHAPTER 29

Continuing Medical Education and Continuing Professional Development in Europe: The New Reality

The most exciting place to be in the world of continuing medical education (CME) is just that: the world. CME is becoming a fact of life—and of continued practice—for physicians in many countries, especially those in the European Union (EU).

Despite a lack of evidence that mandating CME as a requirement to maintain a medical license provides proof that a doctor is competent, an increasing number of European nations have imposed such a requirement. As a result, CME administrative structures, regulations, and courses have been multiplying. Live education, particularly in national and international congresses, is still the norm. However, a clear trend toward electronic CME (eCME) is developing across the EU.

The accepted paradigm for CME in the United States and Canada is slowly becoming adopted in most European countries. That paradigm includes needs assessment of the target audience; development of appropriate content and a delivery method independent of a funding source; and outcomes assessment (though seldom progressing beyond physician satisfaction). The EU is moving rapidly toward acceptance of this paradigm in part because of the work of the European Union of Medical Specialists (UEMS) and its subsidiary body, the European Accreditation Council for CME® (EACCME). Some specialty societies have set up their own CME accreditation boards,

most notably in cardiology and pneumology. Additionally, there is a trend toward going beyond CME and onward to continuing professional development (CPD). The CME structure for general practitioners, as compared to specialists, has been less well defined, though the European Union of General Practitioners (UEMO) and the European division of the World Organization of Family Doctors (WONCA) are making strides to catch up.

The work of the UEMS, the Global Alliance for Medical Education (GAME), and the less formal Rome Group has promoted the concept of CME harmonization in the EU and around the world. The challenge for the future is to implement such a concept and to encourage all nations to join in an effort to improve the quality of health care for their citizens through evidence-based, learner-based, and patient-based CME.

The European Union of Medical Specialists

The European Union of Medical Specialists (UEMS) was established in 1958, following the signing of the Treaty of Rome in 1957 by the six founding countries.[1] In the Treaty of Rome, harmonization and mutual recognition of diplomas is foreseen as a part of the free movement principle. The objective of the UEMS has always been bringing together the medical specialists of the

TABLE **29-1** *UEMS Charters*

Charter Name	Adoption Year	Objective
Charter on Continuing Medical Education	1994	Sets out the basic structure of CME and points the need for the profession to taking a leading role
Charter on Quality Assurance in Specialist Practice	1999	Includes the need for CME to maintain quality assurance
Charter on Visitation of Training Centres	1997	Assesses and improves the quality of graduate training
Charter on Continuing Professional Development (also called the Basel Declaration)	2001	Defines CPD as the educative means of updating, developing, and enhancing how doctors apply the knowledge, skills, and attitudes required in their working lives; categorizes CPD as essential to ongoing specialty training
Declaration on Ensuring the Quality of Medical Care (also called the Budapest Declaration)	2006	Emphasizes the profession's responsibility for regulating physician practice; states that "the continuum of medical education provides the means, at all stages of a doctor's career, of imparting high standards of medical practice"

Source: http://admin.uems.net/uploadedfiles/174.pdf; http://admin.uems.net/uploadedfiles/175.pdf; http://admin.uems .net/uploadedfiles/179.pdf; http://admin.uems.net/uploadedfiles/35.pdf; http://admin.uems.net/uploadedfiles/875.pdf.

member states and reaching consensus on content and quality of medical specialist training and practice. The outcome of this process was meant to serve as the foundation for EU legislation.

The specialist sections—now numbering 52—were established from 1962 onwards, and the UEMS with its sections was instrumental in the shaping of the Doctors Directive in 1975, which established mutual recognition of medical diplomas between the member states of the EU.[2] The start was slow, but in the 1970s the EU moved towards legal provisions in this matter. In the follow-up, however, little attention was paid to the contributions of the UEMS, and quality requirements remained limited. The EU blocked the progress of implementation of quality requirements during the 1980s, and a new approach was required.

In the 1990s, the UEMS emphasis moved toward key issues such as professional training, continuing education, quality assessments, and tools like logbooks and visitations of training centers. The outcome of this process was embodied in UEMS Charters, which were presented to the professional authorities in the EU countries as models and recommendations for national policy (see Table 29-1). Although the UEMS Charters do not have legal value, their influence upon national regulations has been considerable.

By 2007, medical associations of 35 countries were represented in the UEMS, with 30 as full members and five as associate members.[3] In 2008, UEMS celebrated its 50th anniversary with a meeting of the entire constituency, the national medical associations, the UEMS sections and boards, as well as delegates from the National Accreditation Authorities (NAAs) throughout the EU.

CME and CPD Process and Accreditation

CME or CPD is an important part of medical practice in the EU today. The training needed to become a specialist doctor starts with undergraduate and graduate training at the university, followed by postgraduate training that is done ideally in cooperation between the profession and the university. In the past this was the end of the process, but it is more than obvious that lifelong learning for the practitioner is essential to maintain knowledge and skills.

The process started with CME, where mainly theoretical courses and congresses were organized. Nowadays this is moving to CPD by the improvement of communication, information technology, and managerial and social skills and is more concentrated on the practice of each individual practitioner and his or her needs. Several of the Charters referred to, plus other UEMS documents, were prepared by the CME/CPD Working Group chaired by Edwin Borman, MD, of the United Kingdom (UK) from 1999 to 2009.[4]

CME or CPD needs and organization are the duties of the NAA in each EU member state. The NAA has to define how many credits and which kind of credits are needed for each year or time period. A physician cannot gain all of his or her credits by following only one means of CME or CPD; credits may be earned through long-distance learning programs, live events, enduring material like CD-ROMs, or articles, depending on the credit system of each NAA.[5]

During the 1990s, many European countries began taking steps towards mandatory CME together with legal or professional recertification or re-licensing and financial incentives or contracts with insurances and hospitals, even though that was not the position of the UEMS. Table 29-2 indicates the current status of mandatory and voluntary CME in European countries.

To help European medical specialists harmonize and improve the quality of their education, in October 1999, under the direction of the then secretary-general Cees Leibbrandt, MD, the UEMS Council set up the European Accreditation Council for CME (EACCME), with a view to allow the recognition and exchange of CME credits in Europe easily. From the point of view of the providers of events, the accreditation process has become less time-consuming and easier, since providers do not have to apply to each NAA

TABLE 29-2 *Mandatory and Voluntary CME Status in Europe*

Country	Status
Austria	Mandatory
Belgium	Mandatory
Croatia	Mandatory
Czech Republic	Mandatory
Denmark	Voluntary
Finland	Voluntary
France	Mandatory
Germany	Mandatory
Greece	Voluntary
Hungary	Mandatory
Iceland	Voluntary
Ireland	Mandatory
Italy	Mandatory
Luxembourg	Voluntary
Netherlands	Mandatory
Norway (GPs only)	Mandatory
Poland	Mandatory
Portugal	Voluntary
Romania	Mandatory
Slovakia	Mandatory
Slovenia	Mandatory
Spain	Voluntary
Sweden	Voluntary
Switzerland	Mandatory
Turkey	Voluntary
United Kingdom (with revalidation)	Mandatory

in those countries in which physician attendees practice. The CME/CPD activity needs to have an international dimension in order to be considered by EACCME.[6]

The quality control of CME activities is a key element in this process, using the expertise of existing European and national professional bodies involved in accreditation. At the same time, EACCME recognized the political necessity to comply with NAA regulations because these bodies are responsible for registering doctors' CME-CPD and awarding licences to practice.

The governing body of the EACCME structure is a UEMS Council, which is made up of representatives from national associations of each UEMS member country. An advisory council provides recommendations with regard to the management of European accreditation. This body is made up of representatives from national professional CME authorities, including national CME accrediting bodies; UEMS, including its sections and boards; and professional specialist organizations and societies.

Right from the start, it was clear that national professional regulatory bodies would approve a structure such as EACCME. The only condition was that these bodies would remain in charge of events in their own country and would have a major input in the process of EACCME. This is a political reality. The requirements were set in 2003 and Figure 29-1 shows how the process works in practice:

- The final word concerning accreditation of each activity remains the decision of the national regulatory body in the country where the activity takes place.
- The Brussels administration should be as lean as possible.
- Quality assurance and determination of number of credits of separate CME activities would be decentralized, EACCME relying upon the expertise of professional bodies in each specialty (such as the UEMS Sections and/or Boards and European Speciality Accreditation Boards).
- There would be no accreditation of commercially biased activities or Internet activities. (As of 2009, EACCME accredits eCME.)
- Each activity should be judged separately; providers are not accredited for series of activities stretching over years.
- Administrative expenses of EACCME are borne by the providers of activities applying for European accreditation. Expenses would be limited, avoiding duplication in Brussels of work already done by other accreditation bodies.[7]

In 2002 EACCME signed an agreement with the American Medical Association (AMA) to mu-

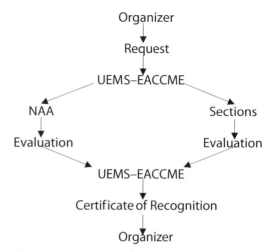

Figure 29-1 Flowchart of the EACCME process. The request process takes more than three months. The evaluation process takes less than three weeks. *Source: Continuing Medical Education and Professional Development in Europe; Development and Structure* (Brussels: Union of European Medical Specialists, 2008), 13.

tually recognize credits.[8] This has been renewed and is valid from July 1, 2006, for a period of four years. In this way, European physicians attending an accredited event in the United States can have these credits recognized in Europe, and US physicians gain the same benefit if attending an accredited event in Europe.

The organizer of an event fills in the Web-based application form with all the relevant and needed documents. The request form is distributed by e-mail to the two partners. The relevant UEMS Section and/or Board assesses the scientific value of the activity. The NAA guarantees the value of the credits allocated to the activity. When both partners approve, the organizer receives a letter confirming European accreditation and mutual recognition of AMA PRA Category 1 credits.

As the different NAAs apply different credit systems, the European CME Credits (ECMEC) were introduced in order to harmonize the number of credits on the following basis: one ECMEC per hour, three ECMEC for half a day, and six ECMEC for a full-day event. National authorities can then convert these credits into national units. The UEMS–EACCME asks a fee for the processing of the applications. This fee is based only on the number of participants and is a sliding scale. The two equal major partners in the system share their part of the fee.

Efforts will soon be concentrated to ask the organizers to prepare an evaluation of the event, answering questions such as was the event well organized, did I learn something from the event, will what I learned from the event change my practice, and did I feel any bias? The principal aim of this evaluation is not to retrospectively throw away the allocated credits but rather to help the organizer plan the next activity of the same kind.

CME Systems in Five European Countries

A legal regulation in France made CME mandatory in 1996 for doctors involved in public, private, and mixed systems. Since that time, four plans have been proposed but none implemented as of 2009. Requirements keep changing but appear to include performance improvement, practice audits, and CPD courses. Some 500 providers had been accredited as of 2008, and physicians do participate in available courses.[9]

CME (CPD) is mandatory in all 16 states of Germany with mutual recognition between their Chambers of Physicians for MDs in offices organized within the National Association of Statutory Health Insurance Physicians (KBV) and those with the qualification of a specialist in hospitals for regular hospitals for acute cases.

Under the federal system, the regional chambers of physicians are primarily responsible for CME, but there is a harmonized structure for mutual recognition of credits. The Senate for Medical Education of the German Federal Medical Association has issued guidelines for the accreditation of CME activities in eight typical categories: lectures and discussions, congresses, workshops with active participation, interactive education (scientific print-media, CD, DVD,

Web), self-study, part-time training on the job ("hospitation"), and work as an author and/or lecturer. The basis for gaining a certificate is a minimum of 250 credits over a period of five years. Failure to do so can result in a reduction in payment for physician services and eventual loss of license.[10]

In 1999, the Italian government passed an Act in Law making CME mandatory both in the National Health System and in private practice. The Italian Ministry of Health started a system for all health-care professionals in April 2002. The health-care professional does not have the full choice of his or her CME; part of it must be obtained according to the national or regional health priorities. Financing is almost solely by the pharmaceutical industry, which therefore has had a major effect.[11]

As of 2009, the system was in disarray because of a reorganization of government ministries and differences among the provinces regarding accreditation of programs versus providers and other issues. It appears that a new system being instituted in 2010 across the country will be based on accreditation of providers and will include CPD and require transparency of commercial sponsorship and clear identification of conflict of interest.[12]

The CME system is voluntary in Spain. CME credits are used for professional career purposes in regional public health services in which most Spanish physicians are employees (salary incentive). It appears that the system will move toward incorporating relicensure and recertification in the future.

By law, the 17 regional governments are responsible for the accreditation of continuing education of heath professions. All of them report to the Central Commission, a subcommittee of the Inter-Territorial Council of the Ministry of Health. The Spanish Medical Association has developed a specific accreditation system for CME, after having been entrusted with doing so by the Ministry of Health and the Ministry of Education. The Spanish Accreditation Council for CME

(SACCME) was created in 2003 in partnership with FACME, the Spanish Assembly of Deans of Medical Schools and the Spanish Council of Medical Specialties. An agreement on mutual recognition has been signed between the Spanish Medical Association–SACCME and the UEMS–EACCME.[13]

In the UK, the term *CPD* is used because CPD includes not only CME but also continuing education in all aspects of a doctor's professional life, both clinical and nonclinical. Meeting the standards for CPD set by the medical Royal Colleges is necessary for a satisfactory annual appraisal and, generally, to remain in good standing with the doctor's college. CPD is virtually mandatory. Appraisal is a contractual obligation, in which a doctor's education and development needs for the following year are agreed upon and learning objectives are documented as part of a personal development plan that is reviewed at the subsequent appraisal to ensure that objectives have been met.

The NAA in the UK is the Academy of Medical Royal Colleges, which is responsible for CPD through a group made up of the directors of CPD of each constituent college or faculty. The General Medical Council (GMC), which serves as the UK's national regulatory authority, has stated that CPD should cover all areas of a doctor's professional practice and all domains of the document "Good Medical Practice."[14]

The most significant change proposed in the UK is the introduction of a compulsory system of revalidation, divided into a process of re-licensure and a second process of specialist recertification that will apply to those on the GMC's Specialist Register and to general practitioners.[15]

The Role of Specialty Accreditation Bodies

Initially EACCME forwarded applications for accreditation of educational events to the NAA of the country where the event was going to take place and also to the relevant UEMS Specialty Section or Board. The NAA frequently had a clerical infrastructure to facilitate its assessment of the event, but this did not apply to the UEMS Sections and Boards, which lacked the resources to employ ancillary staff. In 2001, cardiology, followed by pneumology, tackled this problem by forming joint accreditation boards composed of members nominated by the UEMS Specialty Section and by the corresponding European scientific society. Thus the European Boards for Accreditation in Cardiology (EBAC) and Pneumology (EBAP) were formed. Other specialties that have set up accreditation boards include urology, infectious diseases, oncology, and hematology. These boards are known as European Specialty Accreditation Boards (ESABs).[16] The scientific societies provided financial support to establish the joint boards in the expectation that the boards would eventually become self-financing.

There is a conflict of interest in this system since the main provider in each specialty is the European scientific society that is represented in the ESAB. As ESABs have developed, some (EBAC and EBAP) have sought increased autonomy from UEMS but still abide by the EACCME accreditation principles.[17]

ESABs aim to facilitate the process by which European doctors obtain the CME credits necessary to satisfy the regulatory authorities in their own countries. They also make a judgment on whether proposed educational programs are of sufficient standard to be accredited as suitable CME material. Initially this just meant looking at the program of the event to determine its duration, from which the number of available credits would be calculated. In addition the ESABs attempt to exclude the possibility of bias by the pharmaceutical industry. Specialist reviewers have been recruited by the ESABs, and usually an application for accreditation is sent to two or three of the reviewers.

Some ESABs as well as some NAAs have tried to influence providers to improve the quality of their CME by providing guidelines about delivery of educational material. But fewer than five percent of applications are turned down. This is partly because it is difficult to assess the quality of CME from looking at the program and partly because the event has been fully organized by the time the application is being reviewed and it is too late to make changes that the ESAB may consider to be necessary. In addition to live events, ESABs are now accrediting eCME. At present ESAB reviewers must experience the whole program rather than just checking the people involved and looking at the topics, as happens with live events. Reviewers must commit more time and effort; this raises the possibility that they will have to be paid for their work, thereby further increasing the costs for the providers. So far there is no evidence that the activities of ESABs have resulted in improved CME quality.

The Role of GP Organizations

In most European countries professional organizations are the principal governing bodies that support continuous medical education and continuous professional development (lifelong learning).[18]

The basic principles of CME/CPD for GPs at the European level are largely defined by the European Union of General Practitioners (UEMO) and gradually have become a common strategy internationally as well as within individual European countries.[19] While many Central and Eastern European countries still follow the rule of availability and supply-driven CME/CPD activities, the approach practiced in countries such as UK, Denmark, and Netherlands has developed into activities focusing on needs of the individual doctor, practice, and community. As described in a UEMO statement, "It is the responsibility of the individual general practitioner to make optimal use of resources (time, finance) which in the given national system are set aside for CPD. This is achieved by enabling the GPs themselves to explicitly identify their personal learning needs and select their CPD activities accordingly."

The approach is in line with the joint document of the European Academy of Teachers in General Practice and Family Medicine (EURACT) and the European Association for Quality in General Practice/Family Medicine (EQUIP), two WONCA Europe member networks that developed a common statement of CME/CPD activities in the light of quality assurance.[20] It states that planning professional development should start from perceived needs in individual practices; the goals are set by the physician or the practice team setting up a personal or practice professional development plan. Quality assurance offers various methods to detect, define, and analyze these needs.

The crucial role of professional organizations within Europe is to ensure availability of events and programs in order to fulfill those needs as well as defend basic principles of international practice within individual countries. This includes mutual responsibility for the determination of a minimum amount of time for CPD on an annual basis, which should be reflected in the resources (finances, time, CPD offers) made available nationally for this purpose. As various teaching methods have different strengths and weaknesses, the broadest possible range of learning opportunities should be offered. The individual doctor must be able to choose the methods that (1) are most relevant for him or her in the context of the identified learning needs, (2) include opportunities to have skills updated or learned, and (3) challenge the attitudes that may impede excellent patient care.

A broad array of CPD activities with regard to both form and content is a prerequisite for high quality CPD. Accreditation in accordance with established criteria could be a method for securing quality. Obligatory CME does not guarantee quality. Nonetheless, according to a EURACT survey performed in 2009, 56 percent of CME/CPD activities in Europe go through the mandatory process of accreditation. The principle of voluntary choice is the only way of ensuring that the individual needs are covered in the best possible manner and that the resources earmarked for CPD are used effectively.

While those basic principles of CME/CPD organizational aspects have been developed by UEMO as well as other European organizations and networks mentioned above, the content of the activities for a long time has been based on the sporadic clinical topics, coming from the perceived needs of learners. The situation in Europe started changing dramatically after the publication of a new document that redefined the basic principles of the discipline of the GP/FP. "The European Definition of General Practice/Family Medicine," a document developed by joint efforts of all WONCA Europe member organizations and networks, was launched during the 2002 WONCA Conference in London.[21] The document, which later gained appreciation far beyond the European region, defined or described key features of the discipline of general practice or family medicine, the role of the general practitioner, and core competencies of the general practitioner or family physician. These key changes in the definition of the professional role of GP led to development of the educational document—EURACT Educational Agenda of General Practice/Family Medicine, which defined educational consequences for activities at all levels of the learning process, including CME/CPD activities, aimed at achieving and maintaining the competencies required by the profession.[22] As a consequence of this strategy, the main challenge for CME/CPD in future is expected to move towards the learning and teaching processes based on the competence-oriented approach and dictated by needs of the individual professional and the community.

Role of the Pharmaceutical Industry

In Europe, most CME/CPD activities have been financed by the pharmaceutical industry, which in many cases has paid the travel expenses of selected physicians to attend European or international congresses and provided luxury accommodations and meals. In some instances, companies themselves have served as the developers of CME content, which has then been offered through medical organizations.

The scenario is changing. Norway has long resisted the support of industry for its CME events. The UEMS has stipulated that proof of disclosure of conflict of interest and absence of commercial bias are required for EACCME accreditation. The Royal Colleges of Physicians of the UK requires a declaration that commercial sponsorship does not influence structure or content of CME/CPD, that educational grants must be unrestricted, and that there must be a clear separation of promotion from education. The industry itself, through the International Federation of Pharmaceutical Manufacturers Associations (IFPMA), has promulgated a code of marketing practices that specifies that "companies should avoid using renowned or extravagant venues" for educational events and that "hospitality provided should not exceed what healthcare professional recipients would normally be prepared to pay for themselves."[23]

By EURACT's definition, a GP's choice must be independent of influence from public authorities, insurance systems, and the pharmaceutical industry. This approach has received new meaning after the challenging initiative of the Nordic Colleges, which suggested that "all accredited, approved, continuous medical education must be undertaken without the involvement of the pharmaceutical industry" in order to "secure the doctors' integrity and credibility and to reduce the possibilities of undue influence."[24] It was explicitly discussed during the WONCA Europe Council meeting in 2005, and though no decision was reached, the approach raised awareness that the future CPD activities of primary care professionals may be strongly regulated by professional organizations in regard to conflicts of interest and sponsorship of the events. Although the pharmaceutical industry still has significant influence on the CME/CPD processes in Europe through explicit sponsorship of educational events (up to 71 percent, according to some surveys), the future of the CME/CPD in Europe is likely to be significantly influenced by this ongoing discussion.

Future Implications for CME in Europe

The assurance of high quality CME/CPD must build upon criteria established by the profession in close cooperation with academic organizations and universities. The philosophy of all national professional medical organizations is that patient care is best served when quality and content of medical training and practice are the domain of the medical profession. In each country the profession is defending this position. The establishment of quality requirements must furthermore involve other interested parties: patients, public authorities, insurance systems, and politicians. Unfortunately, it appears that governments, insurances, and commercial interests have been eager to take over the quality agenda.

The UEMS with its sections and boards is by far the largest of all political European medical associations and has extensive grassroots support. It has done much, but more is needed. So far each country is autonomous in health-care matters, but European integration is gaining momentum. The profession must be ready to play its role in a future integrated European health-care policy, starting at the national level, that includes unity of purpose and policy of national organizations, coordination of separate national organizations, and enlargement of investment by national medical organizations in European medical matters, in imagination, and in people, expertise, and financial means.

At the European level, a more unified voice of the medical profession is needed, leaving intact the professional independence of groups like medical specialists and general practitioners. Very likely, the authority of the EU in health-care issues will expand in the future. The medical profession should bring forward its views on the quality issue in one voice. It should prepare itself to provide the EU in the future with constructive and well founded recommendations on key issues.

One key issue, of course, is the future of CME/CPD. Some of the considerations include:

- An emphasis on independent CME, free of bias, whether from commercial or institutional sources, that offers a fair balance to participating physicians.
- Evidence-based lifelong learning not only in clinical areas but also in other areas of professional life that employ adult learning principles.
- Needs assessment as the foundation of programs, based on identifying gaps in individual, group, and community care of patients, particularly those with chronic diseases.
- Use of a variety of media, emphasizing interactivity and small group discussions in a continuum of learning.
- Outcomes measurement not only of physician satisfaction and knowledge change but also of improvement in competence, performance, and patient outcomes.
- A solid relationship with industry based on mutual trust and industry's recognition that CME/CPD needs to be controlled by medical profession providers in terms of topic selection, faculty selection, content development, and outcomes measurement.

The benefit to such a framework should be improved patient care.

Another critical issue is accreditation of events vs. providers. If Europe persists with the system of accrediting individual educational items, more expert reviewers and more time will be involved. The end result may be expensive compliance with bureaucratic regulations without improvement in the quality of CME. If providers themselves are accredited on the basis of a review of their previous activities, this would allow the accrediting authorities to set standards to which the providers must adhere. In addition, the reviewing doctors need not be clinical specialists, since specialist expertise is not necessary to assess provider performance.

Italy has moved in this direction; France had done so in its 2008 national plan—never implemented. The rest of Europe might be wise to consider changing as well to what might be a simpler, cheaper system, which in turn might improve CME quality and result in better clinical practice. In addition, provider accreditation could resolve the conflict of interest between ESABs and the corresponding scientific society and its parent body, UEMS.

Yet another challenge recently introduced in Europe is the evaluation of the impact of the CPD activities on quality of health-care provision, as briefly referred to above in terms of outcomes measures. While CPD activity is part of a common strategy in all countries, assessment of cost-effectiveness of the interventions is not yet a common approach. Continuing professional development for health-care professionals must be cost effective to avoid a waste of resources, and economic studies of such interventions must therefore be of sufficient quality and quantity to allow conclusions to be drawn.[25]

Key Events in Global Harmonization

In theory the health-care professional must participate in CME that is based on individual educational needs, ensure that the needs are relevant to professional practice, evaluate the extent to which the needs have been met, in the context of a change in knowledge, competence, or performance, and finally verify that mechanisms are in place to keep educational activities free of commercial bias.

However, the major problem today is that the various CME systems are very different and fragmented throughout the world. In a perfect world, a health-care professional coming from Germany and attending a conference in Canada would be able to collect his or her CME credits and use them back home. Today this is not the case, but the possibility of this actually happening is no longer a mirage, thanks to the work of the Rome Group and GAME.

The Rome Group

In 2003, Alfonso Negri, MD, then scientific/technical secretary of ICAP, Italian Council for Accreditation in Pneumology, and EAACI, European Allergology and Clinical Immunology, had the idea of trying to bridge the gaps between accreditation systems around the world by getting the various players in CME/CPD together to find common ground.[26]

A first meeting—USA–EU: Sharing the Educational Effort—was held in Milan in March 2003 with representatives of the Union of European Medical Specialists, the American Medical Association, the Italian Ministry of Health's CME Commission, the Italian Federation of Scientific Medical Societies, and other international as well as Italian scientific societies. Serono Symposia International Foundation provided logistical and financial support to this initiative from the beginning.

Starting from the second meeting, in Rome in October of the same year, the foundations were laid to find common ground on reciprocity of credits. During the succeeding years the group expanded to include additional EU countries and Canada. Today it is referred to as the *Rome Group* because these meetings are held annually in Rome. Negri is secretary general.

The Rome Group is currently made up of representatives of the following institutions:

- American Medical Association
- Royal College of Physicians and Surgeons of Canada
- Finnish Medical Association
- Accreditation Council for Continuing Medical Education
- Union of European Medical Specialists
- College of Family Physicians of Canada
- Spanish Accreditation Council for CME
- French National Committees for CME
- Italian Federation of Scientific Medical Societies

- Federation of Royal Colleges of Physicians
- National CME Commission of the Italian Ministry of Health
- Bavarian Chamber of Physicians
- Bulgarian Union of Scientific Medical Societies

The first major work of the Rome Group was a consensus document (appropriately named the Rome Document) on basic values and responsibilities underlying the substantial equivalence of CME and CPD systems. This document was based on the agreement that reasonable uniformity between nations in the principles and outcomes in the accreditation of CME/CPD and providers and organizers and credit systems would be valuable. Physicians could obtain credits for different local, national, and international organizations that require CME/CPD for maintenance of status purposes. In addition, physicians attending activities, and organizations that value accredited CME/CPD, could be assured of education that is of good and predictable quality. Among the many important elements of continuing medical education and professional development (CME/CPD) systems are (1) physician-learners involved in learning projects in support of their personal CPD, (2) providers and organizers of educational activities (or events) that are an educational resource to physicians, and (3) accrediting organizations that certify that the providers and organizers of educational activities meet certain accreditation standards so that credit can be awarded for participation in the activity. The Rome Group has also started a project to develop a common glossary of terms in CME/CPD.

Global Alliance for Medical Education

The Global Alliance for Medical Education (GAME) was established in June 1995 to serve as a forum for the exchange of ideas among leaders of nonprofit and for-profit organizations involved internationally in the development and marketing of CME and health education programs.[27]

GAME was launched in a manner similar to that of the Alliance for Continuing Medical Education (ACME) and shares the same founding father, Lewis Miller. The ACME began in 1975 when Miller, a publisher of clinical journals and other CME enduring materials, brought together a group of 45 persons from several disciplines to discuss the future of CME. While he continued his involvement with the ACME, he began to focus his publishing activities on the international development and distribution of CME. In 1990, he formed Intermedica Partners, a small group of associates in the United States and abroad, to carry out the first of two previously noted objectives.

By 1995, the group recognized a need to open membership to create a forum in which many more people could meet and exchange ideas. Ultimately, 22 people from the United States and seven other countries attended an informal meeting in June 1996, which was the start of GAME as an independent nonprofit organization. Members approved a formal structure and elected nine people to the board of directors.

Attendance at the second annual meeting in 1997 expanded to 50 persons from Europe, Latin America, North America, Australia, and Asia. The topics discussed included the development of CME in Europe, Latin America, and China; the possibility of reciprocal international systems of CME credit; disease management; and the use of new technologies in CME and health education.

A year later, at the third annual meeting in June 1998, some 70 people from around the world joined together in New York City to examine "How the New Media Will Affect CME and Health Education." The director of Columbia University's Center for New Media was the keynoter; presentations followed on changing formats already in use (e.g., online CME) and on pharmaceutical marketers' expectations of the needs for CME and health education in the emerging markets of the Far East, Latin America, and Eastern Europe.

Attendance and enthusiasm have grown, particularly as Europe has moved to its own system of CME through the new EACCME. Recent meetings have taken place in Montreal, Rome, New York, and Lyon, France, with further emphasis on harmonization of CME guidelines around the world.

GAME leaders, using their combined knowledge and experience, hope to be involved as advisors to CME leaders and health ministries in those countries that do not yet have a formal CME accreditation system.

Notes

1. *UEMS Yearbook* (Brussels: Union of European Medical Specialists, 2008), 15.

2. *UEMS Yearbook*, 15–16.

3. Ibid., 17.

4. Ibid., 19.

5. *Continuing Medical Education and Professional Development in Europe; Development and Structure* (Brussels: Union of European Medical Specialists, 2008), 27–30.

6. *Continuing Medical Education*, 9–11.

7. "The European Accreditation Council for Continuing Medical Education (EACCME)," Union of European Medical Specialists Web site, http://www.uems.net/uploadedfiles/48.pdf (accessed July 11, 2010).

8. "Memo to AMA Council on Medical Education," Union of European Medical Specialists Web site, http://www.uems.net/uploadedfiles/57.pdf (accessed July 11, 2010).

9. "Top Priority of the New CME Law in France: Performance Improvement," *The Global CME Newsletter* (November 2009), http://www.wentzmiller.org (accessed July 11, 2010).

10. *Continuing Medical Education*, 27–30.

11. Ibid., 40–42.

12. "Italy's CME System Moving to a Higher Level," *The Global CME Newsletter* (October 2009), http://www.wentzmiller.org (accessed July 25, 2010).

13. *Continuing Medical Education*, 56–57.

14. "Good Medical Practice," General Medical Council Web site, http://www.gmc-uk.org/guidance/good_medical_practice.asp (accessed July 25, 2010).

15. *Continuing Medical Education*, 61–64.

16. "Quality evaluation," European Specialty Accreditation Boards Web site, http://www.cme-european.org/European_CME/Quality_evaluation.php (accessed July 25, 2010).

17. Ibid.

18. R. Saltman and others, eds., *Primary Care in the Driver's Seat? European Observatory on Health Systems and Policies Series* (London: Open University Press, 2006).

19. "UEMO Policy: CPD—Continuing Professional Development of General Practitioners in Europe," European Union of General Practitioners Web site, http://www.uemo.org/text_policy.php?sec=14&cat=64 (accessed July 25, 2010).

20. "Continuing Professional Development Integration of Formal CME and Quality Improvement Initiatives, Policy Document of EQUIP and EURACT," European Academy of Teachers in General Practice and Family Medicine Web site, http://www.euract.org (accessed July 25, 2010).

21. The European Definition of General Practice/Family Medicine. WONCA Europe, 2002.

22. J. Heyrman, ed., *EURACT Educational Agenda of General Practice/Family Medicine* (Leuven: EURACT, 2005).

23. I. Starke, "Industry Support and Conflicts of Interest" (presentation, meeting of Global Alliance for Medical Education, Lyon, France, 2009); International Federation of Pharmaceutical Manufacturers Associations, "IFPMA Code of Pharmaceutical Marketing Practices 2006 Revision" (April 21, 2006).

24. "Continuing Professional Development Integration," European Academy of Teachers in General Practice; G. Roksund, "News from the Nordic Colleges of General Practitioners," *Scandinavian Journal of Primary Health Care* 23 (2005): 195–197.

25. C. A. Brown and others, "Cost Effectiveness of Continuing Professional Development in Health Care: A Critical Review of the Evidence," *British Medical Journal* 324 (2002): 652–655.

26. A. Negri, "The Group of Rome: Harmonization in Action" (presentation, meeting of Global Alliance for Medical Education, Jersey City, N.J., 2008).

27. "History," Global Alliance for Medical Education Web site, http://www.game-cme.org/about (accessed July 25, 2010).

Lewis A. Miller, Saurabh Jain, Sondra Moylan, and Pablo A. Pulido

CHAPTER 30

Continuing Medical Education for the World: Spreading to Latin America, Asia, Africa, and the Middle East

Formal systems of continuing medical education (CME) are expanding rapidly for physicians in Latin America, Asia, the Middle East, and Africa. Mandatory CME is not as prevalent as in the United States and Europe, but it does exist in a number of countries, particularly those that once were part of the far-flung British Empire—with the exception of India, which still has no system at all.

As in the United States and Europe, live education, particularly in national and international congresses, is still the norm. However, a clear trend toward electronic CME (eCME) is developing in many regions. Interprofessional continuing education is a concept that is only recently emerging in a few countries.

More Middle East and Asian representatives are now attending meetings of an international CME membership organization—the Global Alliance for Medical Education (GAME)—than in earlier years, while Latin American participation has declined. However, the Latin American region is beginning to investigate the possibility of creating a Latin American Accreditation Council for CME (LAACCME); the PanAmerican Federation of Associations of Medical Schools (PAFAMS) is taking the lead, rather than the specialty societies, which brought about the creation of the European Accreditation Council for CME (EACCME).

Events in Latin America

As in other parts of the world, CME programs in Latin America started as individual initiatives led by the national professional associations, medical schools, and universities, with support from ministries of health, hospitals, and the private sector (particularly the pharmaceutical industry, which plays a major role in a few countries in the region). Most programs and program providers had no formal accreditation standards. Governments had not developed mandatory or voluntary recertification or revalidation programs for general practitioners and/or specialists.

Latin America, a vast area of the American continents, has a population of close to 600 million (roughly eight percent of the world's population). The region presents extreme contrasts both between and within its countries, not only from socio-economical and political viewpoints but also from the perspective of approaches taken to improve health-care delivery and related education systems. The total number of physicians in Latin America is comparable to that of the United States (approximately 600,000). There is a broad and uneven distribution within each country, and most physicians work in the urban areas. Progress has been made in recent years in average life expectancy: from 50 years after World War II, to 67 in 1990, and to 72.8 today.

TABLE 30-1 *Status of CME in Latin America**

Country	Professional Accreditation	Mandatory for Specialists	Mandatory for GPs	Voluntary	No/Partial Accreditation	Standards for Commercial support
Argentina	X		X			
Bolivia					X	
Brazil	X	X				
Chile	X			X		
Colombia					X	
Costa Rica	X			X		
Mexico	X	X				
Ecuador					X	
Paraguay					X	
Perú	X	X				X
Uruguay	X			X		
Venezuela					X	
Others in Central America					X	

*CME legislation is about to be enacted in Colombia and Venezuela.

The PAFAMS is a nonprofit organization that stimulates programs to improve medical school performance through the national associations. In partnership with other international and national organizations, PAFAMS has facilitated the continuous exchange of experiences and research, geared to improve the quality of medical education.[1] A key component of this continuing exchange has been an emphasis on continuing professional education (CPE) designed to meet societal needs and demands.[2]

As a result of the efforts of PAFAMS, medical associations, and health ministries, in the past 10 years initiatives for CME accreditation and recertification have been formally developed in Colombia, Brazil, Mexico, Peru, and Argentina. A 2006 survey conducted on the status of CME among key representatives from major countries (see Table 30-1) showed that, in spite of many imbalances, there is a positive trend, though with no formal enforcement of the regulations

for accreditation and certification of CME activities and attendees.[3] Furthermore, the newest initiatives pursuing *behavioral changes among physicians* as a result of CME and continuing professional development (CPD) programs and reflected in patient outcomes have not been formally adopted yet in any country in the region. They are, however, generating considerable interest.

A rapid penetration and adoption of information technology has been observed in recent years, and thus e-learning CME initiatives have been put in place in a few countries (Argentina, Brazil, Mexico, and Colombia) and accredited accordingly.

There is an opportunity for an organization such as PAFAMS to work in alignment with the national associations, either professional or academic, and the respective governments to explore the feasibility of creating a regional council for accreditation of CME (i.e., LAACME), taking into consideration the successful developments in the United States and Europe.

In order to explore this possibility, an electronic survey of CME/CPD standards was circulated among 317 key opinion leaders from medical schools, medical societies, and other health and education institutions from the Americas by PAFAMS during the period of May 2007 through September 2007. The areas surveyed included satisfaction with CME systems in the region, intrinsic value of CME, feasibility for harmonization, and the potential role of leadership institutions in this process.

Results of this survey can be summarized as follows: (1) there is dissatisfaction with the current state of CME/CPD and (2) there is a need for harmonization of CME/CPD systems. PAFAMS and other educational stakeholders are expected to play a role in harmonization across Latin America. Although there are significant obstacles to achieving harmonization, there is a need for strong coordination between stakeholders to improve the quality of the population's health care through CME/CPD.

A separate study examined patient care quality and the potential need to improve non-clinical skills among practitioners and leaders from medical schools and medical associations in 13 Latin American countries, including Mexico, Brazil, Venezuela, and Argentina.[4] Results reveal declining patient care quality, satisfaction, and outcomes in all countries and strong global interest in collaboration, knowledge sharing, and co-development of educational programs for use in multiple countries, particularly in the areas of managerial capabilities, information technology, patient-physician interaction, ethics, and health policies.

There are ongoing efforts to align and synergize initiatives between government, academic institutions, professional associations, and the private sector (pharmaceuticals, banking, and other industries) to respond to these needs and develop regional programs aimed to prove the value of CME/CPD in leveraging health care.[5]

Events in the Middle East

Formal CME/CPE is advancing in the Middle East, particularly in the United Arab Emirates (UAE). The Health Authorities of Abu Dhabi and Dubai recognize that CME is a continuous process of acquiring new knowledge and skills throughout one's professional life. The UAE looks towards the American CME system as a benchmark for developing its own CME/CPE criteria. Many hospitals in the UAE are affiliated with American and European academic medical centers such as the Mayo Clinic, Harvard Medical School, and Cleveland Clinic.

Abu Dhabi

In 2007, the Health Authority–Abu Dhabi (HAAD) took major steps to strengthen continuing professional education, linking renewal of licenses for all health professionals to proof that they have been attending CE activities. Physicians are required to participate in 50 hours of CME per year, of which at least 25 must be formal learning opportunities such as lectures, seminars, or workshops provided by recognized educational institutions or professional bodies, and accredited by the HAAD or another internationally recognized body. At least 10 of the 25 hours must be in their specialty.

The CME department of HAAD conducted workshops and on-site visits to explain the importance of the CME process and encourage the health facilities' in-house education departments and pharmaceutical companies to carry out and sponsor CE events. HAAD has incorporated the US Accreditation Council for Continuing Medical Education (ACCME) Essentials and Policies into its requirements. An electronic system enables accurate accounting of credit hours.[6]

Israel

CME in Israel is still voluntary, and obtaining CME credits does not provide for any special recognition. There are no re-licensure or re-accreditation legislation requirements. However, physicians who do not participate in any CME activities for five years will have their names published and must take an examination to be eligible for academic or professional promotion.

The Education Committee of the Scientific Council of the Israel Medical Association (IMA) sets criteria for CME accredited activities and for CME certification. To gain certification, an IMA member must accumulate 500 points in five years from a basket of activities.[7]

The largest Health Management Organization (HMO), Clalit, serves 60 to 70 percent of the population under the governmental National Health Insurance system, employing its physicians on the basis of a collective contract with the physicians union. The strength of the union has enabled every doctor to have CME time that varies with his or her academic seniority from 28 to 52 half-day sessions per year. The doctors are free to choose their own CME activity. In addition the HMO may require its doctors to attend an additional six days of CME a year within the organization—usually used to promote organizational clinical policy goals.

Various contractors offer CME options, the largest being Ben-Gurion University of the Negev, and Tel-Aviv University. The HMO will also cover two-thirds of the cost of university CME programs that doctors choose to attend outside their working hours. The pharmaceutical industry subsidizes some HMO and university programs and also offers its own free lunch activities and conferences, which are however not generally recognized for CME credits.[8]

Iran

Iran has had mandatory CME for all health professionals since 1996, administered by the Ministry of Health and Medical Education and the Medical Council of Iran. Iran has been following US ACCME standards since 2005. Medical

schools are the primary providers, putting on 3,805 live programs in 2007; 680 were provided by medical associations and societies.

For recertification, physicians need 125 credits every five years or 50 credits each year, In addition to live programs, printed courses are eligible for credit, and as of 2007, Internet courses were being considered. The main source of support—80 percent—comes from registration fees paid by participants. Pharmaceutical companies and other sources fund a small amount.[9]

Events in Africa

Many African nations have some form of CME for their physicians, sometimes offered by government health ministries, sometimes by medical schools, often by pharmaceutical companies. But few have organized systems—mandatory or voluntary. The following are descriptions of how CME is organized in Egypt and South Africa.

Egypt

Once licensed, a physician can practice for life without any requirements for CME. There are CME courses marketed for their certificates, issued by a CME organization recognized in the country. Although not a requirement, the Egyptian Medical Association (EMA) has developed an accreditation process, but it serves primarily as a political function, as practicing physicians must be members of the EMA.[10]

South Africa

South Africa has an active and comprehensive system of continuing professional development (CPD), administered through a statutory council: the Health Professions Council of South Africa (HPCSA), working with 12 professional boards and serving 120,000 health professionals. The present system was instituted in January 2007, supplanting a 2000 obligatory system administered by the Medical and Dental Board for 40,000 health professionals.

The previous system required all practitioners to submit proof of CPD attendance, but in the words of one critic, Professor Marietjie de Villiers, deputy dean of education at the University of Stellenbosch, "the system was just a points chasing exercise, focusing on time spent rather than educational benefit."[11] The new system emphasizes greater involvement of the learner, using effective learning strategies that are not always time-related; some may be easy, others more complex, and are measured in units (CEUs). Thirty CEUs are required annually. Learning activities may be a single program, without measurable outcome; a continuing program with a measurable outcome; or a formally structured program with formal assessment.

In the future, the HPCSA hopes to move to a competence-based model, and finally to performance change.

Events in Asia

Countries in Asia are more advanced than in Africa in the development of CME systems, whether mandatory or voluntary. Singapore and Hong Kong are most advanced with mandated CME, but some of the larger nations such as China and Indonesia are moving in the same direction. Pakistan has committed to a mandatory system but is just starting development. Malaysia and Thailand have had voluntary systems and are not likely to convert soon to mandated; India is lagging behind.

Singapore

A CME system was launched in Singapore in 1989, became more formal in 1993, and in 2003 became compulsory and was mandated for license renewal in 2005. The program is conducted by the Singapore Medical Council (SMC), a statutory board under the Ministry of Health, which maintains the Register of Medical Practitioners in Singapore and regulates professional conduct and ethics.

Singapore has a total of 7,841 doctors, of which 4,297 are associated with the public sector and 3,051 with the private sector. To renew their licenses, physicians must obtain 50 points every two years through the usual range of educational activities, including Internet CME.[12] There are no significant restrictions on activities of potential commercial supporters. Commercial interests financially support physicians attending conferences.

The CME Coordinating Committee of the SMC includes representatives from the Singapore Medical Association; Academy of Medicine, Singapore; College of Family Physicians, Singapore; and Division of Graduate Medical Studies and the associate deans of public sector hospitals. According to Eng Hin Lee, MD, chairman of the CME Coordinating Committee of the SMC, the mandated system is now well accepted by doctors in institutional practices but encountered some objections from private practitioners in solo practice. The majority of doctors are fulfilling their requirements. The committee is now studying establishing a maintenance of competency system.[13]

Malaysia

CME/CPD in Malaysia is a voluntary program sponsored by the Malaysia Medical Association (MMA). It was established in 2002 after extensive consultation with the American Medical Association and other organizations. There are about 290 registered CME providers in Malaysia, and more than 5,000 activities are carried out every year for 10,000 registered participants.[14]

Providers of CPD activities include all organizations that conduct medical programs, including lectures, workshops, and conferences. Such organizations register with the MMA CPD secretariat and apply to the secretariat for accreditation of specific CPD activities in advance. When approved, the secretariat will allocate credit points, based on the MMC CPD grading system.

In the Ministry of Health Malaysia, the CPD program can lead to promotion and salary increments. This program covers registered medical practitioners in Ministry of Health hospitals and all categories of health care personnel.[15]

Hong Kong

The Medical Council of Hong Kong, which oversees the licensing of more than 10,000 physicians, is responsible for implementing a mandatory requirement for CME/CPD over a three-year period. The Hong Kong Academy of Medicine is the premier academic organization in Hong Kong, established by statute in 1993. It has the mandate to maintain the standard of specialist training and specialist CME and CPD in Hong Kong. Other organizations offer programs for GPs.

CME, in the conventional sense, is perceived to focus more on updating medical knowledge, while CPD aims to promote development of competencies relevant to the practice profile of a practitioner.

Thailand

In 2000, the Thai Medical Council announced the development of the Center for Continuing Medical Education (CCME) to organize and support the CME system, improve networking, and enhance collaboration among medical institutes, hospitals, and other health care providers. CME in Thailand is presently carried out on a voluntary basis. Most, if not all, physicians clearly demonstrate their commitment to CME and are willing to participate. The system uses a "swipe" card to assist physicians in documenting their participation in the CME activity.[16]

Physicians in Thailand need to collect about 100 CME credits every five years. Currently, 58 percent of the Thai physicians are able to achieve this target.[17]

Indonesia

Indonesia launched its CPD program for all members at the 26th Indonesia Medical Association (IMA) congress December 1, 2006. In 2008, CPD was made mandatory for all physicians. The IMA required credit is 250 units every five years; 10 percent of these credits must be obtained through nonclinical activities such as research, evidence-based medicine, and dedication to the profession and community.

The objectives of the CPD program conducted by IMA and its sub-organizations (Association of Specialist Medical Doctors and Association of Primary Services Medical Doctors) are (1) to maintain and promote the professionalism of doctors according to global standards of competence (upholding quality and ethics) and (2) to guarantee the existence of quality medical services through a certification of doctors program. The organization responsible for conducting the CPD program is IMA's CPD board. Implementation is done by all specialty associations and colleges, private CME providers, and other associations within the IMA.[18]

Events in India

CME has been catching up in India, despite the lack of legal incentives, thanks to the efforts of regional medical associations, pharmaceutical companies, and independent CME providers. But there is much more to be done.

Currently, there is no law in India to regulate medical practice and review the competence levels and skills of medical professionals once they start practicing, despite the Medical Council of India (MCI) urging the Indian parliament to pass such a law. The MCI proposal is "gathering dust," in the words of the leading Indian newspaper.

Until recently, the MCI was the regulatory

body that would eventually decide on whether CME should be compulsory for doctors to retain their licenses to practice, how much CME a doctor should obtain, what is acceptable as CME, etc. The MCI planned to make CME compulsory, and several versions of the legislative framework have been evaluated. While mandatory CME is inevitable, the time frame over which it will happen is unclear. Plans have been set back for some time: the government has dissolved the MCI because of charges of fraud and corruption and has appointed an interim body to take on MCI responsibilities.

In the meantime, however, several individual bodies and associations have taken the initiative to drive CME among doctors, including the Delhi Medical Council and Neurological Society of India. The Association of Physicians of India has also considered this. In 2001, the Indian Medical Association announced that CME of 150 credit hours over a five-year period would be made mandatory for membership, but the plan was not implemented. However, members are often motivated to comply because the associations are the most credible forums for them to exchange ideas with their peers. As time progresses, it seems certain that this culture of mandatory CME for doctors will prevail across the medical community in India.

Events in Pakistan

Pakistan has some 100,000 physicians, including 18,000 specialists, registered. Until recently, the CME system has been described as "not only depressing but also frustrating. Whatever little CME programs exist, they are mostly funded by the pharmaceutical industry . . . and attendance . . . is very thin."[19] A survey taken in 2007 indicated that the most common CPD activities were professional reading and discussion with peers; major barriers were lack of time or interest in the educational activity, and lack of finances.[20]

However, as a result of a series of conferences, in 2009 the first steps were taken to launch a national CPD program under the aegis of the Pakistan Medical and Dental Council (PMDC). The PMDC will be responsible for formulating rules, regulations, and accreditation of CPD programs. The Ministry of Health, the Pakistan Medical Association, and professional specialty organizations are to be involved in the body setting up the system, according to recommendations from the First National Consultation Group meeting.[21]

The group also recommended that a department of medical education be established at all medical institutions and universities to develop CPD programs. Rashid Jooma, Pakistan director general of health and chair of the PMDC CPD/CME committee, has proposed use of professional specialty organizations to evaluate CPD schemes in order to keep their members up to date, and eventually lead to re-registration. It is expected, however, that the CPD system will be voluntary in the beginning.

Events in China

Hospitals and medical institutes usually organize CME activities in China. These are primarily in the form of grand rounds, case reviews, paper presentations, and self-learning activities, for example reading medical journals and books and attending medical conferences and workshops.

In 1991, a "Temporary Regulation of Continuing Medical Education" was issued by the Ministry of Health, which confirmed that CME is the right and the responsibility of the physicians and mandated physicians to join CME activities. In 1996, the Ministry's CME Committee was founded and is currently leading the CME organization in China. This committee comprises representatives from the Ministry of Health, provincial health bureaus, the Chinese Medical Association (CMA), medical schools, and medical research institutions.

Minimum requirement is 25 CME credits each year.[22] There are two types of credits: Category I credits include credits that are acquired through attending the national CME programs; the minimum requirement is five to 10 credits per year. Category II credits include credits acquired through self-learning; the minimum requirement is 15 to 20 credits per year. Category I activities are accredited by the Ministry and provincial CME committees and organized by CME and affiliated medical schools and institutions.[23] Currently, CME credits are necessary for a physician's professional position advancement in China but not mandated by law.

Events in Japan

The Japan Medical Association (JMA) established a voluntary continuing medical education program in 1987 to address basic science and health-care issues, improve physician-patient relations, and improve the quality of medical care.[24] JMA has a membership of 165,000 (as of 2006), representing 60 percent of the total physician population and with a high proportion of GPs. JMA and its related municipal and prefectural associations have CME committees following a curriculum covering not only medical science but also ethics, law health policy, etc. Learning methods include lectures, workshops, academic presentations or articles, and "home learning" through self-assessment in print or Internet-based courses. A CME certificate is awarded to physicians who self-declare that they have completed 10 credit units or more in one year; after three consecutive certificates, physicians are granted the Certificate of Recognition for Completion of CME.[25]

Beginning in 2008, the JMA and 27 specialty societies offer interchangeability of course credits. Specialists have an obligation to attend national congresses of their association and to accumulate 50 or more credits within five years in order to maintain their certification. Each society sets its own curriculum. Attending or giving lectures is the primary method of earning credits. Courses are located in medical schools and hospitals, as well as at the national meetings, many of which gain major support from pharmaceutical companies.

Will Japan develop a mandated system of CME? In 2007, the Ministry of Education and Science recommended that to maintain their qualification, doctors should understand medical research, commit to lifelong learning, and commit to quality improvement. But so far any discussion about a mandated system is in the future.[26]

Events in Australia and New Zealand

An accreditation system focused on CPD in Australia is highly evolved, and accreditation is available to various stakeholders, including commercial organizations. CPD has been compulsory in Australia for primary care physicians since 1989, but not for other physicians. Every GP has to accumulate 130 points every triennium.

The Royal Australian College of General Practitioners (RACGP) governs the CPD program for primary care physicians in Australia. The college has more than 19,000 members, and more than 6,000 members of its National Rural Faculty. The college is the largest general-practice representative body in Australia and the largest representative body for rural general practice.

The RACGP program, the Quality Assurance and Continuing Professional Development Program (QA&CPD), requires that the physician take at least two Category 1 options, which include active learning, clinical audit, evidence-based journal club, developing a learning plan, small group learning, higher education, and more.[27]

The Royal Australasian College of Physicians (RACP), representing more than 9,000 specialty physicians, offers its own CPD programs and credits through MyCPD, developed in consultation with the Royal College of Physicians and Surgeons of Canada.[28] MyCPD offers programs in six categories: educational development, teaching, and research; group learning activities; self-assessment programs; structured learning projects; practice review and appraisal; and other learning activities. All training and education programs of the RACP are accredited by the Australian Medical Council (AMC) and the Medical Council of New Zealand (MCNZ).

As of 2008, there is no commonwealth requirement in Australia for CPD, but some state medical boards and specialty societies do require evidence of participation. In New Zealand, participating in CPD programs is mandatory for recertification and renewal of the annual practicing certificate, per the Health Practitioner's Competence Assurance Act (2003).[29]

Among the problems facing physicians in both Australia and New Zealand is the difficulty of obtaining locum tenens support to take CPD courses. Despite the compulsory requirements, participation levels fall below 100 percent for this and other reasons, and enforcement is difficult.[30]

Implications for the Future outside Europe and the United States

Will there be harmonization of CME/CPD standards around the world? Yes, in this 21st century, but not in the next decade. The first step will be to achieve some regional harmonization, as has been done in Europe. There are stirrings in this direction in Latin America, but not much more. In the Middle East, there is unlikely to be collaboration of any sort between Israel and its Arab neighbors. India and China, as the two economic giants of the future, are still struggling with adoption of any internal system, much less ready to join a regional harmonization effort. While Australia and New Zealand have brought together certain standards of credit systems, there are still major differences between specialty colleges and the GP College.

It is likely that the profession, through medical associations, medical schools, and specialty societies, can move toward harmonization in emphasis on evidence-based clinical content, requirements for nonclinical education in ethics and health policy, and approaches to multimedia learning methodologies.

It is less likely that in the next decade there will be harmonization of techniques of needs assessment and outcomes measurement. It is even less likely that national authorities will seek to align their national policies for assuring health care quality with those of their neighbors. Politics is always a local issue.

Optimism must always be the first word in discussing the global future of CME/CPD. Patience is the second.

Notes

1. P. Pulido and others, "Changes, Trends and Challenges of Medical Education in Latin America," *Medical Teacher* 28, no. 1 (2006): 24–29.

2. H. Silva and others, "Trends, Challenges and Promotion of Clinical and Cardiovascular Research in Latin America and the Caribbean," *CVD Prevention and Control* 2 (2006): 129–135.

3. P. Pulido and others, "Harmonization of CME/CPD in Latin America" (PAFAMS communication at a Global Alliance for Medical Education meeting on the Global CME Harmonization 2.0, Strategies for the Future, New Jersey, June 2008).

4. P. Pulido and others, "Need for Improved Nonclinical Medical Education: A Study in Thirteen Countries," *Health Affairs* (forthcoming).

5. "2008 President's Report," Project Globe Consortium for Continuing Professional Development Web site, http://www.globecpd.org (accessed July 19, 2010).

6. Nawal Khalid, personal communication with the author, 2008.

7. P. Shvartman, "Continuous Medical Education in Israel" (presentation at Global Alliance for Medical Education, June 2008).

8. Michael Weingarten.

9. Aslani A. Personal, personal communication with the author, 2008.

10. Morad Abou-Sabe, personal communication with the author, 2008.

11. M. de Villiers, "Global Challenges in Continuing Professional Development: The South African Perspective," *Journal of Continuing Education in the Health Professions* 28, no. 51 (2008): 25–26.

12. "Statistics, Health Manpower," Ministry of Health Singapore Web site, https://www.moh.gov.sg/mohcorp/statistics.aspx?id=5966 (accessed July 19, 2010).

13. "Continuing Medical Education," Singapore Medical Council Web site, http://www.smc.gov.sg/html/1140055893077.html (accessed July 19, 2010).

14. L. Sullivan, "CME/CPD in Malaysia: 10 years past

to 10 years forward" (presentation at the Global Alliance for Medical Education, Montreal, Canada, June 7, 2010).

15. Ibid.

16. Chairat Shayakul, personal communication with the author, March 2009.

17. Center for Continuing Medical Education, Office of the Permanent Secretary, Ministry of Health Web site, http://www.ccme.or.th (accessed July 19, 2010).

18. *Implementation Manual, Continuing Professional Development Program* (Indonesia Medical Association, 2007).

19. S. Jawaid and others, "Continuing Professional Development and the Role of Specialty Organizations," *Pakistan Journal of Medical Sciences* 91, no. 1 (2003): 5–11.

20. Z. Siddiqui, "Continuous Professional Development of Medical Doctors in Pakistan: Practices, Motivation and Barriers" (AARE Conference Proceedings, 2007).

21. "Formulating Rules and Regulations and Accreditation of CPD Programmes," *Pulse* (August 2009): 15–31.

22. Cao Zeyi, "Physicians' Training and Continuing Medical Education in China" (Hospital Authority Convention, 1997).

23. Chinese Ministry of Health Web site, http://www.moh.gov.cn (accessed July 19, 2010).

24. A. Takaji and others, "Current State of CME in Japan" (presentation at the Alliance of CME, January 21, 2008).

25. M. Ishii, "The Continuing Medical Education Program of the Japan Medical Association," *Journal of the Medical Association of Japan* 51, no. 4 (2008): 219–224.

26. A. Negri, personal notes after visit to Japan, November 12, 2009.

27. "2008–2010 QA&CPD Program," Royal Australasian College of General Practitioners Web site, http://www.racgp.org.au/Content/NavigationMenu/educationandtraining/QACPD/20082010Triennium (accessed December 1, 2009).

28. "Review of the Maintenance of Professional Standards Program," Royal Australasian College of General Practitioners Web site, http://www.racp.edu.au (accessed April 10, 2010).

29. "Continuing Medical Education and Continuing Professional Development: International Comparisons," *British Medical Journal* 320 (2000): 432–435.

30. Barry Taylor, personal communication with the author, 2008.

PART VIII

Reflections on Moving toward the Future

James C. Leist, Joseph S. Green, and
Robert E. Kristofco

CHAPTER 31

The Meaning and Value of Continuing Medical Education

Continuing medical education (CME) has various stakeholders that influence and are influenced by CME. Those stakeholders include individual physicians and the medical profession as a whole, who are the direct beneficiaries of CME; patients and society in general, who are the indirect beneficiaries of CME; and the providers of CME and their organizations that actually provide CME for physicians and their teams. Each has a perspective about the meaning and value of CME that has evolved over time.

Meaning and value are concepts that many have struggled to explain. For the purpose of this chapter, *meaning* is defined as how CME is interpreted by the stakeholder and *value* is defined as the importance of CME to that stakeholder. The authors will review the perspectives of each stakeholder from past to present and conclude with a perspective about the meaning and value of CME that all stakeholders should share for the future.

Perspectives from the Past and Present

The major focus for CME in the past and present is for the physician to learn more in order to keep current. CME providers have had the secondary role of assisting physicians in this effort, while patients and society have played only a minor role in setting expectations.

The Perspective of the Physician and the Medical Profession

The pursuit of meaning and value in lifelong learning is as old as the medical profession. From cave paintings in Lascaux, France, depicting healing with herbs, medicine has valued the development of a knowledge base as a means to learning. Egyptian and Babylonian medicine provide rich archives demonstrating the evolution of medical practice, including a text recording surgical technique and a diagnostic handbook dating from the 2nd millennium BC. Historical records of medical developments in nearly every culture confirm that a high value has been placed on codifying what was known or what was discovered in order to make it available to others.

From another perspective, medicine has always been concerned about beneficence: "Do no harm." Central to this ethical precept is the notion of competence. In order to perform acceptably those duties related to patient care, the professional must commit to lifelong learning. Looking at continuing education in the context of the medical oath is an interesting window on the value that has historically been placed on lifelong learning. In a study that looked at 48 ancient, medieval, modern, and contemporary medical oaths, it was found that 20 (42 percent) referenced lifelong learning. Of these 20, two were of ancient origin and 18 were more modern and contemporary. While most of the oaths studied address acquisition of knowledge and skills, early oaths do not articulate the responsibility to be a lifelong learner.[1]

Sir William Osler exemplifies a medical leader who articulated a strong commitment to lifelong learning. Osler observed that "the hardest conviction to get into the mind of a beginner is that the education upon which he is engaged is not a college course, not a medical course, but a life course, for which the work of a few years under teachers is but a preparation."[2] This individualist perspective prevails today and is reinforced by broader efforts undertaken by the profession to assume greater responsibility for lifelong learning. Now, driven additionally by regulation because of public and government influence, CME has become a more visible and valued professional responsibility; it validates physician competence and performance in practice.

Important public and professional bodies from state legislatures to medical specialty boards and medical professional societies, along with accrediting bodies at every stage of physician learning, have established new expectations for lifelong learning. With the repeated calls for quality improvement from the Institute of Medicine (IOM) and others, contemporary medicine is reexamining its values and its commitment to lifelong learning. Additionally, a growing body of research concludes that continuing education, as it is too often practiced today, provides limited prospects for addressing gaps in practice or improving care.[3]

Educational research has demonstrated that medical education in the model of memorization and lecture fails to adequately provide the student with the functional ability to effectively practice medicine. Medical schools have been taking steps to advance modern curricula that allow for more self-directed learning and correlation of basic and clinical science concepts. Improving the assessment of student performance and incorporating broad-based standards that now include attention to issues of professionalism, systems of care, and communication demonstrate a shift in the thinking about the foundations of physician professional development. Likewise, the meaning and value of CME are being revitalized by many present developments. The focus of CME is shifting to continuing professional development (CPD), reflecting the perspective that learning is continuous and multi-dimensional in the complex milieu of medicine. The formal institution of required competencies for physician trainees harks back to the bedrock values of medicine practiced by practitioners from the earliest times. Competency should be the hallmark of a professional across the ages. The meaning and expectations have not changed. Only the methods have advanced. CME has a rich history, and countless examples have shown that lifelong learning occupies a position of high importance for individual physicians and the medical profession.

The Perspective of the CME Provider and Organizations

Despite intriguing evidence that concern about how well physicians keep up has been around for a long time, the fact is that it has only been recently—in this century—that issues surrounding continuing medical education have received serious attention.[4]

Of course the century referred to in the previous quote is now the last century, but looking backwards will assist in understanding how the meaning and value of CME have changed. The historical development of today's CME can be divided into four stages: (1) in the early 1900s, William Osler advocated for physician lifelong learning; (2) in the 1930s, innovative postgraduate courses were targeted at meeting practicing physicians' needs; (3) after World War II, medical knowledge and specialization grew rapidly; and (4) in the 1960s, professional educators applied the principles of adult learning to CME. This history has led to many of the values tied to CME during the twentiethth century.

The provision of CME originated in the academic settings of medical schools, hospitals, and specialty societies where physicians cared for patients or advocated for improved patient care. Hospital CME providers were usually staff who assisted physicians in creating a weekly or monthly grand rounds activity that allowed specialists to share their knowledge with their primary care colleagues. In addition, mortality and morbidity conference activities developed in most hospitals as a mechanism for the medical staff to review critically their patient care decisions in a safe, collegial, peer-review type activity. (Interestingly, these real practice-linked activities were rarely certified for credit.) The early focus of CME was as an additional benefit of graduate medical education (GME) designed to assist in "repairing" physicians. This was followed in the 1930s and 1940s with a new emphasis—keeping up to date with the ever-expanding medical knowledge. Later in the late 1960s and early 1970s, Clement Brown and Henry Uhl urged the use of a bi-cycle approach to patient care with the physician as the linkage between the evaluation of patient care and the development of CME activities related to identified problems.[5]

Medical schools originally served to provide faculty experts for the CME activities that were being developed for the members of local or specialty medical societies; indeed, in the late 1920s the University of Michigan and the University of North Carolina developed their unique role in CME as Extension Divisions into their surrounding communities and hospitals. This led to more regionalization around the country by linking medical schools with local community hospitals, which had direct implications for affecting referral patterns for the use of specialists. Area health education centers (AHECs) were born of this movement in order to meet the learning needs of physicians and other health-care providers and to address the shortage of health manpower needs in the rural communities. Medical schools valued grand rounds and other educational activities for

their departments, as well as national or regional meetings, to reward their faculty and showcase their medical expertise.

Specialty medical societies began to develop in the early part of the 20th century in response to the expanding specialization in medicine. The foci of these CME activities were national symposia for specialists interacting with each other about the latest developments and often "circuit-riding" courses made up of specialists talking to primary care physicians. Formal medical specialty boards developed around the same time, which led to the specialty certification process and eventually to the need for recertification. After the Flexner Report of 1910, the restructuring of state medical licensing boards created new approaches to the oversight and assessment of medical practice.

Another major development providing insight about the meaning and value of CME relates to mandatory CME, as seen in required hours of CME for physicians for re-licensure, recertification, or credentialing. The American Medical Association Physician's Recognition Award (AMA-PRA) has been used as a benchmark in various mandatory CME efforts. Many require around 50 hours a year or 150 hours over a three-year period. Accreditation of CME providers was formalized in 1977 with the creation of the Liaison Committee on Continuing Medical Education, followed in the 1980s by its successor, the Accreditation Council for CME (ACCME). These developments began to raise the bar on the requirements for becoming and remaining a CME provider. Staff in these organizations began to learn more about the educational processes inherent in the essentials for accreditation.

Most CME providers used the same basic educational formats for their physician audiences. As Phil R. Manning stated in the book *Alliance for CME Primer*, "The strategies that physicians most often use in carrying out their CME activities— and this pattern has not changed appreciably over the years—are: reading professional journals and literature, attending courses and conferences and participating in discussions with colleagues."[6]

Suter et al. in 1984 stated:

> The pressures on the health professions and their continuing education systems are great. These pressures become apparent in exchanges between patients and health professionals, in the activities of consumer groups, and in legislative and fiscal actions of state and federal governments. One manifestation of these pressures is the introduction of mandatory continuing education for many health professions, which has been spearheaded by professional groups, regulatory agencies, and state governments. As a consequence, there is not only greater need for continuing education opportunities in the various professions but also increasing demand for public accountability of the continuing education process.[7]

Towards the end of the twentieth century, continuing education of all health professionals came of age. Although it was still a cottage industry made up of various CME providers and groups, little communication or collaboration occurred among these various providers. Every CME office supported the notion that it was required to do everything for its physician audience, yet few of these providers had clearly articulated who their primary and/or secondary audiences actually were. Several critical events occurred throughout the last quarter of the century that contributed to an evolution of values and meaning for CME. These included such things as the development of new visions for CME; new educational processes, formats, and methods; new organizations of CME professionals; and new resources such as textbooks, a journal, newsletters, and electronic list serves; the beginnings of regulatory oversight; the increased importance of revenue; and finally, the ACCME Standards for Commercial Support.

The CME literature began to focus on new and different futures for CME. In fact, a new CME paradigm was suggested in the late 1980s.[8] This paradigm shift dealt with educational processes for physicians that linked learning with quality

and performance improvement data. The field of CME was urged to adopt new learning technologies such as use of the Internet, video discs, CD-ROMs, audience response systems, and the use of hand-held PDAs. Several textbooks, newsletters, and a journal appeared during this period, outlining the changing nature and extent of CME, each of them with a slightly different way of approaching this burgeoning educational landscape.

Research continually pointed to the need to use smaller group interactive techniques to engage learners and to avoid using passive learning formats such as large lectures. The ACCME accreditation process was silent on its recommendations about educational processes and formats, but adult educators involved in the CME profession provided consistent data that depicted the value of physician learners being more actively involved in their own learning. CME providers began to experiment with many new formats to meet the learning needs of their audiences.

Almost every CME provider type, including hospitals, medical schools, and specialty societies, began to create its own professional organization within, or outside, the Alliance for CME, the largest CME professional association. In addition, new entities began to emerge into the CME world, including publishing companies, medical education companies, communications companies, travel organizations, medical group practices, and technology firms. Each of these had different approaches to meeting the educational needs of a subset of physician learners, and each developed electronic mechanisms to encourage communications among like CME organizations. These resultant electronic "listserves" allowed for more rapid exchange of information, which led to significant changes occurring in these organizations within a very short period of time.

In 1991, a US Senate committee made an initial inquiry into the appropriateness of pharmaceutical and medical device companies' support of CME, claiming that potential conflicts of interest might exist that would not be in the best interests of patient care. The initial reaction to this was a brief period of reduced support for CME offices by the pharmaceutical and device companies; however, it was short-lived, and industry funding began to escalate beyond anyone's wildest imaginations, to the point where total funding from industry was projected at nearly $1.5 billion a year, or between 40 percent and 50 percent of total CME funding, by the turn of the century. The Food and Drug Administration (FDA) was tasked with developing guidelines for the interaction between health-care professionals and the pharmaceutical and medical device companies. Concurrently, the ACCME was modifying a new set of standards of commercial support for the CME profession, insisting that there must be a separation of certified CME from other promotional ventures of supporting industry partners.

At the same time that governmental regulators and the ACCME were placing more importance on documenting appropriate processes and procedures that supported CME organizations, the parent organizations of these CME provider offices began to demand more and more revenue from their efforts of providing learning opportunities to physicians. This set the stage for ever-increasing amounts of financial support for CME from industry and more attempts by industry to influence content of CME.

In a sense, the meaning and value of CME to CME providers have been modified over the years, though practice has not been dramatically changed. To a great degree, CME providers still see enhanced interactive group learning as the major mode of education, though some CME providers are increasingly exploring performance improvement (PI) and point-of-care learning on an individual learner basis to complement the enhanced group learning activities.

The Perspective of the Patient and Society

Historically, the patient and society perspective about the meaning and value of CME was limited. The perception was primarily of the physi-cian always providing the best care possible and assuming that the physician had the appropriate knowledge and skills to provide quality care in a personal manner. Patients had their personal doctor who took care of all their needs. Specialization, with the exception of surgery, was limited. The patient believed that the physician was well trained and knew what was needed to practice quality medicine.

From the perspective of society there was limited focus on continued learning by the physician because medicine, as a profession, was believed to have established high standards that controlled medical practice.

As medicine evolved and became more sophisticated, patients began to utilize more specialized practitioners with the increased use of technology and pharmaceuticals to maintain their health. In a sense, the patient believed that his or her health was still the responsibility of the physician, who had been well trained and maintained his or her knowledge to provide the best patient-centered care possible. The patient trusted the physician to stay current about medical practices but had no real understanding of how the physician did so.

But during the latter part of the 20th century, society's implicit trust of physician competence began to waiver. More knowledge about safety issues and medical errors began to raise a concern for the patient and the public in general. Physicians came under more scrutiny, which resulted in challenges to physician performance and an increase in defensive medicine practices to avoid medical malpractice litigation. As a result of this public awareness of physician competence and performance, patients began to question physician practices. As a result, the profession instituted requirements for new physician competencies that went beyond just clinical knowledge and patient care and led to the maintenance of certification (MOC) and maintenance of licensure (MOL) programs to address these concerns of the patient and the public.[9]

With the increased visibility of the quality and

safety of health care, patients have begun to take an increased interest in the quality of their physician provider. Patients expect the highest quality of care using the most current technology by their physician, including more evidence-based care to address their specific medical needs. Patients still want their physician to be responsible for their care, although more patients are taking more responsibility for their own health. Some examples include better eating habits, less smoking, more exercise, and other behaviors that influence health.

Patients are beginning to understand the need for physicians to maintain their currency as an evidence-based professional and are increasingly raising questions about safety, quality, and current evidence for health-care decisions. But even with these changes, patients are still not aware of the meaning and value of CME as an important issue. However, they expect their personal physician to have the most current knowledge and skills and the best technology, if necessary, and to use that knowledge, skill, and technology in the best interest of the patient.

An article written in the 1990s states that the physician needed to consider four dimensions when making a decision about a patient: quality, cost, legal aspects, and ethics.[10] Patients expect quality at a reasonable cost but did not think about the legal aspects until the 1980s, when physicians began practicing what was described as defensive medicine, i.e., conducting many tests to ensure that no medical issue was missed. To a degree the physicians were protecting themselves against litigation, which increased dramatically in the 1990s and has influenced individual medical practice in many ways, including a significant increase in the cost of malpractice insurance. No longer did all patients completely trust their physicians to provide them with the best quality care, and some were acting on that concern.

From a society perspective these same issues exist. National organizations such as the Agency for Healthcare Research and Quality (AHRQ),

the National Institutes of Health (NIH), the Carnegie Foundation for the Advancement of Teaching, and the IOM have begun to evaluate the quality of medical practice and publicize the need for closer involvement and scrutiny by the patient and the public.

Still, the understanding of the meaning and value of CME by the patient and society has been minimal. Although recent concerns about quality and safety have led to important patient and societal questions about the medical profession and the health-care system overall, neither the patient nor society relates strongly to the concept of CME. They do relate strongly to the meaning and value of their physician and the profession staying current and providing their medical care in a quality manner.

Future Perspectives

Whereas the importance of past and present perspectives of the meaning and value of CME begins with the physician and ends with the care of the patient, in the future that orientation will—and already has begun to—shift. Because patients and society are demanding more accountability from the health-care system and of the physicians who provide care, the meaning and value of CME will be influenced more by patients, society, and the profession and less by those involved directly in the delivery of CME.

The Expectations of the Patient and Society

The expectations of the patient and society are expected to dramatically change in the future. Safe quality care is expected at reasonable cost. The physician and the medical team are expected to be up-to-date practitioners based upon current research, the newest technology, and the highest ethical standards and will be evaluated accordingly. As patients learn about the changes that the medical profession is making with recertification and re-licensing, the expectations will continue to rise.

At the same time, patients may expect something else from the physician that is not limited to medical care. Patients will need to learn to take more responsibility for their own care, and physicians will be expected to provide assistance in making that transition. While patients still will not know much about the meaning and specific value of CME, they will have more-complex and higher-level expectations of their physician and the health-care team. Dealing with such expectations is a challenge for the field of CME.

Additionally, the complexity of the current health-care system and the patient population will create multiple expectations for the physician and the health-care team that will need to be addressed through CME. For example: How do physicians and the health-care team deal with various age groups, or minorities, that have different expectations? How do physicians and the health-care team provide that personal care in a cost-effective and responsible manner?

The public is demanding more accountability, and many more organizations are carefully examining the workings of the CME world. These include the Food and Drug Administration, the Office of the Inspector General (OIG) of the Department of Health and Human Services, the IOM, the US Congress, and many others. All are demanding a better system of educating physicians in practice to keep medical and health care safe, personal, cost effective, and of the highest possible quality.

The Perspective of the Physician and the Medical Profession

One of the expectations of physicians as professionals is a commitment to lifelong learning. Over time, the methods and models have changed along with advances in practice. The future of CME or CPD or continuing professional development and improvement (CPDI) will be shaped by a variety of forces. Practice requirements related to MOC and MOL are examples of developments that link expectations for lifelong learning directly to the practice of medicine. Changes in the health-care system resulting from the new health-care reform legislation will no doubt alter the content and methods of professional development. With concerns about medical errors, cost of care, and regional variation in quality and cost continuing to gain the attention of policy makers, medicine is revisiting its commitment to continuing professional development, linking it as a key ingredient in quality improvement initiatives. Practitioners are getting engaged in quality improvement efforts and beginning to formalize information sharing in practice networks and other communities of practice, where they can share reflections on their experiences. Future CME will take advantage of learning approaches like community based participatory research that can engage practitioners with other stakeholders in a lifelong learning process that uses the office practice setting as the laboratory. The motivations for lifelong learning and the meaning and value derived from them are revolutionized when the center of planned learning is the actual practice and the content of the education is derived directly from the patient in the individual physician practice. In this lifelong learning "revolution scenario," the patient plays the key role, and advanced systems enable true "point of care" learning. Furthermore, with the integration of continuing certification and licensure into this learning matrix, efficiencies will be achieved. This system will allow for resources to be more carefully devoted to learning designed to address gaps in practice and to facilitating translation of research to practice. It is highly likely that academic centers and medical specialty societies will become even more engaged in this effort.

The Perspective of the CME Provider and Organizations

Early in the twenty-first century, the term CPD has been adopted as the new way to describe what has been known as CME. The primary change that was taking place was the commitment to application of knowledge into the practice of physicians. CPD "includes educational methods beyond the didactic, embodies concepts of self-directed learning and personal development, and considers organizational and system factors."[11] The medical establishment is beginning to link physician lifelong learning to such important regulatory functions as physician certification (national), licensure (state), and credentialing (local). In addition to the public, which is demanding more accountability from physicians and the medical profession, many professional organizations are beginning to look anew into the CME world. These include the American Medical Association (AMA), the American Board of Medical Specialties (ABMS), the Association of American Medical Colleges (AAMC), and the Council of Medical Specialty Societies (CMSS), among others. All are now trying to create a better system of educating physicians in practice without the undue influence of the supporting pharmaceutical or medical device companies. In the near future, the AMA PRA credit system will likely be linked tightly with the MOC and MOL movements. Each of these processes is emphasizing the use of practice-based performance data to determine possible gaps in physician knowledge, competence, or performance. CME providers will be helping physicians practice evidence-based, quality care, which may require health-care team learning that will complement individual practice-based learning. In addition, this may replace the practice of defensive medicine, whose costs have not been able to be contained. CME professionals are now struggling to determine what help can be provided to their physicians to aid their navigation through these tricky waters.

CME provider organizations are now or will soon undergo transformational change in order to survive this major shift in their role and mission within the medical education world. According to the IOM, both the health-care system and the education system that has produced our health-care professionals are broken and need to be fixed.[12] Health-care reform has been passed by the US Congress and signed into law. When implemented, it will likely change the landscape of CME forever. Certain currently accredited CME provider groups such as the medical education and communication companies are already moving away from being CME providers. Community hospitals are beginning to look to regional consortia or medical schools. Medical schools are re-tooling their approach and beginning to collaborate more with other CME providers. Specialty societies are focusing their efforts on linking their members together in learning portfolios that allow the learner easy access to practice-related performance data, as well as learning opportunities related to identified competence gaps. All providers are struggling to develop more balanced funding of their educational efforts, establishing much more transparent rules and providing more inclusive data relevant to relationships with industry. CME providers are more willing to work collaboratively, rather than each of them trying to do everything for all of their physicians. The parent organizations behind CME providers are finally dealing with the value propositions that clearly articulate an appropriate role for those involved most directly in educating physicians as they move through their careers. CME provider organizations may become much more integrated into the core business of their parent organizations. In doing so, they may also lose some autonomy.

Assessment-based planning and the use of educational formats that involve the learner have emerged as critical to the survival and relevance of the CME community. CME providers are reviewing the skill sets within their organizations and ensuring they have staff competent in educational assessment and instructional design integrally involved in the design, implementation, and evaluation of the new CME/CPD activities. Competency-based curriculum, self-assessment programs, point-of-care learning, gaming and simulation, team-based training, use of registry QI data, clinical guidelines, performance measures, performance improvement CME, embedding guidelines in electronic medical records, and linking reimbursement to quality performance are a few of the new approaches to meeting the lifelong learning needs of physicians today and into the future.

Summary

The meaning and value of CME have changed significantly during the last hundred years and are moving in a powerful direction toward the future. During the past, the focus was on physician learning, and it was the CME provider's responsibility to provide new knowledge, usually in a group setting, with minimal attention to whether that information or knowledge was subsequently used in practice. The purpose, meaning, and value of CME were to provide current knowledge to as many physicians as possible, while the patient and society perspectives were a minor focus for the CME provider.

The future perspective of the meaning and value of CME is dramatically different. The primary focus is now the impact of CME on the physician and the application of that learning in the practice setting that makes a positive difference in the health of the patient and ultimately of society. This new focus on the health of patients and society will enhance the meaning and value of CME and have the following significant implications for the practice of CME providers in the future:

- *CME provider role change:* CME providers should evolve into CPD providers that require skills beyond meeting planning.
- *Learning into practice:* Learning activities will have to be designed to facilitate translation of knowledge (science) into the practice setting using backwards planning with a focus on assessment and the provision of rules, examples, practice, and feedback, as well as blended formats and long-term, performance-based interventions using registry data.
- *Community health status:* CPD providers should focus on patient outcomes and community health status as appropriate outcome measures of educational interventions.
- *Quality and safety:* CPD providers need to address not just medical knowledge but all physician competencies and the quality and safety of patient care.
- *Leadership in health care:* CPD providers should facilitate and promote leadership training to help physicians and the medical profession provide effective leadership to shape the future of health care.
- *Maintenance of Certification:* CPD offices need to be prepared to assist physicians with whom they work in meeting all their regulatory obligations such as certification, licensure, and credentialing.
- *Patient responsibility:* CPD providers should assist physicians with education that advocates for patient responsibility for the patient's own health care through promotion and prevention.
- *Value propositions and outcome measures:* Leaders of CPD efforts will need to work with their parent organization to agree upon the value proposition required to ensure that their contribution is worth the resources needed to carry it out and will need to document the benefit of their involvement in terms of enhanced patient outcomes, reduced costs, increased safety, decreased inappropriate use of medical resources, etc.
- *Collaboration with outside organizations:* Those who remain involved in the on-going professional development of physicians need to work collaboratively with many other organizations and professionals to accomplish such a task. These CPD offices will no longer be able to work in a vacuum.

Notes

1. A. M. Rancich and others, "Beneficence, Justice, and Lifelong Learning Expressed in Medical Oaths," *Journal of Continuing Education in the Health Professions* 25, no. 3 (2005): 211–220.

2. W. Osler, *The Student Life, Aequanimitas: With Other Addresses to Medical Students,* 3rd ed. (Philadelphia: Blakiston's Son, 1932), 400.

3. S. S. Marinopoulos and others, "Review," *Evid Rep Technol Assess* 149 (2007): 1–69.

4. H. S. M. Uhl, "CME: A Brief History," in *Continuing Medical Education: A Primer,* ed. A. B. Rosof and W. C. Felch, 8–17 (New York: Praeger Publishers, 1986).

5. C. R. Brown, Jr., "The Continuing Education Component of the Bi-Cycle Approach to Quality Assurance," in *Quality Health Care: The Role of Continuing Medical Education,* ed. R. H. Egdahl and P. M. Gertman (Germantown: Aspen Systems Corp., 1977).

6. P. R. Manning, "The Future of CME," in *Continuing Medical Education: A Primer,* ed. A. B. Rosof and W. C. Felch, 180–189 (New York: Praeger Publishers, 1986).

7. E. Suter and others, "Introduction: Defining Quality for Continuing Education," in *Continuing Education for the Health Professions: Developing, Managing and Evaluating Programs for Maximum Impact on Patient Care,* ed. J. S. Green and others, 1–32 (San Francisco: Jossey-Bass Publishers, 1984).

8. D. E. Moore and others, "Creating a New Paradigm for CME: Seizing Opportunities within the Health Care Revolution," *Journal of Continuing Education in the Health Professions* 14 (1994): 261–272.

9. A. C. Greiner and E. Knebel, eds., *Health Professions Education: A Bridge to Quality* (Washington, D.C.: National Academies Press, 2003); M. L. DeKay and D. A. Asch, "Is the Defensive Use of Diagnostic Test Good for Patients, or Bad?" *Medical Decision Making* 18, no. 1 (1998): 19–28; American Board of Medical Specialties, "MOC Competencies and Criteria", http://www.abms.org/Maintenance_of_Certification/MOC_competencies.aspx (accessed January 8, 2010).

10. J. C. Leist and J. C. Konen, "Four Factors of Clinical Decision-making: A Teaching Model," *Academic Medicine* 7, no. 16 (1996): 644–646.

11. D. A. Davis and others, "Commentary: CME and Its Role in the Academic Medical Center: Increasing Integration, Adding Value," *Academic Medicine* 85, no. 1 (2010): 12–15.

12. D. Davis and others, "The Horizon of Continuing Professional Development: Five Questions in Knowledge Translation," in *The Continuing Professional Development of Physicians: From Research to Practice,* ed. D. Davis and others, 9–24 (Chicago: American Medical Association, 2003); D. E. Moore and others, "Creating a New Paradigm for CME: Seizing Opportunities within the Health Care Revolution," *Journal of Continuing Education in the Health Professions* 14 (1994): 261–272.

Mary G. Turco, Richard I. Rothstein, and
Carl S. DeMatteo

CHAPTER 32

Continuing Medical Education in an Era of Health-Care Reform:
A Dartmouth Perspective

We are now faced with the fact my friends, that tomorrow
is today. We are confronted with the fierce urgency of now.
In this unfolding conundrum of life and history there is
such a thing as being too late.
—Dr. Martin Luther King, Jr., quoted in a speech by Jim
Yong Kim, president of Dartmouth College

Profound changes in society, technology, and
the economy of the United States and elsewhere
are driving dramatic and persistent transformation of the practice of medicine and, thus,
the education of physicians. Predicted challenges
for training tomorrow's doctors are here today.
This chapter is a reflection by three members of
the Dartmouth Medical School faculty who are
Dartmouth-Hitchcock Clinic administrators with
responsibility for continuing medical education
(CME) on how our particular institution's broad
and varied initiatives, including the development
of the new health care delivery science, are influencing the education of physicians across the
continuum of their professional lives and medical practice.

In this book's foreword, our colleague C. Ever-
ett Koop, MD, framed the present challenge well:
how can physicians learn to care for patients
"wisely, safely and right" while new knowledge
and technology make previous training obsolete,
and innovations in management and business
make delivery systems outmoded?[1] Stuck in a fee-

for-service practice model that delivers seg-
mented care, and an antiquated education model
that adds reimbursable skills and not value, we
need new ways of paying for care, new ways of
delivering care, and new ways of educating the
health care team. Our argument is that today's
clinicians need twenty-first-century CME that
fits twenty-first-century delivery systems. And, to
know what to do, our educational system needs to
be focused on the model of health care delivery to
which we aspire.

Reflecting its origins in the New Hampshire
hinterlands, the motto of Dartmouth College, a
teaching and research institution located in the
rural river valley between the White and Green
Mountains of New Hampshire and Vermont, is
"vox clamantis in deserto"—a voice calling in the
wilderness.[2] Among the institutions that constitute the whole is Dartmouth Medical School
(DMS), founded in 1797 by Nathan Smith, MD,
DMS is part of a historic and successful partnership with the Mary Hitchcock Memorial Hospital (1893), the Veterans Affairs Medical Center
(VAMC) in White River Junction, Vermont (1938,
affiliated 1946), and the Dartmouth-Hitchcock
Clinic (1927). The original Hitchcock Clinic,
modeled by its four founders on the Mayo Clinic
(where one of them, John Pollard Bowler, MD,
had done his Surgical training), became the
Dartmouth-Hitchcock Clinic (DHC) in 1999.[3]

Today, DHC is one of the largest multispecialty, not-for-profit group practices in the country. Its physicians, like those at Mayo Clinic, are salaried and thus ready to move toward capitation or other non-fee for service reimbursement that would allow professional staff to manage patients over time according to the best methods for reaching institutional goals.

At Dartmouth, we of course do not have all of the answers. And, like other organizations, we make mistakes and are slow to change. However, we do have a unique and different environment, a research-oriented reform agenda, and important shared philosophies that inform and enable our institutional efforts to improve. Our objective is to advance past fragmented, sometimes commercially biased and/or ineffective care *and* education to well-designed, accountable, and patient-centered care *and* education. In our twenty-first-century vision of CME, the reflective physician—working inter-professionally—uses data comprehensively, educates herself or himself and patients effectively, and practices the art, science, evaluation, *and* delivery of medicine successfully and compassionately over a lifetime and with every patient.

Tomorrow is today. This chapter presents our perspective on how one academic medical center and its partnering organizations are learning and doing in a concerted effort to reform *clinical care* and *CME* to transform health care in the "fierce urgency of now."

Research-Oriented Reform

Open academic discourse in a rural academic medical center can be an adventure, particularly when peers cause what Senior Advising Dean for Dartmouth's medical students Joseph O'Donnell, MD, calls "perturbances." Since 1979, DMS faculty member John (Jack) Wennberg, MD, MPH, has been a perturber. Trained in epidemiology as well as internal medicine, Wennberg noticed unexplained variations in patients' health care, outcomes and cost. In the late 1960s, he and col-

league Alan Gittlesohn, MD, started collecting and analyzing health care data in Vermont and discovered that the amount of care patients received depends to a large extent on where they lived and the physicians they saw, *but not on the illnesses they had.*[4] For example, about 60 percent of children living in Stowe, Vermont, had their tonsils removed, while in neighboring Waterbury only about 20 percent of children were so treated. Similar patterns of variation were seen for hysterectomies, gall bladder surgery and other common procedures. Part of the reason for the variation was poor science: no one really knew what the outcomes of such difference in clinical practice really were. But it was also a matter of not knowing what patients truly wanted; among their and various colleagues' discoveries was the finding that many well-meaning providers, trained and socialized to make decisions *for* patients rather than listen *to* patients, were not sensitive to patients' preferences regarding profoundly important health care decisions. In addition to studying the outcomes of care, the research suggested a need for hearing the patient's voice with an emphasis on "shared" decision making.

Through the 1980s, they pursued a series of studies that led to an understanding of the causes and potential remedies for unwarranted variation—variation that couldn't be explained on the basis of illness, medical evidence or patient preference. By the late 1980s, Wennberg and his colleagues needed an academic center at DMS to support their work and launch new graduate programs. Over the next two decades, the Center for the Evaluative Clinical Sciences (CECS) became the source of "disruptive innovation" for changing DMS and the Dartmouth-Hitchcock medical system—and put practice variation on the national agenda for reform through the Dartmouth Atlas of Health Care project.[5]

During this period, as computers simplified data collection and analysis, and the Internet simplified information sharing, CECS faculty Wennberg, Elliott Fisher, MD, MPH, Paul Batalden, MD, H. Gilbert Welch, MD, MPH, James Weinstein, DO, MS, and others, started asking and answering provocative questions: Why, according to the evaluative clinical data, does more health care spending not necessarily yield better patient outcomes? Is there a "right level of care for the right patient" and, consequently, a "right cost of care" to drive better business models? What are the costs, risks and benefits of screening to detect illness early? Why, given the general agreement on the goal of patient centered care, is it so difficult to implement shared decision making? Should payment to providers be based on the value of the care they deliver, and not simply the utilization they cause? Should a health care organization's quality be measured and made transparent via the Internet? And, if an organization's quality is lacking, could it be motivated to use data-driven systems thinking and interdisciplinary interventions to re-engineer care?

In challenging Dartmouth to address this last question, Batalden frequently quoted J. Brian Quinn, PhD, MBA, of the Tuck School of Business at Dartmouth, who famously pointed out that "every system is designed to receive the results it gets."[6] By the early 1990s, Batalden and Eugene Nelson, DSc, MPH, were urging health care organizations to self-assess and form a plan to define their culture. The plan would help identify the organization as a "smart organization," that is, a "learning organization" with a "learning culture."[7] Such an organization would use systems thinking to capture data that interdisciplinary teams could adapt in real time with Plan-Do-Study-Act (PDSA) cycles to improve quality. The visual image is a Value Compass that gives a balanced evaluation of a patient's *functional, satisfaction, technical* and *cost* outcomes. Data published in *The Dartmouth Atlas of Health Care* since 1996 showed there was a wide variation in care and outcomes.[8] The "smart" organization, Dartmouth faculty insisted, would give patient care that is the most effective in providing function, satisfaction, and technology outcomes at the lowest cost.

Like Abraham Flexner's research 100 years

earlier had informed the general public about "the inadequate ways that some medical schools were preparing their students for entry into practice,"[9] CECS researchers' findings informed the public and other stakeholders (government, insurers) about many health care systems' failure to deliver evidence-based, preference-sensitive care—care that works and informed patients want! Needless to say, CECS faculty members' questions and arguments perturbed Dartmouth's status quo. Dartmouth-Hitchcock leaders had to ask themselves hard questions: was the system providing every patient with safe, effective, appropriate care, or were there preventable injuries and deaths, limited access, and spiraling costs? Was Dartmouth-Hitchcock a smart, learning organization capturing data and strengthening interdisciplinary teams? Was Dartmouth-Hitchcock continuously striving for improved quality and the highest value for every patient—or was there waste and commercialism? Many institutional answers were unsatisfactory.

The Challenges to Medical Education

The subsequent challenge to Dartmouth-Hitchcock senior leaders was to develop a comprehensive vision of its own transformation to patient-centered, interdisciplinary and value-based medical practice, using lessons learned from CECS colleagues' research, and to figure out how to embed that vision and its guiding principles in their culture. Part of the dilemma was determining whether traditional CME methods could be helpful in making Dartmouth-Hitchcock a learning organization, or whether new methods and strategies for educating 21st century physicians would be necessary.

In 2007, the Center for Evaluative Clinical Sciences was renamed The Dartmouth Institute for Health Policy and Clinical Practice, usually referred to as "TDI." Informed by our TDI colleagues' work and the research and the example of CME exemplars (e.g. the University of Toronto Faculty of Medicine, Baylor School of Medicine, and University of Michigan Medical School), we decided that the answer was the latter. Traditional CME activities—planned and taught using traditional methods (passivity versus interactivity), static resources (classroom versus computers), and outmoded funding sources (commercial versus independent) would not suffice to make D-H a learning organization and transform the culture. We agreed with Batalden, who directed TDI's Center for Leadership and Improvement and participated in the drafting of the Accreditation Council for Graduate Medical Education (ACGME) competencies, that disruptive innovation was the only logical solution. For too long, CME professionals, including ourselves, in spite of important scholarship on experiential learning by David Davis, MD, and others, had persisted in using ineffective education design emphasizing cognitive recall. In addition, we had enabled industry influence. As a result, most traditional CME remained misaligned with performance in practice and subject to potential bias. Batalden warned that CME as we know it may be on a "path to irrelevance" because much of it (1) pretends nothing has happened to change practice, (2) misses strategic opportunities to be woven together with organizational reform, and (3) makes learning harder because it fails to help physicians meet Maintenance of Certification (MOC) and specialty requirements that the American Board of Medical Specialties (ABMS) and American Board of Internal Medicine (ABIM) soon will impose. He advised us to focus on the inextricably linked arms in the "iron triangle of reform": better professional development, better systems performance, and better outcomes. "CME that acknowledges and strengthens this triangle will be of benefit to physicians and society," Batalden argued, "Otherwise, it is not."[10]

Helping Dartmouth-Hitchcock become a learning organization and transforming the "culture of medicine"—in an era of unprecedented health care reform—while also changing how CME is designed, delivered, and funded are enormous challenges. As mentioned earlier, physicians are stuck in a world of irrational payment models and at times perverse forces. They have little time or incentive to change either their learning habits or practice behavior while knowing that they must in order to improve patient outcomes under new funding mechanisms. Their practice is increasingly interdisciplinary. Their workplace has increasingly tacit, implicit jobs done by more workers.[11] John Parboosingh, MB, ChB, FRCSC, notes that twenty-first-century physicians must use complexity-based models of continuous practice management to reach change, and that clinicians change practice behaviors best in clinical settings that are "complex adaptive systems."[12] However many physicians find themselves in clinical settings that are complex but *not* adaptive. They must learn how to improve themselves and those systems simultaneously by self-assessing and working on systems-based solutions.

The ideal method to meet the challenge of reforming continuing medical education and practice then is to embed lifelong learning, as an institutional strategy for continuous transformation, into everyday patient care in every corner of a medical center, private practice, clinic, nursing home, or other delivery site. Our Dartmouth-Hitchcock vision is patient-centered, directly relevant, evidence-based and unbiased continuing medical education *embedded in practice*. This vision is based on TDI theory and its insistence that measurement informs systems improvement. Dr. James "Jim" Weinstein, now president of the Dartmouth-Hitchcock Clinic in addition to serving as director of The Dartmouth Institute, insists that "people who study what they do are better doctors."[13] We agree. The model for our evolving reforms is Batalden's and Nelson's clinical Value Compass conceptualized to drive value into clinical care. This Compass can give a balanced evaluation of medical care *and* education outcomes in terms of patient functional health, perceptual satisfaction, cost, and clinical/biological status. The operative question regarding education becomes, over the period of time when the physician practices medicine, is she/he sufficiently knowledgeable, competent, skilled, and experienced to perform her/his responsibilities in such a way as to provide each patient with the highest quality of care? Every patient leaves each doctor visit (or procedure) evaluating the four outcomes on the Compass:

1. *Functional Health*: Has my quality of life improved; have my complications decreased; has my overall psychological outlook improved?
2. *Perception*: Am I satisfied with my care; is there respect and trust between me and my doctor; is s/he constantly improving her/his professional abilities, including management skills?
3. *Clinical/Biological Status*: Is my clinical care being coordinated; do I understand and am I benefiting from my medical, surgical, mental health and rehabilitation interventions, examinations, prescribing, medical compliance monitoring, and immunizations?
4. *Cost*: Are my overall hospital expenses appropriate; has my doctor eliminated all unnecessary interventions; is my doctor utilizing options that I do not want, cannot afford, and do not have sufficient time to undertake?

Physicians must understand the measures that constitute high value—from a patient's point of view—in order to provide quality care. And each physician must continue to educate and train her/himself over her/his lifetime of professional practice—and not simply during medical school and residency—to improve each patient's four outcome measures.

Consider the value equation for each patient visit:

$$\text{Value} = \frac{\text{Quality \& Outcomes}}{\text{Cost}} \,/\, \text{Time}$$

The continuous, practical, on-the-job and data-informed education of each practicing physician is critical in the era of health care reform. At one time, continuing medical education was derided by many leaders in the academic community (including some medical school deans) as a secondary, non-essential activity in comparison to the primacy of medical school and residency education. No longer. Over a physician's professional career, on-going education is a factor in every patient outcome. Medical school and residency build a foundation for knowledge and competency. They do not assure a professional career of improved performance in practice. At this point in time, many medical students and residents are not taught the evaluative sciences, the importance of discerning comparative results, or the ethics of involving the patient in decision making. In many ways, the current culture of medical schools and residency programs—in their focus on the hierarchical achievement of individual doctors rather than equal partnerships with multiple patients—work against high evaluation of those doctors' four outcome measures for high value, later in their careers.

Our concept for how lifelong and continuous education influences the value equation is the "ideal contract" between patient and physician (as well as other members of the health care team) realized through the sequence of "ideal patient visits." By "ideal" we are suggesting, in consultation with Jack Wennberg and Jim Weinstein, interactive behavior—over time—that reflects mutual individual and shared responsibility akin to the classic concept of the "social contract" used in normative discussion of obligations of society to individuals. Imagine a sequence of ideal patient visits where *everyone* the patient interacts with, starting with the primary care physician (adult or pediatrician) or nurse practitioner, and moving to the specialist, nurse, pharmacist, and every other person on the team, is a dedicated, learner, committed to knowing not only the current evidence-based and essential best practices, but also uses the tools of the evaluative sciences to learn how to improve. The provider and team member knows how to gather and analyze data to determine what interventions are working for the patient and where and why there are variations. Through continuous education and professional development within the practice setting the provider and team members can narrow unwarranted variations, in such a way as to generate greater value for the patient. Using a Primary Care Provider treating a Diabetic Patient as an example, the provider would know the Clinical Population Health Transformation Pathway to guide care delivery to be reliable (sustainable, patient-informed and measured), efficient (accessible, available, productive, not wasteful), and evidence-based (consensus informed, standardized, committed to highest value). The provider would know the essential best practices that must be managed including medical nutrition therapy, hypertension treatments, aspirin regimens, immunizations, and diabetes retinopathy screening. And the provider would know how to self-assess her or his own practice gaps (e.g. prescribing of hypertension medicine, or knowing when to start or change medicines), and use her or his Diabetic Patient's outcome data to determine what knowledge, skill or competency are needed to learn to give better care.[14] Finally, in fulfilling the responsibility of academic medical centers to be responsible for the scientific basis of clinical medicine, the provider would follow her or his patients over time and contribute her or his outcome experience to evaluate treatment theories and reduce scientific uncertainty about the value of medical care.

Imagine also a sequence of ideal patient visits where the patient-provider relationship is democratized and medicine is practiced based on what the patient wants, and not what the doctor chooses. Wennberg argues that the democratization of medicine is the "ultimate disruptive innovation" and an ethical imperative when, as is so often the case, there are genuine options that depend on patient preference such as whether of patient with early stage breast cancer wants a lumpectomy or a mastectomy.[15] How would this evolve? We imagine medical school admissions committees and faulty search committees prior-

itizing applicants' intangibles including their capacity to communicate and treat patients ethically—as well as their capacity to master science. We imagine patients as voting members of these committees. We imagine students and house staff educated constantly to improve interpersonal interactions as well as skills, procedures and service—and prevented from graduating or advancing if they did not. We imagine clinical faculty trained to communicate with diverse patient populations—in clear language at appropriate literacy levels—and to use decision aides effectively to help patients in making informed choices. We imagine new, junior faculty, prior to receiving their academic appointments, trained to be effective educators of patients, students and house staff. Our colleague Catharine "Kate" Clay, MA, RN, director of D-H's Center for Shared Decision Making, notes that "there's a problem with what we give physicians credit for and allow them to do simply because we let them graduate from medical school and finish residency."[16] What if all physicians, nurses, and pharmacists in training and beyond learned *together* in inter-professional teams using interactive methods, open spaces, and simulation centers? Clay points out that we need inter-professional teams where all providers consistently ask their patients the following questions: What do you think I need to do to be more helpful to you? What do you want from our relationship that would be most useful? We imagine physicians and their teammates always listening carefully to the patient's narrative and empowering the patient in conversation. We imagine patients and hospital leaders no longer settling for the smart doctor with "good skills but a terrible bedside manner." This is generally the same doctor who communicates poorly with colleagues as well, and therefore may be disruptive and disrespectful. There may be a place for this physician in Medicine, but not with patients if the physician cannot honor the social contract that underpins an ideal patient interaction.

These major cultural changes are evolving across the medical education spectrum at Dartmouth informed by TDI theory and championed by TDI and other perturbers, including ourselves. A sampling of examples include the seven-year collaboration of Dr. O'Donnell and Ellen Ceppetelli, MS, RN, CNL, director of Nursing Education, in D-H's Office of Professional Nursing, to have DMS medical students shadow and learn from D-H nurses. This activity advances perhaps *the* most important lesson every first year resident learns, that is to partner with experienced nursing colleagues and master what they teach. Another example is the D-H Orthopaedic Residency Program, directed by Charles Carr, MD, where four residents enter a TDI Masters program and complete interdisciplinary research projects involving and shared with peers and teams. These residents' projects create and embed TDI theory and improve practice.

Shared Decision Making and Informed Choice

TDI scholars understand the value equation and believe the principal health reform goals must include shared decision making and informed patient choice. Their definition of shared decision making is: "the best process for establishing need for a given preference-sensitive treatment option. In a shared decision, a health care provider communicates to the patient personalized information about the options, outcomes, probabilities, and scientific uncertainties of available treatment options, and the patient communicates his or her values and the relative importance he or she places on benefits and harms. The patient and physician work together to decide which treatment option best serves the patient's preferences. The aim of this process is to ensure informed patient choice."[17] The definition for Informed Patient Choice is: "a new normative standard for determining medical necessity based on patient understanding of the harms and benefits of treatment options and participation in a shared decision-making process to ensure that the treatment chosen is in keeping with the patient's own values and preferences."[18]

Wennberg argues in *Tracking Medicine: A Researcher's Quest to Understand Health Care* that the democratization of the doctor-patient relationship through shared decision making is probably the most important element in disruptive innovation: it changes utilization patterns, reduces supplier-induced demand—and saves money while increasing patient satisfaction. He writes, "The democratization of the doctor-patient relationship—the replacement of delegated decision making by shared decision making, and the doctrine of informed consent by a standard of practice based on informed patient choice—represents a transformation in the culture of medicine that will not be easy to achieve."[19] Asking a powerful person to relinquish power and deconstruct his hierarchy is never simple.

Nevertheless the central philosophy that informs all Dartmouth-Hitchcock reforms is patient-centeredness. Chair of Community and Family Medicine and Director of the MD-MBA Program at DMS and the Tuck School of Business, Michael Zubkoff, PhD, states that to be patient-centered, doctors must learn to be self-reflective about two things, first, how effective they are in engaging each patient as a partner in designing her/his own care, and, second, communicating to the team of nurses, social workers, pharmacists, therapists, and so forth, that plan successfully in a community relationship with the patient.[20] Patient engagement means flattening the hierarchy between doctors, patients, *and* colleagues in order to manage a personal relationship with the patient, her/his family, and the team.

Flattening the hierarchy in the practice of medicine is a particularly perturbing professional expectation for many physicians trained to behave otherwise. It is profoundly important, however, to produce care in the best interest of the patient, which, as William J. Mayo, MD, taught at Mayo Clinic, "is the only interest to be considered."[21] In their important theoretical work on transforming the teaching and learning of medicine, medical education researchers Alan Bleakley and John Bligh argue that the "intellectual landscape of critical, interdisciplinary inquiry" about physician behavior is one that, thus far, many medical educators "have not inhabited," and thus premises and ideology that inform practice go unexamined.[22] In considering undergraduate medical education taught by medical faculty, Bleakley and Bligh ask provocatively, "What aspects of the medical curriculum best meet the needs of the patient?"—a question they believe educators across the education continuum fail to answer.[23]

Acknowledging the distinction by Donald Schön, PhD, that medical education is "not a technical-rational strategy but primarily a practice artistry employing technical-rational elements," Bleakley and Bligh argue for "patient-led medical education" with a "process-led approach." Such an approach to learning values is based in social learning theory as well as content outcomes. Rather than framing medical education throughout the continuum as an "individual, heroic endeavor" based in individualistic (and often discredited) adult learning approaches, they argue that medical education for the twenty-first-century physician needs a new research base that explores learning as "socialization constructing a professional identity and providing legitimate entry into communities of practice." To accomplish this transformation, Bleakley and Bligh, call for a richer, interdisciplinary approach to enable students and faculty to learn a narrative-based, as well as scientific, evidence-based, approach to patient care. The narrative-based, interdisciplinary approach requires the study of cultural theory (including anthropology, gender studies, sociology, etc.) to enable active, open conversation with a patient fully engaged in a discourse about her/his own care.[24]

Whereas patient-centeredness is now Dartmouth-Hitchcock's central philosophy, adoption has not come easily. Formidable financial, legal and educational barriers have made institution-wide practice challenging. Nevertheless, individual clinicians, researchers and educators have persevered in pushing this culture change forward. Es-

tablishment started in 1988 with research on decision aids with patients being treated at the Veterans Affairs Medical Center (VAMC), a Dartmouth-Hitchcock affiliated teaching hospital, diagnosed with benign prostatic hyperplasia (BPH). The research resulted in fewer surgeries, which saved the VAMC money but confounded Urology residents' need to perform enough BPH operations to meet minimum requirements for board certification. The research ended when, as Wennberg says, "The needs of medical educators trumped patient preferences."[25]

Nevertheless, Dartmouth theorists, researchers and educators continued to identify problems in the health care delivery system and decided how they would like to see the future unfold. Fundamentally, all future medical care would place the patient at the center of the Value Compass. *Unwarranted variations* in treatment that could not be explained by illness rate differences would be confronted using patient preferences and medical evidence. *Overuse* of effective care would be reduced using training and education to assess which patients could go without a procedure or medicine. The *misuse* of preference-based treatment would be managed with shared decision making and ethical treatment requirements. And, the overuse of care, particularly for the chronically ill and elderly would be mitigated with advance directives, palliative medicine, and compassionate care. But the CECS/TDI faculty had no Dartmouth-Hitchcock Medical Center champion for overall cultural reform.

All that all changed in 1996, however, when Dr. James Weinstein, an Orthopeadic surgeon with conservative views on potentially life-changing surgeries, was recruited from the University of Iowa to be Chair of the Dartmouth-Hitchcock Department of Orthopaedics. Weinstein, who had studied back pain patient outcomes, insisted that shared decision making and informed patient choice become the standard of practice in Orthopaedics. In 1999 the founding of the Center for Shared Decision Making provided a means for integrating shared decision making into everyday practice within the walls of DHMC; it stands as the "first ever" example of the commitment of academic medicine to the democratization of the doctor-patient relationship and the ethic of informed patient choice. University of Toronto researcher Annette O'Connor, PhD, an expert in decision aids, joined the faculty and trained the Center's director Kate Clay to support patients during the decision process while Weinstein persuaded physicians to participate.

Eventually, by applying TDI theory to practice, establishing and sustaining a smart organization, and enabling strategic innovations in education, we envision Dartmouth-Hitchcock's best-in-class providers having lower admission and readmission rates, less fragmentation, more consistency, more transparency, lower cost and greatest value—all in the patient's best interest. No matter where the patient enters our health care delivery system, s/he will encounter a coordinated, interdisciplinary team of skilled clinician-educators and learners who provide care options in a sensitive and democratic manner. The future ideal patient visit, informed by the Value Compass and patient-physician contract, will transform clinicians' education in a simple, affordable way that drives value into CME. It concentrates on performance directly related to the patient, generally in the site of care, and using less time and fewer resources to perform the work of education. Properly designed, the elements of disruptive innovation for improved CME support Batalden's iron triangle for better systems performance, better outcomes, and better professional development.

The Future

An important strength of Dartmouth's differentness is that, by encouraging open discourse, perturbing behavior, and disruptive innovation, it makes progress. In 2007, as CECS was transitioning to TDI, Dartmouth-Hitchcock leaders decided to do strategic planning to make the organization "smart." They started by adopting the following *Mission and Vision Statements.*

Mission—Dartmouth-Hitchcock advances health through research, education, clinical practice and community partnerships, providing each person the best care, in the right place, at the right time, every time.

Vision—We achieve the healthiest population possible, leading the transformation of health care in our region and setting the standard for our nation.[26]

Five strategic Task Forces of over 150 individuals developed strategic imperatives including one for *Education and Research*. They wrote: "Leadership in discovering, applying, and translating approaches for achieving optimum population health requires focused and robust academic endeavors." They also developed a Desired Future State which read: "The concept of distinct units of this academic medical center is replaced by a single, unified health system with a philosophy and structure that represents the result of cohesion of clinical service, teaching and research missions and their support structures and finances."[27]

To reach the Desired Future State and improve collaboration across the entire academic and clinical enterprise, Dartmouth Medical School and Dartmouth-Hitchcock, started jointly to plan for and invest in critical research, education, and clinical services. Integrated planning established a foundation of financial transparency and aligned objectives across institutions with clear expectations for performance.[28] Leaders also resolved to make Dartmouth-Hitchcock a "learning organization" with continuing education programs (accredited and non-accredited) supporting the cultural transformation.

Among the goals for an Desired Future State where health science education supported cultural transformation were: expanding integration of CME with Nursing Continuing Education and other disciplines; linking the CME Program to internal Performance Improvement initiatives (e.g. Simulation Center courses, Joint Commission and Microsystems teams); strengthening educational activities associated with quality measurement initiatives to drive improved patient outcomes; and adding more online education offerings, long distance education, and e-learning opportunities.

With the encouragement of the Trustees and Board, we:

- reorganized the Graduate and Continuing Medical and Nursing Education programs into a strategic partnership to strengthen faculty development, residency and fellowship programs, and Regularly Scheduled Series;
- created a Council for Lifelong Learning in Medical Education (CLLiME) co-chaired by the DMS deans for UME, GME and CME, for the purpose of working together to improve medical education for physicians in every stage of their careers;
- reconstituted the CME Advisory Committee to include institution-wide education and administrative leadership;
- developed an Education Strategic Planning Process to provide a unified vision and governance for DHC and MHMH education programs in collaboration with DMS, TDI and the VAMC;
- and started research projects (with Virginia Reed, PhD, and Karen Schifferdecker, PhD) to understand *why* clinician practice behavior change is so difficult in complex systems, *what* variables are consistently associated with behavior change, and *how* to use comparative effectiveness research to improve patient care.

Reaching our technology goals, including more online education offerings, long distance education and e-learning, is now our highest priority. We have laid the foundation by: implementing an online registration, payment and transcription system; redesigning and maintaining a learner-friendly Web site for professionals wishing to attend conferences and Regularly Scheduled Series (grand rounds, case conferences/ morbidity and mortality rounds, and journal clubs, etc.); and, improving tracking of commercial support relationships with Industry, and conflict of interest (COI), reporting and resolution. Our critical next step, in spite of limited resources is, to find creative ways to finance and implement a Center for Instructional Technology to produce online educational offerings to spread and amplify Dartmouth's outstanding academic resources. Our goal is to support cultural transformation both inside and beyond our campuses.

Technology and information systems are critical for meeting our goals in the era of health care reform, but are also among our greatest challenges. Nevertheless, today many Dartmouth-Hitchcock and regional clinicians assess personal performance data from registries or chart reviews. However, a true institutional transformation is taking place as Dartmouth-Hitchcock transitions to a new electronic health record (EHR), an $80 million Dartmouth-Hitchcock investment. The EHR will enable data-driven self-assessment of performance by every clinician for every patient. Dartmouth-Hitchcock's CME directors are working with the leaders of this appropriately named Clinical Transformation Project (an Epic EHR system) to plan and accredit the training using scenarios based on validated practice gaps.

Shared Philosophies

Dartmouth's different-ness, research-oriented reform agenda, and subsequent initiatives to improve care *and* education have been powerful in driving internal reform. The most important component, however, has been leaders with shared philosophies. In the era of health-care reform, three central philosophies have informed Dartmouth-Hitchcock's progress: a commitment to patient-centeredness, a pledge to improve with data-driven assessment, and a willingness to "shake the foundations." All three apply to improving physician education as well as clinical care.

Patient-Centeredness

In this chapter we have described in detail Dartmouth-Hitchcock's persistent march to patient-centeredness through shared decision making and informed patient choice, along with a variety of faculty members', clinician leaders' and educators' efforts to embed these philosophies. A critical element for widespread adoption is leadership's unwavering commitment to justice. These strategic efforts have prepared Dartmouth-Hitchcock's CME program for the future of health care reform and encouraged our cultural transformation to a smarter organization where every patient will receive "the best care in the right place, at the right time, every time."

Learning the necessary social skills to be patient-centered must happen in what James Reason, PhD, calls a "just culture." This is done, according to Jack Wennberg, "by making the practice the education."[29] From a Dartmouth perspective, we understand that we must not only promote, but study how we reach patient-centeredness through a flattening of the hierarchy, self-assessment and self-reflection, patient-led/narrative-based practice, and doctor-led/evidence-based practice—all of which are important elements in the ideal patient visit and Value Compass.

In addition to the activities already mentioned, we promote patient-centeredness with numerous Dartmouth-Hitchcock education initiatives that teach a just culture across institutions and the education continuum. Two examples come from Dartmouth-Hitchcock.

Patient-Safety directors George Blike, MD, and Polly Campion, MS, RN, lead an institution-wide, interactive education series on Dartmouth-Hitchcock's Culture of Safety. Department directors engage all employees in five 20-minute videos and a 30-minute guided conversation on how and why patient safety is a core value. In a "professionally safe" environment, colleagues discuss flattening the hierarchy and speaking up about errors—against the traditional "authority gradient" in what Lucian Leape, MD, defines as a transformation "from paternalism to partnering."[30] In a related example, Dr. Blike, Frances Todd, MSN, RN, and colleagues reinforce the Dartmouth-Hitchcock culture of patient-centeredness, integrity, and safety in classes and accredited activities in the Dartmouth-Hitchcock Patient Safety Training Center, our simulation center where over-confidence and under-confidence in procedures and patient interactions are remediated.

In the Dartmouth-Hitchcock Center for Continuing Education in the Health Sciences we promote and study self-assessment and self-reflection through the use of *Personal Learning Plans* before and after live educational activities to evaluate physician learners' self-reflection of professional development needs—cultural and scientific. With researchers Reed and Schifferdecker, CME director Mary Turco, EdD, analyzes responses to assist learners with intent-to-change practice, as well as to help course directors and planners improve their needs assessment, topic selection, pedagogical methods, and teaching styles.

In TDI's Center for Informed Choice, directed by E. Dale Collins Vidal, MD, MS and Hilary Llewellyn-Thomas, PhD, researchers study a patients' health-care decision-making and the development and implementation of policy and practice-based solutions. Working with colleagues, faculty develop and evaluate decision aids for patients considering a variety of options affecting health outcomes. Using decision science, they analyze patients' treatment options, decision-making styles, and satisfaction with decisions. While the Center for Informed Choice staff disseminates principles and tools to patients and providers through the Center for Shared Decision-Making within the Medical Center, the faculty disseminate to other clinicians by hosting international research symposia; sharing conceptual frameworks, research, and aids through internal performance improvement (PI) CME courses; and, providing scholarships to Dartmouth-Hitchcock clinicians to obtain a Masters degree through TDI's Center for Education. In addition, D-H promotes and studies inter-professional health sciences education in clinical microsystems courses led by Eugene Nelson, Dartmouth-Hitchcock Director of Quality Administration, and colleagues with teams throughout the organization. Dr. Nelson and his colleagues teach Clinical Microsystems Awareness and Transformational development throughout the organization.

Finally, through the Leadership Preventive Medicine Residency Program (LPMR) in TDI Center for Leadership and Improvement, established by Paul Batalden and now guided by Mark Splaine, MD, LPMR faculty educate practicing clinicians in a range of disciplines about ways to develop, construct, implement, and evaluate innovative models to improve the delivery of care. Residents design and study patient-centered practice models and publish their research.

Data Driven Assessment

A key shared philosophy is the importance of data. Most institutional improvement at Dartmouth-Hitchcock is data-driven. Dartmouth-Hitchcock Co-Presidents Weinstein and Nancy Formella, MSN, RN, challenge every employee to avoid ineffective, disorganized or inappropriate care, preventable injury and death, waste, commercialism, spiraling cost, and limited access. Multiple institutional activities respond to the challenge. Clinical leaders generate their publicly released data on departmental, section and unit *Balanced Scorecards* where data become information for patients. *Dartmouth-Hitchcock Quality Measure Reports* provide accurate, honest information to patients on the Dartmouth-Hitchcock Web site in a variety of performance categories (overall, procedures, cancer care, diseases and conditions, rehabilitation, intensive care, children's care, women's health, and charges for health care services.)[31] Patients can link from the Dartmouth-Hitchcock site to *New Hampshire Quality Care* site of the Foundation for Healthy Communities and

North East Health Care Quality Foundation, the Joint Commission's *Quality Check*, and the Centers for Medicare and Medicaid Service (CMS) *Hospital Compare* data. And, while all individual physicians (and other clinicians) do not routinely disclose practice outcomes, some do now and eventually all will. Among the early champions is Orthopaedic surgeon William Abdu, MD, MS, who works on transparency initiatives and gathers data as Medical Director of Dartmouth-Hitchcock's highly regarded Spine Center. Abdu gives each of his patients his business card with the Web site for the Spine Center results—including his own—good and bad. Abdu insists that a doctor sharing an opinion should no longer be allowed to say "from my experience" but should rather say "from my *measured* experience" and then give the patient specific information appropriate to the patient's literacy level.

The EHR is the disruptive innovation technology that will simplify how all Dartmouth-Hitchcock continuing education and professional development initiatives transition to patient-centered activities by means of data-driven assessment. As we use meaningful data to assess patient-care and education outcomes, we will truly shake the foundation of continuing medical education.

Enlightened colleagues are applying data to re-invent CME. Our argument that "tomorrow is today" and that continuing education will help transform how medicine is practiced, is supported by the work of outstanding Dartmouth-Hitchcock clinician-researcher-educators "doing education right." Sohail Mirza, MD, MPH successor to James Weinstein as Chair of Orthopaedics, has designed the "Dartmouth Back Pain Training Program" for regional Primary Care Physicians (PCP), a Performance Improvement CME Activity. The Program helps PCPs provide evidence-based care for patients with back pain by building and training primary-care based expert teams consisting of a physical therapist, a psychologist, and several PCPs working together to evaluate and treat patients experiencing acute and chronic non-specific axial back pain or pain associated with degenerative changes in the lumbar spine. In addition to seven online electronic CME modules based on AHRQ, ACP, APS, and AAOS guidelines, variations of team members identify barriers to change, read published articles on AHRQ Evidence based Practice Center guidelines, attend six one-hour interactive didactic sessions with experts to discuss applying knowledge and establishing relationships and workflows to coordinate care, evaluate patients in clinic sessions, observe spinal surgery and spinal injections, perform lumbar spine MRI interpretations, observe spinal EMG studies, participate in Dartmouth's Functional Restoration Program, manage baseline functional status measurements three and twelve months from treatment, and demonstrate full performance competence on a prior treatment assessment, physical exam, mental health assessment, appropriate imaging, recommendations for exercise, use of Epidural Steroid injections, surgical timing, patient reassessment, and shared decision making. PCP's receive $1,000 compensation for time devoted to completing interventions. Anthem-WellPoint pays a case manger $100 per patient meeting benchmarks on structural and process measures. A program analyst team evaluates health care utilization, costs, and patient outcomes at 12 and 24 months after program implementation, while Anthem-WellPoint provides funding and access to data to support the work. And, learners receive academic credit and earn status as a "Fellow of the Dartmouth-Hitchcock Spine Center." This remarkable educational opportunity is not, as David Davis likes to say, "your grandfather's or grandmother's CME Program."

Shaking the Foundations

In the spring of 2009, the Dartmouth College Board of Trustees selected Jim Yong Kim, MD, PhD, a physician and anthropologist, as their new president. Kim arrived with significant experience as a medical educator and global health re-

searcher. Six months into his presidency, on January 20, 2010 during the national celebration of the life of Martin Luther King, Jr., Kim gave an address to DMS faculty and students titled "Quality Health Care for All: Why We Can't Wait." During the presentation, Kim advocated that medical school faculty and students "shake the foundations" to improve health care delivery systems and medical education and argued for a "social justice movement around quality of all." Paraphrasing Dartmouth's twelfth president, John Sloan Dickey (1945–1970), Kim said "the world's troubles are our troubles" and called upon his medical school faculty and students to put the world's troubled human beings before themselves. He argued that it was important to admit students who, like Martin Luther King, Jr., who said he felt "maladjusted" to the racial segregation he experienced personally, feel maladjusted to injustices they witness or experience today, and provide those students with a strong liberal arts curriculum. Quoting King's speech at Dartmouth on May 23, 1962, Kim noted that the world is in desperate need of men and women like Abraham Lincoln who, "in the midst of an age amazingly adjusted to slavery, had the vision to see that this nation could not exist half slave and half free."[32] Medical students preparing for careers in medicine in the twenty-first century would complete courses in economics, anthropology, as well as sociology, biology, physics, and chemistry, to acquire an understanding that their life's work will be a partnership with individual human beings, most of who are among the world's most disadvantaged.

Molly Cooke, MD, David Irby, PhD, and Bridget O'Brien, PhD, the authors of the 2010 report *Educating Physicians: A Call for Reform of Medical School and Residency from the Carnegie Foundation of Teaching* (the so-called "Flexner Two Report"), insist that reforming the "ossified curricular structures" of medical education is imperative to prepare these Twenty-first-century physicians. In medical school and residency, the authors recommend: (1) education for the integration of knowledge, experience and reasoning; (2) the development of habits of inquiry and improvement; (3) standardization and individualization; and (4) professional identify formation—values and commitments which support the best interest of patients.[33] They suggest changes in the medical curriculum content and design, pedagogy, and assessment.

CME must change dramatically and quickly to train the faculty who will engage and mentor the medical students whom Dr. Kim and Cooke and others describe, the learners who already face performance expectations for the specific competencies of residency and fellowship training, state licensure requirements, and ABMS and MOC certification. Former Director of TDI's Center for Education and DMS Associate Dean for Health Policy and Clinical Practice Gerald O'Connor, PhD, ScD, states that medical education has a "green-belt curriculum" that must evolve to a "black belt" and that first, this has to happen "at home." We recognize that it is necessary to shake the foundations of medical education across the continuum at our own institutions first to address inequality and injustice in health care as well as flawed delivery and education systems.

Closing

Placing patients at the heart of the enterprise, using data to drive health-care strategy, and confidently shaking foundations, are central Dartmouth philosophies for reform. They and many others underpin Dartmouth-Hitchcock's persistent effort to establish an integrated academic system that measurably improves the health of the population of our region and the nation. During the tempestuous health care reform debates of the late twentieth and early twenty-first centuries, strong voices from Dartmouth's rural university and health system, recognizing documented problems in safety, quality, access, and affordability, have called for new health-care delivery systems and improved medical education led by skilled and compassionate physicians. Our

shared belief is that there can be no health-care reform without education reform across the continuum and with patients as partners.

We at Dartmouth believe that current continuing education methods are inadequate and must be replaced by models emphasizing patient-centeredness. Physician learners must prioritize the quality equation and generate the outcome measures required for an ideal patient-physician relationship leading to sequences of ideal patient visits. It has been said, Jack Wennberg reminds us, that "statistics are people with the tears wiped off."[34] Educators must help physicians democratize the doctor-patient relationship, flatten the hierarchy of medicine, and sustain a just institutional culture. We must help clinicians embed education into practice to ensure high competence over a lifetime of practice. At Dartmouth-Hitchcock, CME, in partnership with nursing and allied health, will ultimately be the engine that helps our institution achieve its vision for the healthiest population possible, providing effective, efficient, timely, safe, and equitable patient- and family-centered care to all. It is an exciting time to embrace change.

Theologian Paul Tillich, whose work has strongly influenced Dartmouth President Kim, has written: "Perhaps man will use the power to shake the foundations for creative purposes, for progress, for peace and happiness. The future lies in man's hands, in our hands."[35] Kim and his newly appointed (October 2010) Medical School Dean Wiley "Chip" Souba, MD, ScD, MBA, now lead a unique academic community where the voices of perturbers, reformers, and educators "calling in the wilderness" share a commitment to help improve health-care delivery and education to address the world's troubles. With faith in members of the health care professions we believe that through our creative purposes to reform continuing medical education and change the culture of medicine, we can contribute to the progress that will lead to patients' improved health and subsequent well-being— our ultimate goal.

Acknowledgment

The authors gratefully acknowledge Dartmouth colleague John "Jack" Wennberg, MD, MPH, for his significant contributions to the chapter and for his important insights on the centrality of patient centeredness and shared decision making in reforming medical education and healthcare delivery for all.

Notes

M. L. King Jr, "Beyond Vietnam—A Time to Break Silence" (speech, New York City, April 4, 1967), quoted by President J. Y. Kim in "Quality Health Care for All: Why We Can't Wait" (speech to the Dartmouth Community, Hanover, N.H., January 20, 2010).

1. See the foreword to this book.
2. "What is the Translation of Dartmouth's Motto?" Dartmouth Web site, http://www.dartmouth.edu/~ask/categories/misc/42.html (accessed November 19, 2009).
3. C. E. Putnam, "A Long Running Hit. Dartmouth Medicine," *DMS Publications* 27, no. 2 (2002): 28–39.
4. J. E. Wennberg and A. Gittelsohn, "Small Area Variations in Health Care Delivery: A Population-based Health Information System Can Guide Planning and Regulatory Decision-Making," *Science*, 182 (1973): 1102–1108.
5. C. M. Christensen and others, *The Innovator's Prescription: A Disruptive Solution for Health Care* (New York: McGraw-Hill, 2009).
6. J. B. Quinn, *The Intelligent Enterprise* (New York: The Free Press, 1992).
7. E. C. Nelson and P. B. Batalden, "Patient Based Quality Measurement Systems," *Quality Management in Health Care* 2 (1993): 18–30.
8. J. E. Wennberg and M. M. Cooper, eds., *Dartmouth Atlas of Health Care in the United States* (Chicago: American Hospital Publishing, Inc., 1996).
9. M. E. Whitcomb and D. Nutter, "Learning Medicine in the 21st Century" (The Carnegie Foundation for the Advancement of Teaching, 2002), http://www.carnegiefoundation.org/medical-education/resources (accessed September 1, 2009).
10. P. B. Batalden, discussion with the authors, January 12, 2010.
11. B. C. Johnson and others, "The Next Revolution in Interactions," *The McKinsey Quarterly* 4 (2005): 20–33.
12. J. Parboosingh, "Embedding Practice Improvement Strategies in the Clinical Setting" (presentation, Lebanon, N.H., 2009).
13. J. Weinstein, discussion with the authors, January 15, 2010.

14. S. A. Berry, Clinical Population Health Transformation Pathway Development: Diabetes, presentation to Dartmouth-Hitchcock Department Directors, October 12, 2010.
15. J. E. Wennberg, discussion with the authors, September and October 2010.
16. C. Clay, October, 2010.
17. J. E. Wennberg, *Tracking Medicine: A Researcher's Quest to Understand Health Care* (New York: Oxford University Press, 2010), 225.
18. Ibid.
19. Ibid.
20. M. Zubkoff, discussion with the authors, December 13, 2009.
21. D. Cortese, "Cornerstone of Reforms," presentation at the National Symposium on Medicaid and Health Care Education Reform, Rochester, Minn., April 26, 2009.
22. A. Bleakley, and J. Bligh, "Looking Forward—Looking Back: Aspects of the Contemporary Debate about Teaching and Learning Medicine," *Medical Teacher* 29 (2007): 79–82.
23. Ibid.
24. Ibid.
25. J. E. Wennberg, *Tracking Medicine: A Researcher's Quest to Understand Health Care* (New York: Oxford University Press, 2010), 225.
26. "Dartmouth-Hitchcock Long Range Strategic Plan," executive summary, Dartmouth-Hitchcock Medical Center, Lebanon, N.H., 2008.
27. Ibid.
28. Ibid.
29. "Delivering Patient Safety Series," video (East Sussex, U.K.: TVC Films Ltd., 2009).
30. Ibid.
31. "Dartmouth-Hitchcock Medical Center Quality Reports," Dartmouth-Hitchcock Medical Center Web site, http://www.dhmc.org/webpage.cfm?site_id=2&org_id=459&gsec_id=0&sec_id=0&item_id=20534 (accessed December 15, 2009).
32. M. L. King, Jr, "Towards Freedom" (speech to the Dartmouth Community, Hanover, N.H., May 23, 1962) http://www.dartmouth.edu/~towardsfreedom/transcript.html (accessed February, 2010).
33. M. Cooke and others, *Educating Physicians: A Call for Reform of Medical School and Residency* (San Francisco: Jossey-Bass, 2010).
34. J. E. Wennberg *Tracking Medicine: A Researcher's Quest to Understand Health Care* (New York: Oxford University Press, 2010), 264
35. P. Tillich, *The Shaking of the Foundations* (New York: Scribner's, 1948).

About the Editor and Contributors

Errol R. Alden, MD, is executive director and chief executive officer of the American Academy of Pediatrics and a clinical professor in the department of pediatrics at the Uniformed Services University of the Health Sciences in Bethesda, Maryland.

Susan Alpert, PhD, MD, is senior vice president of global regulatory affairs at Medtronic, Inc.

M. Brownell Anderson, MEd, is senior director of educational affairs in academic affairs at the Association of American Medical Colleges.

Alejandro Aparicio, MD, FACP, is director of the division of continuing physician professional development at the American Medical Association and clinical assistant professor of medicine and assistant professor of medical education at the University of Illinois at Chicago College of Medicine.

DeWitt C. Baldwin, Jr., MD, is professor emeritus at University of Nevada School of Medicine and scholar-in-residence for the Accreditation Council for Graduate Medical Education.

Barbara Barnes, MD, MS, is vice president of contracts, grants, intellectual property, and continuing medical education at the University of Pittsburgh Medical Center.

Mary Jane Bell, BSc, MSc, MD, FRCPC, is director of CE/KTE in the department of medicine at the University of Toronto.

Bruce Bellande, PhD, CCMEP, is president of CME Enterprise, Inc.

Nancy Bennett, PhD, is assistant professor in the department of psychiatry at Harvard Medical School.

Diane Burkhart, PhD, is director of the department of education at the American Osteopathic Association.

Craig M. Campbell, MD, FRCPC, is associate professor, faculty of medicine at the University of Ottawa and director of the Office of Professional Affairs of the Royal College of Physicians and Surgeons of Canada.

Richard M. Caplan, MD, is professor emeritus of dermatology and the program in medical ethics and humanities at the University of Iowa, where he served for 21 years as associate dean for continuing medical education.

W. Dale Dauphinee, MD, FRCPC, FCAHS, is adjunct professor of the division of clinical epidemiology in the Department of Medicine, Faculty of Medicine at McGill University and senior scholar and institute senior mentor at the Foundation for Advancement of International Medical Education and Research

Dave Davis, MD, FCFP, is senior director of continuing education and performance improvement for the Association of American Medical Colleges and adjunct professor of family and community medicine and of health policy, management, and evaluation at the University of Toronto.

Nancy L. Davis, PhD, CCMEP, is executive director of the National Institute for Quality Improvement and Education.

Lois DeBakey, PhD, is professor of scientific communication at Baylor College of Medicine.

Carl S. DeMatteo, MD, is chief quality and compliance officer of Dartmouth-Hitchcock Medical Center and assistant professor of medicine and infectious diseases at Dartmouth Medical School.

Jill Donahue, HBa, MAdEd, is founder of the consulting firm Excellerate and an executive committee member for the Canadian Association of Continuing Health Education.

Maureen Doyle-Scharff, MBA, FACME, CCMEP, leads the medical education group at Pfizer Inc.

Lynn G. Dunikowski, MLS, is director of library services for the College of Family Physicians of Canada.

Robert D. Fox, EdD, is professor emeritus of adult and higher education at the University of Oklahoma.

Harry A. Gallis, MD, is president of CME for Improved Performance and consulting professor of medicine at Duke University and chair of subcommittees on continuing medical education accreditation for the Infectious Diseases Society of America and the North Carolina Medical Society.

Elaine Kierl Gangel is the manager of the CME resources department at the American Academy of Family Physicians.

Thomas C. Gentile, Jr., MSA, is on the Michigan State Medical Society Committee for CME, a member of the Association for Medical Education's Council on CME, and retired as chief academic officer of St. John Providence Health.

Joseph S. Green, PhD, is the senior vice president for professional development and the chief learning officer for the American College of Cardiology.

Leonard Harvey, MD, is past president of the Union of European Medical Specialists and a retired obstetrician/gynecologist in the United Kingdom.

Carol Havens, MD, is director of clinical education for Kaiser Permanente Northern California.

Richard E. Hawkins, MD, is senior vice president for professional and scientific affairs at the American Board of Medical Specialties.

Sheldon D. Horowitz, MD, is special advisor to the president at the American Board of Medical Specialties.

Tamar Hosansky is director of communications of the Accreditation Council for Continuing Medical Education.

Marcia Jackson, PhD, is president of the consulting group CME by Design, chair of the Medscape CME advisory board, and a member of the advisory group for the Coalition to Reduce Racial and Ethnic Disparities in (CV) Outcomes.

Saurabh Jain, MD, is director of continuing medical education solutions for Indegene Lifesystems in Bangalore, India.

Norman B. Kahn, Jr., MD, is executive vice president and chief executive officer of the Council of Medical Specialty Societies.

Theresa Kanya, MBA, is vice president of medical edu-

cation in the medical education and publishing division at the American College of Physicians.

Hans Karle, MD, is the past-president of the World Federation for Medical Education, the Panum Institute, Copenhagen, Denmark.

Murray Kopelow, MD, MS(Comm), FRCPC, is chief executive of the Accreditation Council for Continuing Medical Education.

Robert E. Kristofco, MSW, is director of medical education for Pfizer Inc.

John R. Kues, PhD, CCMEP, is assistant senior vice president of continuous professional development and professor emeritus at the University of Cincinnati Academic Health Center.

Paul J. Lambiase is director of continuing professional education at the University of Rochester School of Medicine and Dentistry.

Penelope L. LaRocque, MA, is a senior associate editor in the division of continuing medical education of the American Academy of Family Physicians.

James C. Leist, EdD, is a professor of health administration at Pfeiffer University, an associate consulting professor of community/family medicine at Duke University School of Medicine, and a staff consultant for the Alliance for Continuing Medical Education.

Brian W. Little, MD, PhD, is the chief academic officer at Christiana Care Health Services, past president of AHME, and past chair of the ACCME.

Bernard Maillet, MD, is secretary general of the Union of European Medical Specialists and a practicing pathologist in Brussels.

Karen V. Mann, BN, MSc, PhD, is professor emeritus at Dalhousie University Faculty of Medicine, Canada, and professor and chair in medical education at Manchester Medical School, the University of Manchester, United Kingdom.

Phil R. Manning, MD, is emeritus professor of medicine and formerly Paul Ingalls Hoagland-Hastings Foundation Professor of Continuing Medical Education at the Keck School of Medicine of the University of Southern California, Los Angeles.

Bernard A. Marlow, MD, CCFP, FCFP, FACME, is the director of continuing professional development for the College of Family Physicians of Canada and past president of the Canadian Association for Continuing Health Education.

Pamela M. Mazmanian, MA, is chief operating officer of Continuing Professional Education, Inc., and provides consulting services to the Medical Society of Virginia Intrastate Accreditation Committee.

Mindi K. McKenna, PhD, MBA, is director of the division of continuing medical education and staff executive for the Commission on Continuing Professional Development for the American Academy of Family Physicians.

Lewis A. Miller, MS, CCMEP, is principal of WentzMiller & Associates, chairman of BestPractice CPD, co-founder of the Alliance for Continuing Medical Education, and founder of the Global Alliance for Medical Education.

Steven Minnick, MD, is the director of medical education for St. John Hospital and Medical Center in Detroit, Michigan, and an assistant clinical dean for the Wayne State University School of Medicine.

Donald E. Moore, Jr., PhD, is currently director of the division of continuing medical education; director of evaluation and education in the office of graduate medical education; professor of medical education and administration; and a faculty associate in the office of teaching and learning in medicine at Vanderbilt University School of Medicine.

Sondra Moylan, MS, is president of the American Academy of Continuing Medical Education.

Alfonso Negri, MD, is secretary general of the Rome CME-CPD Group and technical secretary of the accreditation committee for the European Academy of Allergology and Clinical Immunology.

Robert F. Orsetti, MA, CCMEP, is chief executive officer of Blackwood CME, a member of the National Task Force on CME Provider/Industry Collaboration, a member of the executive committee of the Global Alliance for Medical Education, and an advisor to the National Commission for Certification of CME Professionals.

Daniel J. Ostergaard, MD, is vice president of professional activities at the American Academy of Family Physicians, an alternate delegate to the American Medical Association House of Delegates, and a member of the World Organization of Family Doctors Executive Committee.

Karen M. Overstreet, EdD, RPh, FACME, CCMEP, is president of Indicia Medical Education, LLC.

I. John Parboosingh, MB, FRCSC, is professor emeritus at University of Calgary and a consultant in community learning.

Greg Paulos, MBA, is the chief executive officer of GenLife Institute in Phoenix, Arizona, and was associate director of the division of CPPD at the American Medical Association.

David R. Pieper, PhD, is assistant dean of continuing medical education at Wayne State University School of Medicine and executive director at the Southeast Michigan Center for Medical Education, a graduate medical education consortium previously known as the Oakland Health Education Program.

David Price, MD, FAAFP, is director of medical education with the Colorado Permanente Medical Group, a clinical researcher with Kaiser Colorado's Institute for Health Research, physician lead for continuing education and for depression guidelines for the Kaiser Permanente Care Management Institute in Oakland, California, and a member of Kaiser Permanente's national continuing medical education committee.

Pablo A. Pulido, MD, is president of the PanAmerican Federation of Associations of Medical Schools and president of Project Globe Consortium for CPD in Caracas, Venezuela.

Scott Reeves, PhD, is a scientist with the Keenan Research Centre, Li Ka Shing Knowledge Institute of St. Michael's Hospital, Toronto; the director of research at the Centre for Faculty Development, St. Michael's Hospital; a scientist with the Wilson Centre for Research in Education; and an associate professor in the Department of Psychiatry at the University of Toronto Keenan Research Centre, Li Ka Shing Knowledge Institute of St. Michael's Hospital.

Kate Regnier, MA, MBA, is deputy chief executive and chief operating officer of the Accreditation Council for Continuing Medical Education.

Judith G. Ribble, PhD, CCMEP, is executive director and founding president of the National Commission for Certification of CME Professionals and a member of the Medscape CME advisory board.

Robert K. Richards, PhD, is a consultant to Metropolitan Hospital and formerly served as continuing medical education director for the University of Michigan Medical School and the American College of Cardiology; assistant dean for Michigan State University's Grand Rapids Campus; and president and chief executive officer of GRAMEC.

Delores J. Rodgers, BS, is director of continuing medical education in the department of education at the American Osteopathic Association, where she also serves as secretary to the council on continuing medical education.

Richard I. Rothstein, MD, is chief of the section of gastroenterology and hepatology at Dartmouth-Hitchcock Medical Center and professor of medicine and of surgery and associate dean for continuing medical education at Dartmouth Medical School.

Michael Saxton, MEd, CCMEP, was the former team leader and senior director of the medical education group at Pfizer, Inc.

Madeline H. Schmitt, PhD, RN, is professor emerita at University of Rochester Medical Center.

M. Roy Schwarz, MD, is the past president of the China Medical Board, an adjunct professor in the department of community and public health of Johns Hopkins School of Nursing, and an affiliate professor in the department of medical education and biomedical informatics at the University of Washington School of Medicine.

Bruce Spivey, MD, MS, MEd, is president of the International Council of Ophthalmology.

Robin Stevenson, MD, is president of the European Board for Accreditation in Pneumology and a retired respiratory medicine consultant in Glasgow, Scotland.

Robert L. Tupper, MD, is retired as vice president for medical education at Spectrum Health in Grand Rapids, Michigan, and emeritus professor of internal medicine at Michigan State University College of Medicine, former president of AHME, former chair of the ACCME review committee, and former chairman of the ACCME Council.

Mary G. Turco, EdD, MA, is director of the Center for Continuing Education in the Health Sciences and of Continuing Medical Education at Dartmouth-Hitchcock Medical Center and assistant professor of medicine at Dartmouth Medical School.

W. Douglas Ward, PhD, is an advisor in international and educational affairs for the American Osteopathic Association (AOA), a retired AOA associate executive director and director of education, and former independent consultant on osteopathic medical education accreditation.

Dennis K. Wentz, MD, FACPE, CCMEP, is the former director of the Division of Continuing Physician Professional Development at the American Medical Association (1988–2004). His interest in compiling a history of continuing medical education began when he was associate dean at Vanderbilt University School of Medicine (1980–1988), and he is deeply indebted to his colleagues in CME for helping to create this book.

Richard S. Wilbur, MD, JD, FACP, FCLM, FACPE, FRSM, is chairman of the American Medical Foundation for Peer Review and Education.

Charles E. Willis, MBA, is vice president of education and training at the American Gastroenterological Association.

Robert Woollard, MD, CCFP, FCFP, is professor of family practice at the University of British Columbia.

Egle Zebiene, MD, is president of the European Academy of Teachers in General Practice and a general practitioner in Lithuania.

Index

LIBRARY OF CONGRESS CATALOGING-IN-PUBLICATION DATA

Continuing medical education : looking back, planning
ahead / edited by Dennis K. Wentz.
   p. ; cm.
Includes bibliographical references and index.
ISBN 978-1-58465-988-4 (cloth : alk. paper)
ISBN 978-1-61168-020-1 (e-book)
1. Medicine—Study and teaching (Continuing education)—Canada. 2. Medicine—Study and teaching (Continuing education)—United States. I. Wentz, Dennis K.
[DNLM: 1. Education, Medical, Continuing—Canada.
2. Education, Medical, Continuing—United States.
3. Societies, Medical—Canada. 4. Societies, Medical—
United States. W 20]
R845.C6496 2011
610.71—dc22   2011000073